Eicosanoids and Reproduction

ADVANCES IN EICOSANOID RESEARCH

Series Editor Keith Hillier

Eicosanoids and Reproduction

Edited by

Keith Hillier

Senior Lecturer
Clinical Pharmacology Group
Medical Faculty
University of Southampton
UK

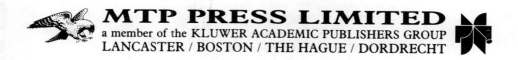

MTP PRESS LIMITED

a member of the KLUWER ACADEMIC PUBLISHERS GROUP
LANCASTER / BOSTON / THE HAGUE / DORDRECHT

Published in the UK and Europe by
MTP Press Limited
Falcon House
Lancaster, England

British Library Cataloguing in Publication Data

Eicosanoids and reproduction.—(Advances
in eicosanoid research series).
1. Human reproduction   2. Acids, Fatty
I. Hillier, K.   II. Series
612'.6   QP251

ISBN 0-85200-956-9
ISBN 0-85200-825-2 series

Published in the USA by
MTP Press
A division of Kluwer Academic Publishers
101 Philip Drive
Norwell, MA 02061, USA

Library of Congress Cataloging in Publication Data

Eicosanoids and reproduction.

(Advances in eicosanoid research series)
Includes bibliographies and index.
1. Prostaglandins.   2. Arachidonic acid—
Derivatives.   3. Endocrine gynecology. I. Hillier, K. (Keith), 1943–   .   II. Series.
[DNLM: 1. Prostaglandins—pharmacodynamics.   2. Prostaglandins—physiology.
WQ 205 E34]
RG129.P7E37 1987   612'.6   87-3092
ISBN 0-85200-956-9

Typeset by Lasertext, Stretford, Manchester
Printed by Butler and Tanner, Frome and London

Contents

List of Contributors

M. Bygdeman
Department of Obstetrics and Gynecology
Karolinska Institute
Box 60500
S-104 01 Stockholm
Sweden

A. Calder
Centre for Reproductive Biology
Department of Obstetrics and Gynaecology
University of Edinburgh
37 Chalmers Street
Edinburgh EH3 9EW
UK

G. Ekman
Research Laboratory of Obstetrics and
   Gynecology
The Bartholin Building
University of Aarhus
DK-8000 Aarhus C
Denmark

I. S. Fraser
Department of Obstetrics and Gynaecology
University of Sydney
New South Wales 2006
Australia

M. A. Heymann
School of Medicine
Cardiovascular Research Institute
University of California
San Francisco
California 94143
USA

T. G. Kennedy
MRC Group in Reproductive Biology
Department of Obstetrics and Gynaecology
   and of Physiology
University of Western Ontario
London, Ontario
Canada N6A 5A5

I. Z. Mackenzie
Nuffield Department of Obstetrics and
   Gynaecology
John Radcliffe Hospital
Oxford
UK

M. D. Mitchell
Department of Reproductive Medicine
   (T-002)
UCSD Medical Center
225 Dickinson Street (H-898)
San Diego
California 92093
USA

N. L. Poyser
Department of Pharmacology
University of Edinburgh Medical School
1 George Square
Edinburgh EH8 9JZ
UK

N. Uldbjerg
Research Laboratory of Obstetrics and
   Gynecology
The Bartholin Building
University of Aarhus
DK-8000 Aarhus C
Denmark

U. Ulmsten
Research Laboratory of Obstetrics and
  Gynecology
The Bartholin Building
University of Aarhus
DK-8000 Aarhus C
Denmark

S. W. Walsh
The University of Texas Medical School
  at Houston
Departments of Obstetrics, Gynecology
  and Reproductive Sciences
6431 Fannin, Suite 3.204
Houston, Texas 77030
USA

Series Editor's Foreword

The original series, *Advances in Prostaglandin Research*, edited by Sultan M. M. Karim, was published by MTP Press in three volumes in 1975 and 1976. A glance at those books illustrates the progress that has been made since then. The thromboxanes were mentioned twice (first publication 1975) and prostacyclin not once (first publication 1976); leukotrienes were only on the horizon.

The amazing generation of research data in the last 10–15 years has given new, broad insights into many areas, including asthma, inflammation, renal, cardiovascular and gastrointestinal diseases and in reproduction, and has led in some instances to real clinical benefit.

This series, *Advances in Eicosanoid Research*, reflects the current understanding of prostaglandins , thromboxanes and leukotrienes. The aim is to provide an introductory background to each topic and the most up-to-date information available.

Although each book stands alone, the eicosanoids cut across many boundaries in their basic actions; selected chapters from each book in the series will provide illuminating and productive information for all readers which will advance their education and research.

In the production of this series, I must acknowledge with pleasure my collaboration with editors and authors and the patient endeavours of Dr Michael Brewis and the staff at MTP Press.

KEITH HILLIER
University of Southampton
England

Preface

This book is an appraisal of areas in human reproduction where eicosanoid studies (prostaglandins, leukotrienes and thromboxanes) are contributing to physiological and pathological awareness and clinical advances.

Currently, patients are reaping the therapeutic benefits of the original observations, made 15–20 years ago by Karim, Embrey, Bydgeman and Wiqvist and their colleagues, that prostaglandins could be used safely and effectively for terminating pregnancy and inducing labour. Benefits from investigations of the effects of prostaglandins in the circulation of neonates have also materialized.

Eicosanoid studies form an integral part of many areas of research in reproduction; pregnancy-related hypertension, cervix form and function, ovulation, the onset of labour, the fetal and neonatal circulation, menstruation and abortion are such topics.

As yet, the eicosanoids have an equivocal place in several of these areas. This is not surprising for a number of reasons: they may, in fact, play only a minor role; there are many closely related eicosanoids and only one may be important; also that their place may be one of a link in a complex of events. The unequivocal proof or denial of their role will only come from improved techniques of identification and reliability of measurement; a new vision of researchers in reproduction is required, broadening the base of their investigations, and embracing more effectively studies of the eicosanoids and their interactions with other bioactive substances.

It may be hypothesized that biological research consists of many small advances providing the springboard for a quantum leap forward in understanding. Almost 50 years passed between the discovery of slow-reacting substance of anaphylaxis and the finding that it is composed of leukotrienes; this discovery strengthened the important links between leukotrienes, asthma and inflammation, and as a result great efforts are being made in research in this area. Leukotrienes have not yet been seen to be as dramatically important in areas of reproductrion and thus the signal for a concerted effort has not yet been triggered.

It is hoped that this book will provide interest and a sound base of knowledge for all readers and a platform for further research studies.

On a personal note, I wish to acknowledge the friendship and collaboration of Sultan Karim who introduced me to prostaglandins in 1967. I also wish to remember with affection my former colleague, the late Mostyn Embrey.

KEITH HILLIER

1
Prostaglandins and ovarian function

N. L. Poyser

INTRODUCTION

The ovary is concerned with the secretion of steroid hormones and with the release of a mature ovum (ovulation). Ovarian function is controlled by hormones secreted by the anterior pituitary gland, namely follicle-stimulating hormone (FSH), luteinizing hormone (LH), and, to a greater or lesser extent depending upon the species, prolactin. A surge of oestradiol from the ovary at oestrus (or mid-cycle in women) stimulates a surge of LH from the pituitary gland which causes final maturation of the ovum and ovulation. An ovulated follicle is transformed by LH into a corpus luteum which secretes progesterone for 10 to 12 days, although in some species, such as the rat, a fully functional corpus luteum is only formed following the additional release of prolactin as a result of coitus. Regression of the corpus luteum (luteolysis) terminates progesterone production, and a new cycle begins. The temporal relationship between oestradiol, LH and progesterone is shown in Figure 1.1. There is much evidence that prostaglandins and, to a more limited extent, leukotrienes are involved in these processes.

LUTEINIZING HORMONE (LH) RELEASE

Rat studies

Effect of inhibitors of prostaglandin (PG) synthesis and action

Ovulation is prevented in immature rats treated with pregnant mare's serum gonadotropin (PMSG) by the administration of indomethacin or aspirin several hours before the expected surge of LH. This inhibition is overcome by administering LH indicating that the inhibitors of PG synthesis are not acting on the ovary to inhibit ovulation[1,2]. The infusion of indomethacin or aspirin into the pre-optic area or the anterior hypothalamus of pro-oestrous rats a few hours before the expected LH surge also blocks ovulation, and this

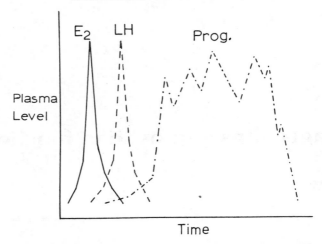

Figure 1.1 The time-course relationship between the increase in plasma levels of oestradiol (E_2), luteinizing hormone (LH) and progesterone (Prog.)

blockade is overcome by luteinizing hormone-releasing hormone (LHRH) administration[3]. The treatment of ovariectomized rats, in which plasma LH levels are raised, with indomethacin given into the third ventricle of the brain or systemically, lowers the concentration of LH in the plasma[4,5]. Ovulation is prevented in intact rats by the administration of a prostaglandin antagonist (N-0164) into the third ventricle[6]. These studies suggest that PGs are involved in the oestradiol-induced surge of LH at ovulation, by an action in the brain rather than by a direct action on the anterior pituitary gland. However, indomethacin administered systemically to cyclic rats failed to prevent the pre-ovulatory LH surge[7,8]. The indomethacin may not have been given in sufficient dosage or at the optimum time, especially as indomethacin is not readily taken up into the rat brain[9]. Flurbiprofen, a potent antipyretic drug (indicating that it can readily penetrate the brain), given systemically inhibited the ovulatory surge of LH in 33% of treated rats and delayed the LH surge by 2 h in the remainder[10] indicating that inhibitors of PG synthesis can interfere with the timing of the LH surge in cyclic rats.

Effect of PGs on LH release

PGE_2 stimulates LH release in pro-oestrous rats and in ovariectomized rats treated with oestradiol. PGE_1 and PGI_2 also stimulate LH release, but $PGF_{2\alpha}$ is ineffective[7,11]. PGE_2 stimulates LH release in ovariectomized rats when injected into the third ventricle but not when administered directly into the anterior pituitary gland[12]. LH release induced by PGE_2 is not blocked by drugs[13-15] which are antagonists at α- or β-adrenoceptors, dopaminergic, serotinergic or muscarinic receptors. LHRH release is increased by PGE_2 administration[16,17] and PGE_2-induced LH release is prevented by treatment with LHRH antiserum[18,19]. These studies indicate that PGE_2 acts directly on

2

the LHRH-containing neurones in the median eminence to stimulate LHRH release, and hence LH release. Its action in the median eminence depends upon both the uptake of extracellular Ca^{2+} and the release of intracellular[20] Ca^{2+}. It is well-documented that there is a noradrenaline link in the brain in oestradiol-induced LH release since the pre-ovulatory surge of LH is prevented by α-adrenoceptor antagonists. PGD_2 injected into the third ventricle of the brain suppresses LH release, apparently by stimulating the release of an opiate agonist (probably β-endorphin) which in turn prevents noradrenaline release and hence LHRH and LH release[21–23]. In contrast to this indirect inhibitory effect, PGD_2 increases LH output when administered directly into the anterior pituitary gland[24].

PG synthesis by the median emigence

PGE_2 is the major PG produced by the median eminence[10,25,26]. Flurbiprofen administered systemically inhibits PG synthesis by the median eminence[10]. Noradrenaline stimulates PGE_2 production by the median eminence[10,27] and this stimulation is inhibited by α_1-, but not by α_2- or β-, adrenoceptor antagonists[28,29]. Indomethacin inhibits LHRH release from the median eminence induced by noradrenaline but not by PGE_2[22].

Effect of leukotrienes

Leukotriene (LT) C_4, but not LTB_4, stimulates LH release from anterior pituitary cells cultured *in vitro*[30]. LTC_4 has a quicker action than LHRH in this respect[31]. Immunohistochemical analysis has revealed that, not only is LTC_4 present in the median eminence, but it is present in the same neurones which contain LHRH[31].

Conclusions

It is clear that, in the rat, increased PGE_2 production by the median eminence is an essential step in the oestradiol-induced ovulatory surge of LH. PGE_2 forms an essential link between noradrenaline release and the stimulation of LHRH-containing neurones (Figure 1.2). Apart from the oestradiol-induced surge of LH on the day of pro-oestrus, during the rest of the cycle the ovarian steroid hormones suppress LH release. Further study is required to see whether this involves increased PGD_2 production by the brain. The discovery that LTC_4 stimulates LH release directly from the anterior pituitary gland and is present in the same neurones as LHRH may mean that LHRH is not the only substance controlling LH release. It will be interesting to see whether PGE_2 stimulates LTC_4 release from neurones in the median eminence.

Studies on other non-primate species

The systemic administration of $PGF_{2\alpha}$ to sheep during the luteal phase of the cycle causes an increase in the plasma concentration of LH[32]. The release of LH induced by oestradiol in the anoestrous ewe is prevented by indomethacin treatment[33]; oestradiol-induced increase in LH release is associated with an

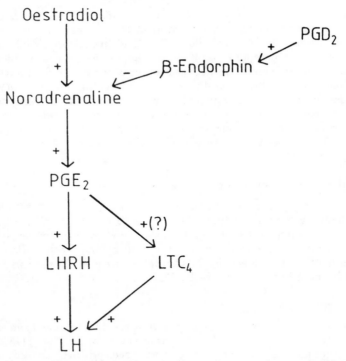

Figure 1.2 Diagrammatic representation of the involvement of prostaglandin (PG) E$_2$ in oestradiol-induced release of luteinizing hormone-releasing hormone (LHRH) and hence of luteinizing hormone (LH) in the rat. Actions of PGD$_2$ and leukotriene (LT) C$_4$ on LH release are also shown

increase in PGF$_{2\alpha}$ from the brain[34]. This output of PGF$_{2\alpha}$ is pulsatile, like the outputs of LHRH and LH.

In the rabbit, PGF$_{2\alpha}$ and, to a lesser extent, PGE$_2$ cause an increase in plasma LH concentration[35]. Ovulation in rabbits induced by vaginal stimulation is associated with an increase in the level of PGE$_2$ in the cerebrospinal fluid[36]. PGF$_{2\alpha}$ stimulates LH release in ovariectomized, oestrogen-treated hamsters[37]. In deermice, the magnitude of the pre-ovulatory surge of LH is considerably reduced by treatment with indomethacin[38]. These studies suggest that PGs are involved in LH release in these four species.

Studies in the monkey

The systemic administration of PGF$_{2\alpha}$ or PGE$_2$ during the last half of the menstrual cycle results in variable increases in LH release, with several small peaks occurring shortly after the administration[39]. PGF$_{2\alpha}$ and PGE$_2$ also stimulate LH release in the male monkey[40]. In ovariectomized monkeys treated with oestradiol, PGE$_2$, but not PGF$_{2\alpha}$, stimulates LH release[41]. The increase in LH release due to oestradiol administration on days 3, 4 and 5 of the cycle is significantly reduced by indomethacin treatment[39]. These studies suggest that PGs play a role in the mechanisms responsible for the pre-ovulatory release of LH in the rat. However, since indomethacin fails to alter basal LH levels in ovariectomized monkeys and to prevent the stimulatory effect of oestradiol on LH release in ovariectomized monkeys, it is suggested[42] that the effect of indomethacin on LH release in the intact monkey[30] is mediated through ovarian mechanisms.

Human studies

Studies on the involvement of PGs in LH release in women are very limited. The intra-amniotic administration of $PGF_{2\alpha}$ for mid-trimester abortion had no effect on LH release[43], whereas $PGF_{2\alpha}$ administered during the late secretory phase causes a small transient increase in plasma LH levels[44]. The effect of PGE_2 or PGI_2 on LH release in women has not been studied. PGD_2 stimulates LH release from the superfused pituitary gland *in vitro*[45], but its effect *in vivo* also needs studying. The administration of aspirin (2.4–6.5 g daily) to three women during the middle part of the cycle failed to inhibit the pre-ovulatory LH surge in two women, while the third woman who was taking the largest dose had her LH surge delayed by 10 days[46].

Summary

There is much convincing evidence in several non-primate species (particularly the rat) that PGs are involved in the pre-ovulatory surge of LH, by acting as a mediator between the release of noradrenaline and the stimulation of neurones containing LHRH in the median eminence (Figure 1.2). The evidence for a similar role of PGs in LH release in primate species (including women) is not so well defined. This may be due to the fact that studies in monkeys have revealed that oestradiol can induce LH release by a direct stimulatory effect on the anterior pituitary gland[47]. However, other studies have shown that increased LHRH secretion occurs in oestradiol-treated, ovariectomized monkeys, and that this is associated with a surge of LH[48]. In women, plasma LHRH levels do increase in the peri-ovulatory period[49,50], suggesting that the ovulatory LH surge in women is dependent upon increased LHRH secretion. Consequently, further study is required to investigate whether increased PG production by the median eminence in women is necessary for the ovulatory LH surge as appears to be the case in several non-primate, mammalian species.

OVULATION

Effect of inhibitors of PG synthesis

Indomethacin administered to rats at about the time of the LH surge prevents ovulation, and the administration of exogenous LH does not overcome this blockade[51]. Indomethacin also prevents ovulation in rabbits[52–54], pigs[55], mice[56], sheep[57] and monkeys[58]. This block of ovulation by indomethacin is overcome by PGE_2 in rats[59] and by $PGF_{2\alpha}$ in rabbits[60], pigs[55] and monkeys[61]. Ovulation is also prevented in 90% of rabbit follicles following an intrafollicular injection of $PGF_{2\alpha}$ antiserum, whereas a similar injection of PGE_2 antiserum prevents ovulation in about 40% of treated follicles[53]. These studies suggest that PGs have a role in ovulation.

In humans, the systemic administration of aspirin fails to prevent ovulation[62]. However, aspirin also fails to prevent ovulation in rabbits in contrast to the inhibitory action of indomethacin[63]. Aspirin is only a weak inhibitor of the cyclo-oxygenase enzyme present in rabbit follicles, whereas indomethacin is a potent inhibitor of this enzyme[63]. Consequently, a more potent inhibitor of PG synthesis needs to be tested on the ovulatory process in women.

PG levels in the ovary

Figure 1.3 shows the mean concentrations of PGE_2, $PGF_{2\alpha}$ and 6-oxo-$PGF_{1\alpha}$ in pig follicular fluid during the peri-ovulatory period. Ovulation occurs about 42 h after oestrus in this species, and it is seen that, in the 2 h period immediately preceding ovulation, there is a rapid rise in the concentration of all three PGs[64]. During the period of study, there is a reversal of the PGE_2 to $PGF_{2\alpha}$ ratio in favour of PGE_2. However, although PGE_2 is the major PG formed, the blockade of ovulation by indomethacin in pigs is overcome by $PGF_{2\alpha}$ and not by PGE_2[55].

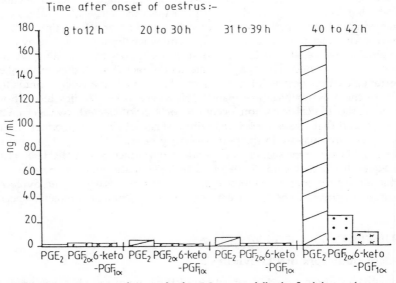

Figure 1.3 Concentrations of prostaglandin (PGs) in pig follicular fluid during the immediate pre-ovulatory period. Time from the onset of oestrus to ovulation is approximately 42 h, and none of the follicles included had undergone ovulation (64)

PGE_2 and $PGF_{2\alpha}$ levels in rat and sheep follicular fluid also increase after the LH surge up to the time of ovulation, with again a reversal of the PGE_2 to $PGF_{2\alpha}$ ratio in favour of PGE_2[65,66]. The levels of 6-oxo-$PGF_{1\alpha}$ have not been measured in the follicular fluid of either species, but the concentration of 6-oxo-$PGF_{1\alpha}$ in the ovary does increase prior to ovulation in the rat[67]. In rabbit follicles the levels of PGE_2 and $PGF_{2\alpha}$ increase after an ovulatory dose of human chorionic gonadotropin (HCG) or LH, or after mating[68,69]. In contrast to the other species, $PGF_{2\alpha}$ levels increase at a faster rate than PGE_2 levels although the ratio of PGE_2 to $PGF_{2\alpha}$ never falls below unity. In the guinea-pig, the levels of $PGF_{2\alpha}$ and PGE_2 in the ovary increase at the end of the oestrous cycle prior to ovulation[70].

In women, the mean concentration of $PGF_{2\alpha}$ in follicular fluid on day 14 of the menstrual cycle (i.e. around the time of ovulation) is from 2 to 5-fold higher than on any other day of the cycle in either the follicular or secretory stages[71]. Another study has shown that $PGF_{2\alpha}$ levels in the follicular fluid of women are increased 30 h after the LH surge[72]. However, follicular PGE_2 levels behave rather oddly since they are relatively high at the time of the LH surge, have fallen at 30 h and then increase again up to similar levels[72].

It is clear that in a number of mammalian species, including the human, there is an increase in the concentration of PGs in ovarian follicular fluid following the ovulatory LH surge up to the time of ovulation. Furthermore, studies in rabbits and pigs have shown that PG levels only increase in those follicles which actually ovulate[64,73].

Control of PG synthesis in ovarian follicles

LH is the stimulus for increased PG in ovarian follicles prior to ovulation[74-76] and its action is mediated by cyclic-AMP[77,78] (c-AMP). *In vitro*, increased PG production by isolated rat and rabbit follicles in response to LH or c-AMP is first apparent only after 3 h, and does not become maximal until after 5 h. Inhibitors of protein synthesis prevent the increase in PG production induced by LH or c-AMP in rat follicles[79,80]. *In vivo*, cycloheximide prevents increased protein synthesis in hamster ovaries following the LH surge[81], and this and other inhibitors of protein synthesis prevent ovulation in hamsters and rabbits by an action in the ovary[81-84]. These inhibitors are most effective up to 3 to 5 h following the ovulatory LH surge, which is exactly the time period during which increased PG synthesis in the follicles occurs.

There is an increase in PG synthetase levels in the rat ovary following the LH surge up to the time of ovulation; this increase is prevented by treating the rats with LH antiserum[85]. The amounts of PGE_2, $PGF_{2\alpha}$, 6-oxo-$PGF_{1\alpha}$ and TXB_2 produced by rat ovarian homogenates *in vitro* increase 5-, 1.6-, 1.7- and 1.7-fold respectively between 18:00 h on the day of pro-oestrus (i.e. shortly after the LH surge) up to 02:00 h on the day of oestrus (i.e. about the time of ovulation)[66]. This preferential increase in PGE_2 synthesizing capacity is probably responsible for the preferential increase in PGE_2 levels in rat follicular fluid. It is not due to an increase in PGH_2 to PGE_2 isomerase activity[66], so it appears that there is an increase in PGH synthetase (cyclo-oxygenase) levels with a greater proportion of the PGH_2 synthesized being directed into the PGE_2-forming pathway. There is also an increase in PG synthetase levels in guinea-pig ovaries prior to ovulation[70,86].

In cultured rat ovarian granulosa cells pre-incubated for 2 h with radioactive arachidonic acid, LH causes a 5-fold increase in PG synthetase levels and an increase in PGE_2 synthesis without stimulating the release of radioactivity from intracellular-bound sites into the incubating medium[87]. These findings were interpreted as meaning that the release of arachidonic acid is not rate-limiting for PG synthesis in ovarian follicles (unlike every other tissue), and that the increase in follicular PG synthesis is due entirely to an increase in PG synthetase levels[87]. This is unlikely since it would mean that arachidonic acid would be freely available to the lower levels of PG synthetase present in ovarian follicles during the rest of the cycle. Consequently, the ovary would have a very much higher production rate of PGs compared with other tissues, and the PGs would have to be rapidly cleared to prevent their accumulation at times other than in the peri-ovulatory period. However, total body synthesis of PGE and PGF is lower in women than in men[88]. The results of Clark *et al.*[87] can be interpreted in other ways which could mean that the release of arachidonic acid is rate-limiting, i.e. (i) pre-labelling for 2 h may not result in a distribution of radioactive arachidonic acid among the various lipid classes in the same proportions as the distribution of endogenous arachidonic acid, and LH may stimulate arachidonic acid release from a 'poorly labelled' source, or (ii) LH may cause a release of radioactive arachidonic acid but it is re-esterified before it can pass out of the cell into the incubation medium. Surely, the release of arachidonic acid has to be rate-limiting, which would mean that LH has to cause an increase in arachidonic acid release as well as increasing PG synthetase levels. Since protein synthesis inhibitors prevent follicular PG synthesis, this would infer that the release of arachidonic acid, as well as the increase in PG synthetase levels, is dependent upon increased protein synthesis. Consequently, one can speculate that LH causes the synthesis of a protein (a 'lipostimulin') which stimulates phospholipase A_2 to release arachidonic acid from phospholipids, and the increase in PG synthetase levels ensures that a greater proportion of the arachidonic acid released is converted into PGs. Obviously, this suggestion requires further study.

As regards which cell type in the follicle is responsible for increased follicular PG production, the overall picture is somewhat confusing. Cultured granulosa cells obtained from the rat ovaries show an increase in PGE_2 synthesis on exposure to LH. PG synthetase levels in rat granulosa cells increase following HCG treatment of PMSG-primed, immature rats and are also increased 4 to 8 h after the ovulatory LH surge in mature rats[87]. The granulosa cells are apparently the major site of PG synthesis in rat follicles. In pig follicles, the granulosa cells and the thecal cells have the ability to synthesize PGE_2, $PGF_{2\alpha}$ and PGI_2, with PG synthesis by both cell types increasing in the peri-ovulatory period[89-91]. PGE_2 tends to be the major PG produced by each type of cell, and thecal cells tend to produce more PGs than the granulosa cells[90,91]. Rabbit granulosa cells and thecal tissue both produce PGF in tissue culture, with production being greater in the former type[92,93]. However, PGF production by either cell type is not stimulated *in vitro* by LH or FSH. Studies in these three species indicate that both granulosa cells and thecal cells are involved in PG production in the peri-ovulatory period, but which cell type is actually involved may be species-dependent.

Mechanism by which PGs cause ovulation

Contractions of rabbit ovaries are reduced by indomethacin and are restored by $PGF_{2\alpha}$. Consequently, ovarian PGs could cause ovulation by increasing ovarian contractility, which exerts pressure on the large pre-ovulatory follicles causing them to burst. However, there is no correlation between ovarian contractility and ovulation in rabbit ovaries[94]. Also, verapamil, a calcium channel blocker, inhibits ovarian smooth muscle contractions without preventing ovulation[95]. Consequently, an increase in general ovarian smooth muscle activity is not responsible for ovulation. The theca externa cells in rat follicles contain smooth muscle fibres[96] and PGs produced within the follicles may cause these fibres in individual follicles to contract, thereby increasing follicular pressure and causing the follicle to rupture. This hypothesis requires further testing.

Rat granulosa cells obtained from those follicles predetermined to ovulate produce increased amounts of plasminogen activator immediately prior to ovulation. FSH, LH, PGE_1, PGE_2 and c-AMP all stimulate production of this enzyme. $PGF_{1\alpha}$ and $PGF_{2\alpha}$ are inactive[97]. Plasminogen activator converts plasminogen to plasmin, and plasmin is capable of weakening bovine follicular wall tissue *in vitro*[98]. PGs may, therefore, initiate ovulation by causing the synthesis of plasminogen activator. However, $PGF_{2\alpha}$ is without effect on plasminogen activator activity, yet, in some species, this is the principal PG involved in ovulation. Also indomethacin, although preventing LH-induced increases in follicular PG levels and ovulation, does not prevent LH- or FSH-induced increases in follicular levels of plasminogen activator[97,99–101]. Consequently PGs do not cause ovulation by stimulating the synthesis of plasminogen activator.

The apex of rabbit follicles destined to ovulate begins to 'thin out' by 9 h after mating (near the time of ovulation). Indomethacin prevents this 'thinning' process[102]. Similar findings have been reported for mouse ovaries[103]. Fibroblasts in rabbit follicles treated with indomethacin fail to undergo a normal ovulatory transition from a quiescent to a proliferative state[102]. It has been suggested that stimulation of collagenase activity in fibroblasts may cause 'thinning' of the follicular wall at the apex of the follicle with eventual rupture of the follicle and the shedding of the ovum[102]. Talopeptin and cysteine, inhibitors of collagenase, prevent ovulation in the hamster[104] and rat[105] ovary respectively. There is increased collagenolysis in rat follicles immediately preceding ovulation, and this increase in collagenolysis and ovulation is blocked by indomethacin[105]. In human pre-ovulatory follicles, PGE_2 significantly reduces radioactive proline incorporation into proteins at the apex of the follicle but not in other areas[106]. This was taken as an indication of a reduced net synthesis of collagen, which is consistent with PGE_2 stimulating collagenase activity. Consequently, in those species studied, it appears that PGs cause ovulation by stimulating collagenase activity at the apex of the follicle which results in the weakening of the follicular wall in that area and its eventual rupture. Thus the ovum is released.

Ovum maturation and progesterone secretion

As well as inducing ovulation, PGE_2 can also cause final maturation of the ovum. However, in rats treated with indomethacin following the LH surge, ovum maturation proceeds normally even though ovulation is prevented. This indicates that PGs are not essential mediators in the former process[59]. PGs of the 'E' series stimulate progesterone secretion *in vitro* by ovarian slices or isolated corpora lutea obtained from a variety of mammalian species including women. Their action is probably mediated by c-AMP. It has been suggested that PGE_2 is the 'second messenger' in LH-induced steroidogenesis in the corpus luteum. However, indomethacin, although blocking ovulation and the increase in follicular fluid levels of PGs, does not prevent luteinization, c-AMP production and steroidogenesis in those species studied[57,58,107–110]. A detailed study in sheep has shown that the intrafollicular injection of indomethacin prevents ovulation, but does not prevent luteinization of the follicle into a structure which secretes normal amounts of progesterone. Oestrous-cycle length is not altered[57], indicating that a luteinized follicle behaves identically to a corpus luteum except that it has an ovum trapped inside. Consequently, PGs are not involved in luteinization or progesterone secretion.

Summary

There is overwhelming evidence that in several mammalian species PGs produced by the follicles in response to LH are essential for ovulation. Their role in ovulation in women has still to be proven beyond doubt, and a detailed study of the effects of indomethacin on ovulation in women would go a long way to removing this doubt. PGs apparently cause ovulation by stimulating collagenase activity, which results in weakening and eventual rupture of the follicle at its apex. LH-induced ovum maturation, luteinization and progesterone secretion are independent of PG involvement. In addition, aminoglutethimide, an inhibitor of steroidogenesis, prevents progesterone production without interfering with follicular PG production and ovulation, indicating that these last two processes are not dependent on steroidogenesis[74,111]. This is outlined in Figure 1.4 where LH increases c-AMP levels, which in turn stimulate PG synthesis and ovulation, and steroidogenesis independently of each other. Consequently, one process can be blocked without affecting the other, so the measurement of plasma progesterone levels is not necessarily an indication that ovulation has taken place.

Finally, ovulation in rats is blocked by nordihydroguaiaretic acid (NDGA), a lipoxygenase inhibitor[112]. Rat ovarian follicles contain 5-lipoxygenase, which converts arachidonic acid into 5-hydroxy-eicosatetraenoic acid (5-HETE),

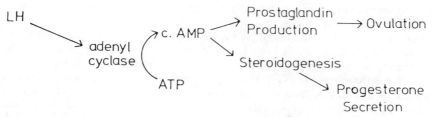

Figure 1.4 An outline of the biochemical processes involved in ovulation and progesterone secretion induced by LH

LTB$_4$, LTD$_4$ and LTE$_4$[113]. Stimulation of LH receptors causes a 5-fold increase in 5-lipoxygenase activity within 6 h[113]. These findings suggest that leukotrienes, as well as PGs, may be involved in ovulation.

LUTEOLYSIS

The length of an oestrous cycle, a menstrual cycle and, in some species such as the rat and rabbit, a pseudopregnancy is determined by the lifespan of the corpus luteum. Consequently, regression of the corpus luteum (luteolysis) is an important process, since its failure results in infertility for a prolonged period. Luteolysis can be divided into two processes, termed functional luteolysis (in which ovarian progesterone output declines) and structural luteolysis (in which morphological changes take place in the corpus luteum causing it to regress). In 1969, the first reports appeared showing that PGF$_{2\alpha}$ was luteolytic in several mammalian species. Since that time the role of PGF$_{2\alpha}$ in luteolysis has been studied extensively.

Studies in non-primates

Susceptibility of the corpus luteum to PGF$_{2\alpha}$

PGF$_{2\alpha}$ will cause premature luteolysis when injected into many non-primate, mammalian species, such as the sheep, cow, pig, guinea-pig, mare, and the pseudopregnant rat, rabbit, mouse and hamster. However, the corpus luteum is not susceptible to the luteolytic action of PGF$_{2\alpha}$ during the early part of its life. PGF$_{2\alpha}$ only causes luteolysis from day 4 in the hamster, day 5 in the cow, sheep, mare and rat, day 10 in the guinea-pig, and day 12 in the pig. In the pig, though, PGF$_{2\alpha}$ administration before day 12 causes plasma progesterone levels to fall to some extent, but the levels return to normal after the infusion has stopped[114]. Therefore, before day 12, PGF$_{2\alpha}$ causes a reversible functional luteolysis, but is incapable of causing structural luteolysis. The corpus luteum in the pig, as in other species, has to acquire 'something' during its lifespan which makes it 'susceptible' to PGF$_{2\alpha}$ in so far as PGF$_{2\alpha}$ causes structural luteolysis.

Binding sites (receptors) for PGF$_{2\alpha}$ are present in the luteal cell membranes in the sheep, cow, mare and rat. The number of $PGF_{2\alpha}$ receptors in corpora lutea obtained from mares varied during the cycle, but no consistent trends were noted[115]. The binding of $PGF_{2\alpha}$ to corpora lutea of the cow increases during the oestrous cycle (due to an increase in affinity of $PGF_{2\alpha}$ for the receptor), reaching its peak when the corpora lutea are regressing[116]. In the pseudopregnant rat, the $PGF_{2\alpha}$ binding capacity of the corpora lutea increases from day 1 to day 4, reaches a maximum on day 7, and then slowly declines from day 9 before luteolysis takes place[117]. It is clear that among these three species there is no consistent trend in $PGF_{2\alpha}$ binding to corpora lutea which could account for the 'something' which makes the corpora lutea 'susceptible' to structural luteolysis induced by $PGF_{2\alpha}$. In fact, $PGF_{2\alpha}$ receptors are present in the corpora lutea before the corpora lutea become 'susceptible'. It is assumed that $PGF_{2\alpha}$ has to combine with its receptor in order to cause luteolysis, although receptors for $PGF_{2\alpha}$ in pig corpora lutea have not been detected[118].

Effect of $PGF_{2\alpha}$ on LH

After combining with its receptor, LH causes an increase in c-AMP production (by activating adenyl cyclase) which in turn stimulates progesterone formation and output. $PGF_{2\alpha}$ prevents the LH-induced increase in c-AMP production in rat corpora lutea[119] and sheep luteal cells[120]. Hence increases in progesterone formation and output are prevented. How is this achieved? LH binds randomly to LH receptors distributed randomly on the surface of luteal cells. As binding increases, the LH receptors group to form micro-aggregates due to lateral movement of the 'bound' LH receptors in the luteal cell membrane. It is considered that this grouping of LH receptors is necessary for the activation of adenyl cyclase[121]. Dibutyryl c-AMP causes massive clumping of LH receptors to occur, indicating that LH-induced c-AMP production has a positive feedback effect on the aggregation of LH receptors. LH receptor movement may therefore be related to c-AMP levels[121]. $PGF_{2\alpha}$ inhibits LH receptor movement in the luteal cell membrane, thereby preventing LH from stimulating adenyl cyclase[121]. The formation of c-AMP and of progesterone is therefore reduced. $PGF_{2\alpha}$ does not inhibit the stimulation of adenyl cyclase by LH in rat isolated luteal membranes, indicating that $PGF_{2\alpha}$ does not affect the cell membrane directly and that the intact cell is necessary for its action[122]. The effect of $PGF_{2\alpha}$ on c-AMP production is rapid (within 15 min in rats).

$PGF_{2\alpha}$ also reduces LH binding to its receptor and eventually causes a loss of LH receptors in the corpora lutea of the rat, sheep and pig[123–125]. The reduction of LH binding in rat corpora lutea is not due to a change in the rate of hormone internalization and degradation, nor to changes in the receptor binding constants for LH[126]. When luteal cells are briefly treated with a pulse of LH, LH binding to these cells is increased by 20 to 30% within 2 h ('up-regulation'). This is due to the appearance of cryptic LH receptors (i.e. receptors present in the membrane but which are not available initially for the binding of LH). $PGF_{2\alpha}$ prevents this 'up-regulation' by preventing the appearance of cryptic LH receptors. Consequently, while $PGF_{2\alpha}$

does not prevent the initial binding of LH to its receptor, the lack of 'up-regulation' results in an overall reduction in LH binding[126]. Furthermore, the eventual loss of LH receptor binding is due, presumably, to the lack of appearance of new LH receptors. Can the effects of $PGF_{2\alpha}$ on LH receptor movement (and hence c-AMP production) and the binding of LH to its receptor be attributable to a common mechanism?

An increase in the intracellular Ca^{2+} concentration in rat luteal cells by the calcium ionophore, A23187, inhibits the LH-stimulated increase in c-AMP production[127]. Raising the Ca^{2+} concentrations also directly inhibits LH-sensitive adenyl cyclase in rat luteal membranes[127]. These findings suggest that $PGF_{2\alpha}$ exerts its inhibitory effect on LH-induced c-AMP formation by increasing the intracellular free Ca^{2+} concentration. The action of $PGF_{2\alpha}$ is not blocked by the calcium-channel blocking drug verapamil[127], suggesting that $PGF_{2\alpha}$ mobilises intracellular Ca^{2+}. $PGF_{2\alpha}$ stimulates the phosphatidylinositol (PI) cycle in rat luteal membranes[128], which presumably results in the formation of inositol-1,4,5-triphosphate (IP_3)[129]. IP_3 causes the release of intracellular[129] Ca^{2+}, so stimulation of the PI cycle by $PGF_{2\alpha}$ provides the mechanism by which $PGF_{2\alpha}$ could liberate intracellular Ca^{2+} within the luteal cell. It has been proposed that Ca^{2+} released by IP_3 can cause the phosphorylation (and thereby the activation) of proteins[129]. Consequently, how is this related to the luteolytic action of $PGF_{2\alpha}$? Studies on corpora lutea from the rat and cow have shown that spontaneous and $PGF_{2\alpha}$-induced luteal regression is associated with a change of the membrane lipid in luteal cells from a liquid-crystalline phase to a gel phase, i.e. the membrane becomes more rigid[130-132]. This change is calcium, calmodulin and protein dependent[133]. The proposed increase in free intracellular Ca^{2+} concentration occurring in the luteal cell as a result of stimulation of the PI cycle by $PGF_{2\alpha}$ would appear, after combining with calmodulin, to cause phosphorylation of proteins in the luteal cell membrane resulting in rigidification of the membrane. Presumably, this change in consistency of the luteal cell membrane prevents LH receptor movement, prevents the appearance of cryptic LH receptors and, eventually, the loss of LH receptors, since the old ones will be used up and new ones will be able to appear (see Figure 1.5). These actions of $PGF_{2\alpha}$ on LH receptors, via stimulation of the PI cycle and rigidification of the luteal cell membrane, would appear to explain the luteolytic action of $PGF_{2\alpha}$. But do they?

Studies on small and large luteal cells

Luteal cells obtained from the corpora lutea of pig[134], cow[135] and sheep[136] are classified into two types depending upon their size, namely *small* and *large*. Both types of cell secrete progesterone, but one large cell secretes more progesterone than one small cell. However, studies in the sheep have shown that progesterone secretion per unit volume is the same for small and large cells and, if the total number of small and large luteal cells is taken into account, total progesterone secretion by the two types of cell does not differ significantly[137]. But differences do exist between the two types of cell. LH greatly stimulates progesterone production by the small luteal cells, but has only a weak effect in this respect on large luteal cells[135,136]. In fact, progesterone

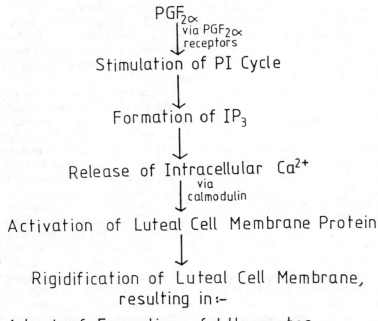

$PGF_{2\alpha}$

via $PGF_{2\alpha}$ receptors

↓

Stimulation of PI Cycle

↓

Formation of IP_3

↓

Release of Intracellular Ca^{2+}

via calmodulin

↓

Activation of Luteal Cell Membrane Protein

↓

Rigidification of Luteal Cell Membrane, resulting in :-

1. Lack of Formation of LH receptor Aggregates

2. Loss of LH binding to its Receptors

3. Loss of LH Receptors

Figure 1.5   Schematic diagram of the initial processes involved in $PGF_{2\alpha}$-induced luteolysis in the rat

production by large luteal cells appears to be LH and c-AMP independent[138]. Since the LH receptors are mainly located on the small luteal cells, from the previous section one would expect $PGF_{2\alpha}$ to act predominantly on the small luteal cells to prevent LH-induced increases in c-AMP production and progesterone secretion. However, small luteal cells contain very few receptors for $PGF_{2\alpha}$, and the majority of the $PGF_{2\alpha}$ receptors in sheep corpora lutea are on the large luteal cells[136]. This is consistent with the finding in cows that the large luteal cells are more sensitive than the small luteal cells to the luteolytic action of $PGF_{2\alpha}$[139]. The treatment of large luteal cells from sheep with $PGF_{2\alpha}$ results in morphological changes, including a retraction of the cell cytoplasm and an apparent extrusion of the cytoplasmic components[140]. Progesterone production by these $PGF_{2\alpha}$-treated large luteal cells is also decreased[140], which cannot be due to an inhibition of LH-induced c-AMP production. It has been suggested[140] that 'PGF$_{2\alpha}$ induces the large luteal cells to release a toxin which must accumulate to critical levels before exhibiting its inhibitory influence on large luteal cell morphology and function'. Presumably this toxin can pass from the large luteal cells to the small luteal cells. Thus the secretion of a substance from the large cells in response to $PGF_{2\alpha}$ could explain both the cytotoxicity for large cells and the reduced response to LH in small cells[140]. How the production of a toxin by large luteal cells in response to $PGF_{2\alpha}$ relates to the findings in the previous section on the rat corpus luteum, where $PGF_{2\alpha}$ causes stimulation of the PI cycle and rigidification of the luteal cell membrane, requires further study. Figure 1.5 is probably an oversimplification of the processes involved.

There is a gradual evolution of the bimodal pattern of distribution of the luteal cells in sheep corpora lutea. Small luteal cells predominate early in the oestrous cycle, but there is a preponderance of large luteal cells late in the luteal phase at the time of luteal regression[141]. Thus the relative lack of large luteal cells early in the cycle may explain why young corpora lutea are not susceptible to the luteolytic action of $PGF_{2\alpha}$, particularly as regards structural luteolysis.

Direct inhibitory actions of $PGF_{2\alpha}$ on progesterone production

Progesterone production by large luteal cells, which is LH and c-AMP independent, is inhibited by $PGF_{2\alpha}$. Also, $PGF_{2\alpha}$ inhibits increased progesterone production induced by c-AMP in a mixed population of luteal cells from the rat[142] and cow[143]. These observations suggest that $PGF_{2\alpha}$ may inhibit some of the enzymes involved in progesterone synthesis. $PGF_{2\alpha}$ treatment of the rat ovary reduces both cholesterol esterase activity and, to a greater extent, cholesterol ester synthetase activity[144]. In the pig, $PGF_{2\alpha}$ may suppress ovarian progesterone production by decreasing the supply of cholesterol P_{450} side-chain cleavage enzyme[145]. In the hysterectomized guinea-pig, $PGF_{2\alpha}$ causes a 50 % inhibition in the conversion of pregnenolone to progesterone and the activities of cholesterol esterase (but not of cholesterol ester synthetase) and of 3β-hydroxy-steroid dehydrogenase are reduced by $PGF_{2\alpha}$[146]. $PGF_{2\alpha}$ also inhibits the conversion of pregnenolone to progesterone in the sheep ovary[147]. $PGF_{2\alpha}$ reduces, therefore, the activities of several enzymes involved in the synthesis of progesterone from cholesterol. Whether these are direct actions of $PGF_{2\alpha}$ on enzyme activity or occur as a result of $PGF_{2\alpha}$-induced morphological changes in the luteal cells requires further study.

$PGF_{2\alpha}$ and oestradiol interaction

Destruction of the follicles in sheep ovaries by X-irradiation prevents $PGF_{2\alpha}$-induced luteolysis, suggesting that oestradiol is necessary for the luteolytic action of $PGF_{2\alpha}$[148]. The treatment of hysterectomized sheep with $PGF_{2\alpha}$, in doses below the threshold for inducing luteolysis, causes luteolysis if given together with oestradiol[149]. Specific receptors for oestradiol are present in the cytosolic fraction of sheep corpora lutea. The concentration of oestradiol receptors is lowest on day 4, is maximum on day 8, and is also high at the time of luteal regression. The concentration of oestradiol receptors is 3.5 times higher in large luteal cells than in small luteal cells[150]. These findings suggest that oestradiol produced by the follicles acts on the large luteal cells in some way so as to permit the luteolytic action of $PGF_{2\alpha}$.

Uterine luteolytic hormone

In several non-primate mammalian species (such as the cyclical sheep, guinea-pig, cow and pig, and the pseudopregnant rat, rabbit, mouse and hamster) hysterectomy prevents luteal regression from occurring at the normal time. The uterus of these species secretes a luteolytic hormone which has been identified as $PGF_{2\alpha}$[151]. The $PGF_{2\alpha}$ secreted by one uterine horn only affects the ipsilateral ovary, indicating that there is a local pathway for transferring $PGF_{2\alpha}$ between a uterine horn and its adjacent ovary. Since there are no direct vascular connections between the uterus and ovary, a countercurrent mechanism of transfer of $PGF_{2\alpha}$ between the utero-ovarian vein and the ovarian artery has been proposed[152]. However, a pathway involving the uterine venous blood alone, as the means by which $PGF_{2\alpha}$ leaves the sheep uterus, does not result in luteolysis[153]. Consequently, based on additional experimental evidence in sheep[154–156], it has been proposed that there is a countercurrent transfer of $PGF_{2\alpha}$ between the uterine lymph vessels and the ovarian artery, and that this is the main route for transfer of $PGF_{2\alpha}$ from the uterus to the ovary.

Studies in several species have shown that oestradiol acting on a progesterone-primed uterus is the optimum combination of ovarian steroids for increasing endometrial $PGF_{2\alpha}$ production[151]. This combination of steroid hormones may form the physiological stimulus in this respect. However, the immunization of sheep against oxytocin delays luteal regression[157], indicating that oxytocin of ovarian origin also forms part of the physiological stimulus which increases endometrial $PGF_{2\alpha}$ production. However, the endometrium only becomes responsive to oxytocin after plasma progesterone levels have started to fall[158,159], since progesterone prevents the increase in numbers of oxytocin receptors in the endometrium induced by oestradiol. Thus it appears that in the sheep, oestradiol acting on the progesterone-primed uterus causes an initial increase in $PGF_{2\alpha}$ output from the uterus. Once plasma progesterone levels have started to fall, the endometrium becomes responsive to oxytocin, so that oxytocin causes a secondary release of $PGF_{2\alpha}$ which is responsible for finally terminating luteal function. Oxytocin of ovarian origin is also necessary for increasing uterine $PGF_{2\alpha}$ output in relation to the goat[160,161], and probably the cow[162].

Effects of $PGF_{2\alpha}$ on the outputs of oxytocin and $PGF_{2\alpha}$ from the ovary

In sheep ovaries, oxytocin is produced by the large luteal cells[163], which also contain the receptors for $PGF_{2\alpha}$. Ovarian oxytocin secretion is increased by $PGF_{2\alpha}$ in the sheep[164] and cow[165]. In the goat, indomethacin treatment reduces uterine $PGF_{2\alpha}$ output and the secretion of oxytocin by the ovary[166]. These studies suggest that increased $PGF_{2\alpha}$ output from the uterus increases oxytocin output from the ovary. However, as the corpora lutea regress, oxytocin output from the ovary falls[167]. Furthermore, ovarian oxytocin output and luteal cell oxytocin concentrations decrease in early pregnant sheep and in hysterectomized sheep at about the same time as occurs in the oestrous cycle[168-170], indicating that oxytocin production by the large luteal cells declines in these two situations despite the lack of luteal regression and, certainly in hysterectomized sheep, the lack of uterine $PGF_{2\alpha}$ secretion.

All cells in the body (except red blood cells) have the ability to synthesize PGs, so it is not surprising that the luteal cells can synthesize $PGF_{2\alpha}$. It has been proposed[171] that $PGF_{2\alpha}$ produced by the ovary may be of importance in luteal regression. In pigs, luteolysis induced by cloprostenol (a $PGF_{2\alpha}$ analogue) is associated with increased $PGF_{2\alpha}$ production by the luteal cells. However, indomethacin does not prevent cloprostenol-induced luteal regression in pigs, even though luteal cell $PGF_{2\alpha}$ synthesis is suppressed[172]. This study indicates that $PGF_{2\alpha}$ produced by the ovary is not necessary for luteal regression. However, further study is required in this respect in other species. What is not disputed is that increased $PGF_{2\alpha}$ production by the uterus is necessary for luteolysis to occur in many non-primate mammalian species.

Luteolysis in primates

Hysterectomy in primates does not prevent regression of the corpus luteum from occurring at the normal time. Hence there is no uterine luteolytic hormone in primates and, therefore, $PGF_{2\alpha}$ produced by the uterus is not necessary for luteolysis. Nevertheless, the question is raised as to whether $PGF_{2\alpha}$ produced by the ovary is responsible for the demise of the corpus luteum in primates, including women.

Studies on non-human primates

Oestradiol administration to monkeys during the luteal phase of the cycle will cause luteolysis, as indicated by a premature decline in plasma progesterone levels and a shortening of the menstrual cycle. It has been proposed that oestradiol produced by the corpus luteum is responsible for luteal regression[173]. The treatment of rhesus monkeys with oestradiol on days 2 to 6 following the LH peak results in plasma progesterone levels being lower than normal during the rest of the cycle, but cycle length is not reduced. The same treatment with oestradiol on days 6 to 10 following the LH surge promptly induces luteolysis as indicated by a fall in plasma progesterone levels and shortening of the cycle[174]. Thus there is a receptive period for the luteolytic action of oestradiol in the rhesus monkey as there is for $PGF_{2\alpha}$ in non-primate mammalian species. Consequently, is oestradiol-induced luteal regression in monkeys mediated by $PGF_{2\alpha}$?

In an early study[175], the systemic administration of $PGF_{2\alpha}$ to monkeys during the mid-luteal phase caused a decline in plasma progesterone levels and premature menstrual bleeding; nevertheless, normal menstrual bleeding occurred at the expected time. However, the menstrual cycle was shortened if oestradiol was given with the $PGF_{2\alpha}$. In a later study[176], $PGF_{2\alpha}$ was infused directly into the corpus luteum of rhesus monkeys commencing 5 to 7 days following the ovulatory oestradiol surge. Premature luteolysis occurred, as determined by a significant fall in plasma progesterone levels and the early onset of menstruation. Cloprostenol administered to marmoset monkeys as a single dose which was not luteolytic when administered on days 6 or 7 of the luteal phase, caused premature luteolysis in some monkeys when administered on days 8 or 9, and induced premature luteolysis in all monkeys when administered between days 10 and 17[177]. These studies indicate that $PGF_{2\alpha}$ is truly luteolytic in the monkey and, as in non-primate mammalian species, young corpora lutea are not susceptible to the luteolytic action of $PGF_{2\alpha}$. Luteolysis induced by $PGF_{2\alpha}$ and oestradiol in the rhesus monkey is associated with a decrease in LH receptor-binding capacity in the corpus luteum[178].

The output of $PGF_{2\alpha}$ (as indicated by measuring its metabolite 13,14-dihydro-15-keto-$PGF_{2\alpha}$) was higher from the ovary bearing the corpus luteum than from the opposite ovary without a corpus luteum, in rhesus monkeys during the late luteal phase and menstruation[179]. Thus luteal regression in the rhesus monkey is associated with an increase in ovarian $PGF_{2\alpha}$ output. Whether this increase in ovarian $PGF_{2\alpha}$ production is the result of stimulation by oestradiol and is the cause of luteolysis requires further investigation. Indomethacin treatment of rhesus monkeys during the luteal phase did not prevent the decline in plasma progesterone levels and menstruation from occurring at the normal time[180]. However, it was not shown that the dose of indomethacin used inhibited ovarian PG synthesis.

Oxytocin infused into the corpus luteum of rhesus monkeys also causes a premature decline in plasma progesterone levels and early menstruation[181]. Since oxytocin is present in the monkey corpus luteum[182], a role for oxytocin in luteolysis in the monkey cannot be disregarded.

Studies in women

The administration of oestradiol into the ovary bearing the corpus luteum shortens the length of the menstrual cycle[173]. Diethylstilboestrol administration for 5 days from day 7 of the luteal phase causes a premature decline in plasma progesterone levels and menstrual cycle length to be shortened by 2 to 4 days[183]. Consequently, as in the monkey, oestradiol produced by the corpus luteum has been proposed as the stimulus for luteal regression[173]. Is its action mediated by $PGF_{2\alpha}$?

$PGF_{2\alpha}$ receptors are present in human corpora lutea[184]. $PGF_{2\alpha}$ inhibits LH-stimulated progesterone output from human granulosa cells in culture[185]. This is probably due to inhibition of c-AMP production. However, $PGF_{2\alpha}$ only has this inhibitory action in corpora lutea that are older than 6 days[186]. The superfusion in vitro of human luteal slices with cloprostenol causes a drop in progesterone output but this inhibition is not maintained and progesterone output returns to control levels or even higher during the cloprostenol treatment[187]. As with pig luteal tissue, cloprostenol stimulates $PGF_{2\alpha}$ output from human luteal slices[187].

Several studies have shown that the administration of $PGF_{2\alpha}$ to women causes slight to moderate falls in plasma progesterone levels. After $PGF_{2\alpha}$ treatment, plasma progesterone levels return to pre-treatment values and menstrual cycle length is unaffected. In a more detailed study[188], $PGF_{2\alpha}$ was injected directly into the corpus luteum between days 5 and 8 following the ovulatory LH surge. There was a rapid fall in plasma progesterone levels, the nadir coinciding with the onset of uterine bleeding which occurred 24 h after the $PGF_{2\alpha}$ injection and lasted up to seven days. However, plasma progesterone levels quickly returned to normal (despite the uterine bleeding) and fell again at the 'normal' time. The human corpus luteum appears particularly resistant to $PGF_{2\alpha}$. Although functional luteolysis can be demonstrated with $PGF_{2\alpha}$, it is only temporary and progesterone production quickly recovers. The human corpus luteum does not seem to acquire that 'something' which makes it 'susceptible' to the $PGF_{2\alpha}$-induced morphological changes which result in structural luteolysis. Perhaps, as in the pig, structural luteolysis is not induced in the human until two to three days before the corpus luteum would normally regress. The effect of $PGF_{2\alpha}$ injected directly into the corpus luteum on day 10 or 11 of the luteal phase may be worth studying. Notwithstanding, there is one report where the IV infusion of $PGF_{2\alpha}$ over a 5 h period into a woman on day 21 of the cycle (presumably about day 7 of the luteal phase) resulted in a premature and permanent decline in plasma progesterone levels, and early menstruation. This treatment cycle was shorter than normal[189]. However, this study appears to be an exception rather than the rule.

Despite the general lack of a complete luteolytic action of $PGF_{2\alpha}$ in women, several studies have measured $PGF_{2\alpha}$ in the human corpora lutea during the luteal phase to see if there is an increase prior to luteal regression. One study reported that luteal $PGF_{2\alpha}$ levels increased in the late luteal phase[190], one study reported that the levels did not change[191], and a third study reported that $PGF_{2\alpha}$ levels were lower in the late luteal phase[192]. A fourth study reported that luteal $PGF_{2\alpha}$ levels increased 6-fold between the early and mid-luteal phases but then decreased by 50 % during the late luteal phase[193]. Consequently, there is no consistent agreement as to whether luteal $PGF_{2\alpha}$ levels do increase prior to luteal regression. Plasma from the ovary containing the corpus luteum contains significantly higher levels of oestradiol, proge-sterone and $PGF_{2\alpha}$ than plasma from the ovary without a corpus luteum[194]. A positive relationship existed between the elevated oestradiol and $PGF_{2\alpha}$ levels in the luteal phase. However, it was not shown whether this was a cause and effect relationship or whether these increases were necessary for luteolysis.

There have been no systematic studies reporting the effects of the administration of inhibitors of PG synthesis (e.g. aspirin, indomethacin) on plasma progesterone levels and menstrual cycle length in women. However, as such drugs are in widespread use for treating pain and inflammatory conditions, one would have thought that any adverse effects on menstrual cycle length would have been reported by now. It would appear that $PGF_{2\alpha}$ produced by the ovary is not involved in luteal regression in women. Nevertheless, this conclusion must remain open, until it has been shown that the non-steroidal anti-inflammatory drugs in the doses used completely inhibit ovarian $PGF_{2\alpha}$ synthesis without affecting the lifespan of the corpus luteum.

Overall, it still remains a mystery as to what causes luteolysis in women, especially if $PGF_{2\alpha}$ is not involved. Perhaps oestradiol inhibits luteal function directly, but it has still to be proven that oestradiol is the physiological stimulus for luteolysis in women. Oestrogen treatment does reduce LH receptor number in human corpora lutea which is consistent with its luteolytic action[195]. On the other hand, $PGF_{2\alpha}$ increases the number of LH receptors in human corpora lutea, which is not consistent with its luteolytic action in other species[195]. Perhaps this is why $PGF_{2\alpha}$ does not cause structural luteolysis in women. Other possible stimuli for luteolysis cannot be overlooked. It has been reported that oxytocin is present in the human corpus luteum[196], but oxytocin in vitro did not have an inhibitory effect on progesterone production by cultured luteal cells obtained from human corpus luteum[197]. The effect of oxytocin infused into the human corpus luteum in vivo on luteal function merits investigation. In rats, LHRH acts directly on the corpus luteum to decrease progesterone production in a similar manner to $PGF_{2\alpha}$, i.e. it prevents LH-induced increases in c-AMP production and stimulates the PI cycle[198]. Perhaps LHRH is present in the human corpus luteum and is responsible for luteal regression; or there may be an as yet unidentified luteolytic peptide in the human ovary waiting to be discovered.

GENERAL CONCLUSIONS

There is much evidence from studies in non-primate mammalian species that (a) PGs are involved in the release of LH by acting as a mediator between the release of noradrenaline and the stimulation of LHRH-containing neurones in the median eminence, (b) PGs are the mediators in LH-induced ovulation and (c) $PGF_{2\alpha}$ is the uterine luteolytic hormone. It is likely, though still not proven, that PGs are involved in LH release and ovulation in women. In contrast to many non-primate mammalian species, the uterus does not control the life span of the corpus luteum in women, so $PGF_{2\alpha}$ produced by the uterus is not involved in luteolysis in women. In addition, there is no convincing evidence that $PGF_{2\alpha}$ produced by the ovary is responsible for luteolysis in women, especially as the human corpus luteum appears particularly resistant to the luteolytic action of $PGF_{2\alpha}$, particularly as regards $PGF_{2\alpha}$ inducing structural luteolysis. The cause of luteolysis in women remains unclear. Since PGs are apparently involved in several reproductive processes concerned with ovarian function, it might be expected that the prolonged use of non-steroidal anti-inflammatory drugs, especially in high doses, would result in reduced fertility. Indeed, the chronic treatment of deermice with indomethacin reduces litter size by 50%[199]. Whether fertility is reduced in women who are receiving chronic treatment with non-steroidal anti-inflammatory drugs is not known, but it would seem to merit investigation.

REFERENCES

1. Orczyk, S. and Behrman, H.R. (1972). Ovulation blockade by aspirin or indomethacin in vivo – evidence for a role of prostaglandins in gonadotrophin secretion. Prostaglandins, 1, 3–20
2. Behrman, H.R., Orczyk, G.P. and Greep, R.O. (1972). Effect of synthetic gonadotrophin-releasing hormone (GN-RH) on ovulation blockade by aspirin and indomethacin. Prostaglandins, 1, 245–258

3. Linton, E.A. and Whitehead, S.A. (1980). Role of arachidonic acid metabolites in the hypothalamic control of ovulation in the rat. *Biol. Reprod.*, **23**, 726–732

4. Ojeda, S.R., Harms, P.G. and McCann, S.M. (1975). Effect of inhibitors of prostaglandin synthesis on gonadotrophin release in the rat. *Endocrinology*, **97**, 843–854

5. Sato, T., Tyujo, T., Hirono, M. and Iesaka, T. (1975). Effects of indomethacin, an inhibitor of prostaglandin synthesis, on the hypothalamic-pituitary system in rats. *J. Endocrinol.*, **64**, 395–396

6. Botting, J.H., Linton, E.A. and Whitehead, S.A. (1977). Blockade of ovulation in the rat by a prostaglandin antagonist (N-0164). *J. Endocrinol.*, **75**, 335–336

7. Tsafriri, A., Koch, Y. and Lindner, H.R. (1973). Ovulation rate and serum LH levels in rats treated with indomethacin or prostaglandin E_2. *Prostaglandins*, **3**, 461–468

8. Sato, T., Taya, K., Tjujo, T. and Igarashi, M. (1974). Ovulation block by indomethacin, an inhibitor of prostaglandin synthesis: a study of its site of action in rats. *J. Reprod. Fertil.*, **39**, 33–40

9. Hucker, H.B., Zacchei, A.G., Cox, S.V., Brodie, D.A. and Cartwell, N.H.R. (1966). Studies on the absorption, distribution and excretion of indomethacin in various species. *J. Pharmacol. Exp. Ther.*, **153**, 237–249

10. Brown, C.G. and Poyser, N.L. (1984). Studies on the control of prostaglandin production by the hypothalamus in relation to LH release in the rat. *J. Endocrinol.*, **103**, 155–164

11. Kimball, F.H., Porteus, S.E., Kirton, K.T., Frielink, R.D., Creasy, D.M. and Dayan, A.R. (1979). Prostaglandin (PGI_2) effects on anterior pituitary hormones *in vivo*. *Prostaglandins*, **18**, 377–386

12. Harms, P.G., Ojeda, S.R. and McCann, S.M. (1974). Prostaglandin-induced release of pituitary gonadotrophins: central nervous system and pituitary sites of action. *Endocrinology*, **94**, 1459–1464

13. Spies, H.G. and Norman, R.L. (1973). Luteinizing hormone release and ovulation induced by the intraventricular infusion of prostaglandin E_1 into pentobarbital blocked rats. *Prostaglandins*, **4**, 131–141

14. Harms, P.G., Ojeda, S.R. and McCann, S.M. (1976). Failure of monoaminergic and cholinergic receptor blockers to prevent prostaglandin E_2-induced luteinizing hormone release. *Endocrinology*, **98**, 318–323

15. Linton, E.A., Perkins, M.N. and Whitehead, S.A. (1977). Catecholamines and prostaglandins in the central control of ovulation. *J. Physiol. (Lond.)*, **266**, 61P

16. Eskay, R.L., Warberg, J., Mical, R.S. and Porter, J.C. (1975). Prostaglandin E_2-induced release of LH-RH into hypophysial portal blood. *Endocrinology*, **97**, 816–824

17. Ojeda, S.R., Wheaton, J.E. and McCann, S.M. (1975). Prostaglandin E_2-induced release of luteinizing hormone-releasing factor. *Neuroendocrinology*, **17**, 283–287

18. Chobsieng, P., Naor, Z., Koch, Y., Zor, U. and Lindner, H.R. (1975). Effect of prostaglandin E_2 on LH release in the rat: evidence for hypothalamic site of action. *Neuroendocrinology*, **17**, 12–17

19. Drouin, J., Ferland, L., Bernard, J. and Labrie, F. (1976). Site of the *in vivo* stimulatory effect of prostaglandin on LH release. *Prostaglandins*, **11**, 367–376

20. Ojeda, S.R. and Negro-Vilar, A. (1985). Prostaglandin E_2-induced luteinizing hormone-release involves mobilization of intracellular Ca^{2+}. *Endocrinology*, **116**, 1763–1771

21. Kinoshita, F., Nakai, Y., Katakami, H., Imura, H., Shimizu, T. and Hayaishi, D. (1982). Suppressive effect of prostaglandin (PG) D_2 on pulsatile luteinizing hormone release in conscious castrated rats. *Endocrinology*, **110**, 2207–2209

22. Kalra, S.P. and Crawley, W.R. (1982). Epinephrine synthesis inhibitors block naloxone-induced LH release. *Endocrinology*, **111**, 1403–1405

23. Leaden, C.A. and Kalra, S.P. (1985). Reversal of β-endorphin-induced blockade of ovulation and luteinizing hormone surge with prostaglandin E_2. *Endocrinology*, **117**, 684–689

24. Tasaka, K., Miyake, A., Sakumoto, T., Aona, T. and Kurachi, K. (1983). Prostaglandin D_2 induces release of luteinizing hormone from the rat pituitary gland without the modulation of hypothalamic luteinizing hormone releasing hormone. *J. Endocrinol.*, **99**, 289–292

25. Ojeda, S.R., Naor, Z. and McCann, S.M. (1978). Prostaglandin E levels in hypothalamus, median eminence and anterior pituitary of rats of both sexes. *Brain Res.*, **149**, 274–277

26. Cseh, G., Szabo, I.K., Lang, T. and Pulkovitz, M. (1978). Distribution of prostaglandins E and F in different regions of the rat brain. *Brain Res. Bull.*, **3**, 293–298

27. Ojeda, S.R., Negro-Vilar, A. and McCann, S.M. (1979). Release of prostaglandin Es by

hypothalamic tissue – Evidence for their involvement in catecholamine-induced luteinizing hormone-releasing hormone release. *Endocrinology*, **104**, 617–624

28. Ojeda, S.R., Negro-Vilar, A. and McCann, S.M. (1982). Evidence for the involvement of α-adrenergic receptors in norepinephrine-induced prostaglandin E$_2$ and luteinizing hormone-releasing hormone release from the median eminence. *Endocrinology*, **110**, 409–412

29. Heaulme, M. and Dray, F. (1984). Noradrenaline and prostaglandin E$_2$ stimulate LH-RH release from rat median eminence through distinct α-adrenergic and PGE$_2$ receptors. *Neuroendocrinology*, **39**, 403–407

30. Hulting, A.-L., Lingren J.A., Hokfelt, T., Heidvall, K., Eneroth, P., Werner, S., Patrono, C. and Samuelsson, B. (1984). Leukotriene C$_4$ stimulates LH secretion from rat pituitary cells *in vitro*. *Eur. J. Pharmacol.*, **106**, 459–460

31. Hulting, A.-L., Lindgren, J.A., Hokfelt, T., Eneroth, P., Werner, S., Patrono, C. and Samuelsson, B. (1985). Leukotriene C$_4$ as a mediator of luteinizing hormone release from rat anterior pituitary cells. *Proc. Natl. Acad. Sci. USA*, **82**, 3834–3838

32. Carlson, J.C., Barcikowski, B. and McCracken, J.A. (1973). Prostaglandin F$_{2\alpha}$ and the release of LH in sheep. *J. Reprod. Fertil.*, **34**, 357–362

33. Carlson, J.C., Barcikowski, B., Cargill, V. and McCracken, J.A. (1974). The blockade of LH release by indomethacin. *J. Clin. Endocrinol. Metab.*, **39**, 399–402

34. Roberts, J.S. and McCracken, J.A. (1975). Prostaglandin F$_{2\alpha}$ production by the brain during estrogen-induced secretion of luteinizing hormone. *Science*, **190**, 894–896

35. Carlson, J.C., Wong, A.P. and Perrin, D.G. (1977). The effects of prostaglandins and mating on release of LH in the female rabbit. *J. Reprod. Fertil.*, **51**, 87–92

36. Leach, C.M., Reynoldson, J.A. and Thorburn, G.D. (1982). Release of E prostaglandins into the cerebrospinal fluid and its inhibition by melatonin after cervical stimulation in the rabbit. *Endocrinology*, **110**, 1320–1324

37. Saksena, S.K., Lau, I.F. and Chang, M.C. (1974). Prostaglandin F$_{2\alpha}$ and LH release in female hamsters. *J. Reprod. Fertil.*, **41**, 215–217

38. Meeuvsen, K. and Seeley, R.R. (1979). Effects of indomethacin on plasma LH levels in female and male deermice (*Peromyscus maniculatus*). *Prostaglandins*, **18**, 639–646

39. Carlson, J.C., Wong, A.P. and Perrin, D.G. (1977). Luteinizing hormone secretion in the rhesus monkey and a possible role for prostaglandins. *Biol. Reprod.*, **16**, 622–626

40. Kimball, F.A., Kirton, K.T., Forbes, A.D., Frielink, R.D., Porteus, S.F., Wilks, J.W., Mohberg, N.R. and Turner, L.F. (1979). Serum FSH, LH and testosterone in the male rhesus following prostaglandin injection. *Prostaglandins*, **18**, 117–126

41. Batta, S.K., Niswender, G.D. and Brackett, B.G. (1978). Elevation of rhesus monkey plasma luteinizing hormone levels in response to E-series prostaglandins. *Prostaglandins*, **16**, 835–846

42. Steger, R.W., Balmaceda, J.P., Sclerkhodr, T.M. and Asch, R.H. (1982). Failure of indomethacin to block the estrogen-induced luteinizing hormone surge in the ovariectomized rhesus monkey. *J. Clin. Endocrinol. Metab.*, **54**, 845–848

43. Sowers, J.R., Fayez, J., Colantino, M. and Jonas, H. (1978). The effect of intra-amniotic prostaglandin F$_{2\alpha}$ on anterior pituitary hormone release during midtrimester abortion. *Fertil. Steril.*, **30**, 403–407

44. Hillier, K., Dutton, A. and Corker, C.S. (1973). The effect of prostaglandin F$_{2\alpha}$ administration on plasma steroid and LH levels in the luteal phase of the menstrual cycle. In Bergstrom, S. (ed.) *Advances in the Biosciences*, Vol. 9, pp. 673–678 (Braunschweig:Vieweg).

45. Miyake, A., Tasake, K., Mori, S., Saito, Y. and Aono, T. (1983). Prostaglandin D$_2$ stimulates secretion of luteinizing hormone from pituitary gland *in vitro*. *Acta. Endocrinol.*, **104**, 164–166

46. Greenway, F.L. and Swerdloff, R.S. (1978). Effect of aspirin (prostaglandin synthetase inhibitor) on ovulation. *Fertil. Steril.*, **30**, 364–365

47. Nakai, Y., Plant, T.M., Hess, D.L., Keogh, E.J. and Knobil, E. (1978). Sites of negative and positive feedback actions of estradiol in control of gonadotrophin secretion in rhesus monkey. *Endocrinology*, **102**, 1008–1014

48. Levine, J.E., Norman, R.L., Gliessman, P.M., Oyama, T.T., Bangsberg, D.R. and Spies, H.G. (1985). *In vivo* gonadotropin-releasing hormone release and serum luteinizing hormone measurements in ovariectomized, estrogen-treated rhesus macaques. *Endocrinology*, **117**, 711–721

49. Arimura, A., Kastin, A.J. and Schally, A.V. (1974). Immunoreactive LH-releasing hormone in plasma: midcycle elevation in women. *J. Clin. Endocrinol. Metab.*, **38**, 510–513
50. Elkind-Hirsch, K., Ravnikar, V., Tulchinsky, D., Schiff, I. and Ryan, K.J. (1984). Episodic secretion patterns of immunoreactive luteinizing hormone-releasing hormone (IR-LH-RH) in the systemic circulation of normal women throughout the menstrual cycle. *Fertil. Steril.*, **41**, 56–61
51. Armstrong, D.T. and Grinwich, D.L. (1972). Blockade of spontaneous and LH-induced ovulation in rats by indomethacin, an inhibitor of prostaglandin synthesis. *Prostaglandins*, **1**, 21–28
52. Grinwich, D.L., Kennedy, T.G. and Armstrong, D.T. (1972). Dissociation of ovulatory and steroidogenic actions of luteinizing hormone in rabbits with indomethacin, an inhibitor of prostaglandin synthesis. *Prostaglandins*, **1**, 89–96
53. Armstrong, D.T., Grinwich, D.L., Moon, Y.S. and Zamecnik, J. (1974). Inhibition of ovulation in rabbits by intrafollicular injection of indomethacin and prostaglandin F antiserum. *Life Sci.*, **14**, 129–140
54. O'Grady, J.P., Caldwell, B.V., Auletta, F.J. and Speroff, L. (1972). The effects of an inhibitor of prostaglandin synthesis (indomethacin) on ovulation, pregnancy and pseudopregnancy in the rabbit. *Prostaglandins*, **1**, 97–106
55. Downey, B.R. and Ainsworth, L. (1980). Reversal of indomethacin blockade of ovulation in gilts by prostaglandins. *Prostaglandins*, **19**, 17–22
56. Downs, S.M. and Congo, F.J. (1982). Effects of indomethacin on preovulatory follicles in immature, superovulated mice. *Am. J. Anat.*, **164**, 265–274
57. Murdoch, W.J. and Dunn, T.G. (1983). Luteal function after ovulation blockade by intrafollicular injection of indomethacin in the ewe. *J. Reprod. Fertil.*, **69**, 671–675
58. Wallach, E.E., de la Cruz, A., Hunt, J., Wright, K.H. and Stevens, V.C. (1975). The effect of indomethacin on HMG-HCG induced ovulation in the rhesus monkey. *Prostaglandins*, **9**, 645–658
59. Tsafriri, A., Lindner, H.R., Zor, U. and Lamprecht, S.A. (1972). Physiological role of prostaglandins in the induction of ovulation. *Prostaglandins*, **2**, 1–10
60. Diaz-Infante, A., Jr., Wright, K.H. and Wallach, E.E. (1974). Effects of indomethacin and prostaglandin $F_{2\alpha}$ on ovulation and ovarian contractility. *Prostaglandins*, **5**, 567–581
61. Wallach, E.E., Bronson R., Hamada, Y., Wright, K.H. and Stevens, V.C. (1975). Effectiveness of prostaglandin $F_{2\alpha}$ in restoration of HMG-HCG induced ovulation in indomethacin-treated rhesus monkeys. *Prostaglandins*, **10**, 129–138
62. Chaudhuri, G. and Elder, M.G. (1976). Lack of evidence for inhibition of ovulation by aspirin in women. *Prostaglandins*, **11**, 727–735
63. Espey, L.L. (1983). Comparison of the effect of nonsteroidal anti-inflammatory agents on prostaglandin production during ovulation in the rabbit. *Prostaglandins*, **26**, 71–78
64. Hunter, R.H.F. and Poyser, N.L. (1985). Ovarian follicular fluid concentrations of prosta-glandins E_2, $F_{2\alpha}$ and I_2 during the pre-ovulatory period in pigs. *Reprod. Nutr. Dev.*, **25**, 909–918
65. LeMaire, W.J., Leidner, R. and Marsh, J.M. (1975). Pre and post ovulatory changes in the concentration of prostaglandins in rat Graafian follicles. *Prostaglandins*, **9**, 221–229
66. Murdoch, W.J., Dailey, R.A. and Inskeep, E.K. (1981). Pre-ovulatory changes in prostaglan-dins E_2 and $F_{2\alpha}$ in ovine follicles. *J. Anim. Sci.*, **53**, 192–205
67. Brown, C.G. and Poyser, N.L. (1984). Studies on ovarian prostaglandin production in relation to ovulation in the rat. *J. Reprod. Fertil.*, **72**, 407–414
68. LeMaire, W.J., Yang, N.S.T., Behrman, H.H. and Marsh, J.M. (1973). Preovulatory changes in the concentration of prostaglandins in rabbit Graafian follicles. *Prostaglandins*, **3**, 367–376
69. Yang, N.S.T., Marsh, J.M. and LeMaire, W.J. (1974). Prostaglandin changes induced by ovulatory stimuli in rabbit Graafian follicles. The effect of indomethacin. *Prostaglandins*, **4**, 395–404
70. Sharma, S.C., Wilson, C.M.W. and Pugh, D.M. (1976). *In vitro* production of prostaglandins E and F by the guinea–pig ovarian tissue. *Prostaglandins*, **11**, 555–568
71. Darling, M.R.N., Jogee, M. and Elder, M.G. (1982). Prostaglandin $F_{2\alpha}$ levels in the human ovarian follicle. *Prostaglandins*, **23**, 551–556
72. Sechel, M.M., Swartz, S.L., Smith, D., Levesque, L. and Taymor, M.L. (1984). *In vivo* prostaglandin concentrations in human preovulatory follicles. *Fertil. Steril.*, **42**, 482–485

73. Yang, N.S.T., Marsh, J.M. and LeMaire, W.J. (1974). Post ovulatory changes in the concentration of prostaglandins in rabbit Graafian follicles. *Prostaglandins*, **6**, 37–44

74. Moon, Y.S., Zamecnik, J. and Armstrong, D.T. (1974). Stimulation of prostaglandin F synthesis by luteinizing hormone in rabbit ovarian follicles grown in organ culture. *Life Sci.*, **15**, 1731–1738

75. Bauminger, S., Lieberman, M.E. and Lindner, H.R. (1975). Steroid-independent effect of gonadotropins on prostaglandin synthesis in rat Graafian follicles. *Prostaglandins*, **9**, 753–764

76. Shemesh, M. and Hansel, W. (1975). Stimulation of prostaglandin synthesis in bovine ovarian tissues by arachidonic acid and luteinizing hormone. *Biol. Reprod.*, **13**, 448–452

77. Marsh, J.M., Yang, N.S.T. and LeMaire, W.J. (1974). Prostaglandin synthesis in rabbit Graafian follicles *in vitro*. Effect of luteinizing hormone and cylic AMP. *Prostaglandins*, **7**, 269–283

78. Clark, M.R., Marsh, J.M. and LeMaire, W.J. (1978). Stimulation of prostaglandin accumulation in pre-ovulatory rat follicles by adenosine-3', 5'-monophosphate. *Endocrinology*, **102**, 39–44

79. Clark, M.R., Marsh, J.M. and LeMaire, W.J. (1976). The role of protein synthesis in the stimulation by LH of prostaglandin accumulation in rat preovulatory follicles *in vitro*. *Prostaglandins*, **12**, 209–216

80. Zor, U., Strulovici, B., Nimrod, A. and Lindner, H.R. (1977). Stimulation by cyclic nucleotides of prostaglandin-E production in isolated Graafian follicles. *Prostaglandins*, **14**, 947–961

81. Wang, S.-C. and Greenwald, G.S. (1985). Effect of cycloheximide injected at proestrus on ovarian protein synthesis, peptide and steroid hormone levels, and ovulation in the hamster. *Biol. Reprod.*, **33**, 201–212

82. Pool, W.R. and Lipner, H. (1966). Inhibition of ovulation by antibiotics. *Endocrinology*, **79**, 858–864

83. Barros, C. and Austin, C.R. (1968). Inhibition of ovulation by systemically administered actinomycin D in the hamster. *Endocrinology*, **83**, 177–179

84. Alleva, J.J., Bonventre, P.F. and Lamanna, C. (1979). Inhibition of ovulation in hamsters by the protein synthesis inhibitors diphtheria toxin and cycloheximide. *Proc. Soc. Exp. Biol. Med.*, **162**, 170–174

85. Bauminger, S. and Lindner, H.R. (1975). Periovulatory changes in ovarian prostaglandin formation and their hormonal control in the rat. *Prostaglandins*, **9**, 737–751

86. Poyser, N.L. (1983). Differential stimulation of prostaglandin and thromboxane synthesizing capacities in guinea-pig uterus and ovary. *Prostaglandins, Leuk. Med.*, **10**, 163–177

87. Clark, M.R., Marsh, J.M. and LeMaire, W.J. (1978). Mechanism of luteinizing hormone regulation of prostaglandin synthesis in rat granulosa cells. *J. Biol. Chem.*, **253**, 7757–7761

88. Samuelsson, B. (1973). Quantitative aspects of prostaglandin synthesis in man. In Bergstrom, S. (ed.) *Advances in the Biosciences*, Vol.9, pp. 7–14, (Braunschweig: Vieweg).

89. Veldhuis, J.D., Klase, P. and Demers, L. (1982). Luteinizing hormone stimulates the production of prostacyclin by isolated ovarian cells *in vitro*. *Prostaglandins*, **22**, 319–327

90. Evans, G., Dobias, M., King, G.J. and Armstrong, D.T. (1983). Production of prostaglandins by porcine preovulatory tissue and their roles in intrafollicular function. *Biol. Reprod.*, **28**, 322–328

91. Ainsworth, L., Tsang, B.K., Marcus, G. and Downey, B.R. (1984). Prostaglandin production by dispersed granulosa cells and theca internal cells from porcine preovulatory follicles. *Biol. Reprod.*, **31**, 115–121

92. Erickson, G.F., Challis, J.R.G. and Ryan, K.J. (1977). Production of prostaglandin F by rabbit granulosa cells and thecal tissue. *J. Reprod. Fertil.*, **49**, 133–134

93. Triebwasser, W.F., Clark M.R., LeMaire, W.J. and Marsh, J.M. (1978). Localization and *in vitro* synthesis of prostaglandins in components of rabbit preovulatory Graafian follicles. *Prostaglandins*, **16**, 621–632

94. Hamada, Y., Bronson, R.A., Wright, K.H. and Wallach, E.E. (1977). Ovulation in the perfused rabbit ovary: the influence of prostaglandins and prostaglandin inhibitors. *Biol. Reprod.*, **17**, 58–63

95. Kitai, H., Santulf, R., Wright, K.H. and Wallach, E.E. (1985). Examination of the role of

calcium in ovulation in the *in vitro* perfused rabbit ovary with the use of ethyleneglycol-bis (β-aminoethyl ether)-n,n'-tetraacetic acid and verapamil. *Am. J. Obstet, Gynecol.*, **152**, 705−708

96. Lindner, H.R., Amsterdam, A., Salomon, Y., Tsafriri, A., Nimrod, A., Lamprecht, S.A., Zor, U. and Koch, Y. (1977). Intraovarian factors in ovulation: determinantes of follicular responses to gonadotrophins. *J. Reprod. Fertil.*, **51**, 215−235

97. Strickland, S. and Beers, W.H. (1976). Studies on the role of plasminogen activator in ovulation. *In vitro* response of granulosa cells to gonadotropins, cyclic nucleotides, and prostaglandins. *J. Biol. Chem.*, **251**, 5694−5702

98. Beers, W.H. (1975). Follicular plasminogen and plasminogen activator and the effect of plasmin on ovarian follicle wall. *Cell*, **6**, 379−386

99. Shimada, H., Okamura, H., Noda, Y., Suzuki, A., Tojo, S. and Takado, A. (1983). Plasminogen activator in rat ovary during the ovulatory process − independence of prostaglandin mediation. *J. Endocrinol.*, **97**, 201−206

100. Espey, L., Shimada, H., Okamura, H. and Mori, T. (1985). Effect of various agents on ovarian plasminogen activator activity during ovulation in pregnant mare's serum gonadotropin-primed immature rats. *Biol. Reprod.*, **32**, 1087−1094

101. Reich, R., Miskin, R. and Tsafriri, A. (1985). Follicular plasminogen activator: in ovulation. *Endocrinology*, **116**, 516−521

102. Espey, L.L., Coons, P.J., Marsh, J.M. and LeMaire, W.J. (1981). Effect of indomethacin on preovulatory changes in the ultrastructure of rabbit Graafian follicles. *Endocrinology*, **108**, 1040−1048

103. Downs, S.M. and Longo, F.J. (1983). An ultrastructure study of preovulatory apical development in mouse ovarian follicles. Effects of indomethacin. *Anat. Rec.*, **205**, 159−168

104. Ichikawara, S., Ohta, M., Morioka, H. and Murao, S. (1983). Blockage of ovulation in the explanted hamster ovary by a collagenase inhibitor. *J. Reprod. Fertil.*, **68**, 17−19

105. Reich, R., Tsafriri, A. and Mechanic, G.L. (1985). The involvement of collagenolysis in ovulation in the rat. *Endocrinology*, **116**, 522−527

106. Dennefors, B., Tjugum, J., Norstrom, A., Janson, P.O., Nillson, L., Hamberger, L. and Wilhelmsson, L. (1982). Collagen synthesis inhibition by PGE_2 within human follicular wall − one possible mechanism underlying ovulation. *Prostaglandins*, **24**, 295−302

107. Lindner, H.R., Tsafriri, A., Lieberman, M.E., Zor, U, Koch, Y., Bauminger, S. and Barnea, A. (1974). Gonadotropin action on cultured Graafian follicles: induction of maturation division of the mammalian oocyte and differentiation of the luteal cell. *Rec. Prog. Horm. Res.*, **30**, 79−138

108. Phi, L.T., Moon, Y.S. and Armstrong, D.T. (1977). Effects of systemic and intrafollicular injections of LH, prostaglandins, and indomethacin on luteinization of rabbit Graafian follicles. *Prostaglandins*, **13**, 543−552

109. Ainsworth, L., Tsang, B.K., Downey, B.R., Baker, R.D., Marcus, G.J. and Armstrong, D.T. (1979). Effects of indomethacin on ovulation and luteal function. *Biol. Reprod.*, **21**, 401−411

110. Barbosa, I., Maia, H., Jr., Lopes, T., Elder, M.G. and Coutinho, E.M. (1979). Effect of indomethacin on prostaglandin and steroid synthesis by the marmoset ovary *in vivo*. *Int. J. Fertil.*, **24**, 142−144

111. Armstrong, D.T., Dorrington, J.H. and Robinson, J. (1976). Effects of indomethacin and aminoglutethimide phosphate *in vivo* on luteinizing hormone-induced alterations of cylic adenosine monophosphate, prostaglandin F, and steroid levels in preovulatory rat ovaries. *Can. J. Biochem.*, **54**, 796−802

112. Reich, R., Kohen, F., Naor, Z. and Tsafriri, A. (1983). Possible involvement of lipoxygenase products of arachidonic acid pathway in ovulation. *Prostaglandins*, **26**, 1011−1020

113. Reich, R., Kohen, F., Slager, R. and Tsafriri, A. (1985). Ovarian lipoxygenase activity and its regulation by gonadotropin in the rat. *Prostaglandins*, **30**, 5813−5900

114. Kyzymowski, T., Kotwica, J., Okrasa, S., Doboszynska, T. and Ziecik, A. (1978). Luteal function in sows after unilateral infusion of $PGF_{2\alpha}$ into the anterior uterine vein on different days of the oestrous cycle. *J. Reprod. Fertil.*, **54**, 21−27

115. Kimball, F.A. and Wyngarden, L.J. (1977). Prostaglandin $F_{2\alpha}$ specific binding in equine corpora lutea. *Prostaglandins*, **13**, 553−564

116. Rao, Ch.V., Estergreen, V.L., Carmon, F.R., Jr. and Mass, G.E. (1979). Receptors for

gonadotropin and prostaglandin $F_{2\alpha}$ in bovine corpora lutea of early, mid and late luteal phase. *Acta. Endocrinol.*, **91**, 529–537

117. Brambaifa, N. and Schillinger, E. (1984). Binding of prostaglandin $F_{2\alpha}$ and 20α-hydroxysteroid dehydrogenase activity of immature rat ovaries throughout pseudopregnancy. *Prostaglandins, Leuk. Med.*, **14**, 225–234

118. Mattiolo, M., Galeati, G., Prandi, A. and Seren, E. (1985). Effect of $PGF_{2\alpha}$ on progesterone production in swine luteal cells at different stages of the luteal phase. *Prostaglandins, Leuk. Med.*, **17**, 43–54

119. Lahav, M., Freud, A. and Lindner, H.R. (1976). Abrogation by prostaglandin $F_{2\alpha}$ of LH-stimulated cyclic-AMP accumulation in isolated rat corpora lutea of pregnancy. *Biochem. Biophys. Res. Commun.*, **68**, 1294–1300

120. Fletcher, P.W. and Niswender, G.D. (1982). Effect of $PGF_{2\alpha}$ on progesterone secretion and adenylate cyclase activity in ovine luteal tissue. *Prostaglandins*, **23**, 803–816

121. Luborsky, J.L., Slater, W.T. and Behrman, H.R. (1984). Luteinizing hormone (LH) receptor aggregation: modification of ferritin-LH binding and aggregation by prostaglandin $F_{2\alpha}$ and ferritin-LH. *Endocrinology*, **115**, 2217–2227

122. Behrman, H.R. (1979). Prostaglandins in hypothalamo-pituitary and ovarian function. *Annu. Rev. Physiol.*, **41**, 685–700

123. Behrman, H.R., Grinwich, D.L., Hichens, M. and MacDonald, G.J. (1978). Effect of hypophysectomy, prolactin, and prostaglandin $F_{2\alpha}$ on gonadotropin binding *in vivo* and *in vitro* in corpus luteum. *Endocrinology*, **103**, 349–357

124. Diekman, M.A., O'Callaghan, P., Nett, T.M. and Niswender, G.D. (1978). Effect of prostaglandin $F_{2\alpha}$ on the number of LH receptors in ovine corpora lutea. *Biol. Reprod.*, **19**, 1010–1013

125. Barb, C.R., Kraeling, R.R., Rampacek, G.B. and Pinkert, C.A. (1984). Luteinizing hormone receptors and progesterone content in porcine corpora lutea after prostaglandin $F_{2\alpha}$. *Biol. Reprod.*, **31**, 913–919

126. Luborsky, J.L., Dorflinger, L.J., Wright, K. and Behrman, H.R. (1984). Prostaglandin $F_{2\alpha}$ inhibits luteinizing hormone (LH)-induced increase in LH receptor binding to isolated rat luteal cells. *Endocrinology*, **115**, 2210–2216

127. Dorflinger, L.J., Albert, P.J., Williams, A.T. and Behrman, H.R. (1984). Calcium is an inhibitor of LH sensitive adenylate cyclase in the luteal cell. *Endocrinology*, **114**, 1208–1218

128. Raymond, V., Leung, P.C.K. and Labrie, F. (1983). Stimulation by prostaglandin $F_{2\alpha}$ of phosphatidic acid: phosphatidylinositol turnover in rat luteal cells. *Biochem. Biophys. Res. Commun.*, **116**, 39–46

129. Berridge, M.J. and Irvine, R.F. (1984). Inositol triphosphate, a novel second messenger in cellular signal transduction. *Nature (Lond.)*, **312**, 315–321

130. Buhr, M.M., Carlson, J.C. and Thompson, J.E. (1979). A new perspective on the mechanism of corpus luteum regression. *Endocrinology*, **105**, 1330–1335

131. Carlson, J.C., Buhr, M.M., Gruber, M.Y. and Thompson, J.E. (1981). Compositional and physical properties of microsomal membrane lipids from regressing rat corpora lutea. *Endocrinology*, **108**, 2124–2128

132. Carlson, J.C., Buhr, M.M., Wentworth, R. and Hansel, W. (1982). Evidence of membrane changes during regression in the bovine corpus luteum. *Endocrinology*, **110**, 1472–1476

133. Riley, J.C.M. and Carlson, J.C. (1985). Calcium-regulated plasma membrane rigidification during corpus luteum regression in the rat. *Biol. Reprod.*, **32**, 77–82

134. Lemon, M. and Moir, L. (1977). Steroid release *in vitro* by two luteal cell types in the corpus luteum of the pregnant sow. *J. Endocrinol.*, **72**, 351–359

135. Ursely, J. and Leymarie, P. (1979). Varying responses to luteinizing hormone of two luteal cell types isolated from bovine corpus luteum. *J. Endocrinol.*, **83**, 303–310

136. Fitz, T.A., Mayan, M.H., Sawyer, H.R. and Niswender, G.D. (1982). Characterization of two steroidogenic cell types in the ovine corpus luteum. *Biol. Reprod.*, **27**, 703–711

137. Rodgers, R.J., O'Shea, J.D. and Findlay, J.K. (1983). Progesterone production *in vitro* by small and large ovine luteal cells. *J. Reprod. Fertil.*, **69**, 113–124

138. Hayer, P.B., Fitz, T.A. and Niswender, G.D. (1984). Hormone-independent activation of adenylate cyclase in large steroidogenic ovine luteal cells does not result in increased progesterone secretion. *Endocrinology*, **114**, 604–608

139. Heath, E., Weinstein, P., Merritt, B., Shanks, R. and Hixon, J. (1983). Effects of prostaglandins on the bovine corpus luteum: granules, lipid inclusions and progesterone secretion. *Biol. Reprod.*, **29**, 977–986

140. Fitz, T.A., Mock, E.J., Mayan, M.H. and Niswender, G.D. (1984). Interactions of prostaglandins with subpopulations of ovine luteal cells. 2. Inhibitory effects of $PGF_{2\alpha}$ and protection by PGE_2. *Prostaglandins*, **28**, 127–138

141. Fitz, T.A. and Sawyer, H.R. (1982). Changes in the quantity and size of steroidogenic cells in ovine corpora lutea during the oestrous cycle and early pregnancy. *Biol. Reprod.*, **26**, Suppl. 1, 54A

142. Jordan, A.W. (1981). Effects of prostaglandin $F_{2\alpha}$ treatment on LH and dibutyryl cyclic AMP-stimulated progesterone secretion by isolated rat luteal cells. *Biol. Reprod.*, **25**, 327–331

143. Pate, J.L. and Condon, W.A. (1984). Effects of prostaglandin $F_{2\alpha}$ on agonist-induced progesterone production in cultured bovine luteal cells. *Biol. Reprod.*, **31**, 427–435

144. Behrman, H.R., MacDonald, G.J. and Greep, R.O. (1971). Regulation of ovarian cholesterol esters: evidence for the enzymatic sites of prostaglandin-induced loss of corpus luteum function. *Lipids*, **6**, 791–796

145. Torday, J.S., Jefcoate, C.R. and First, N.L. (1980). Effect of prostaglandin F-2α on steroidogenesis by porcine corpora lutea. *J. Reprod. Fertil.*, **58**, 301–310

146. Dwyer, R.J. and Church, R.B. (1979). Effect of prostaglandin F-2α on ovarian enzyme activity in the hysterectomized guinea-pig. *J. Reprod. Fertil.*, **56**, 85–88

147. Hoppen, H.O., Williams, D.M. and Findlay, K.I. (1976). The influence of prostaglandin F-2α on pregnenolone metabolism by the autotransplanted ovary of the ewe. *J. Reprod. Fertil.*, **47**, 275–281

148. Hixon, J.E., Gengenbach, D.R. and Hansel, W. (1975). Failure of prostaglandin $F_{2\alpha}$ to cause luteal regression in ewes after destruction of ovarian follicles by x-irradiation. *Biol. Reprod.*, **13**, 126–135

149. Gegenbach, D.R., Hixon, J.E. and Hansel, W. (1977). A luteolytic interaction between estradiol and prostaglandin $F_{2\alpha}$ in hysterectomized ewes. *Biol. Reprod.*, **16**, 571–579

150. Glass, J.D., Fitz, T.A. and Niswender, G.D. (1984). Cytosolic receptor for estradiol in the corpus luteum of the ewe: variation throughout the estrous cycle and distribution between large and small steroidogenic cell types. *Biol. Reprod.*, **31**, 967–974

151. Horton, E.W. and Poyser, N.L. (1976). Uterine luteolytic hormone: a physiological role for prostaglandin $F_{2\alpha}$. *Physiol. Rev.*, **56**, 595–651

152. McCracken, J.A., Carlson, J.C., Glew, M.E., Goding, J.R., Baird, D.T., Green, K. and Samuelsson, B. (1972). Prostaglandin $F_{2\alpha}$ identified as a luteolytic hormone in sheep. *Nature New Biol. (Lond.)*, **238**, 129–134

153. Abdel Rahim, S.E.A., Bland, K.P. and Poyser, N.L. (1984). Surgical separation of the uterus and ovaries with simultaneous cannulation of the uterine vein extends luteal function in the sheep. *J. Reprod. Fertil.*, **72**, 231–235

154. Abdel Rahim, S.E.A., Bland, K.P. and Poyser, N.L. (1984). Sequential changes in the concentration of prostaglandins and steroids in uterine lymph in sheep during the oestrous cycle. *Prostaglandins, Leuk. Med.*, **14**, 403–409

155. Abdel Rahim, S.E.A. and Bland, K.P. (1985). The lymphatic drainage of the cranial part of the sheep's uterus and its possible functional significance. *J. Anat.*, **140**, 705–709

156. Heap, R.B., Fleet, I.R. and Hamon, M. (1985). Prostaglandin F-2α is transferred from the uterus to the ovary in the sheep by lymphatic and blood vascular pathways. *J. Reprod. Fertil.*, 645–656

157. Sheldrick, E.L., Mitchell, M.D. and Flint, A.P.F. (1980). Delayed luteal regression in ewes immunized against oxytocin. *J. Reprod. Fertil.*, **59**, 37–42

158. Roberts, J.S., McCracken, J.A., Gavagan, J.E. and Soloff, M.S. (1976). Oxytocin-stimulated release of prostaglandin $F_{2\alpha}$ from ovine endometrium *in vivo*-Correlation with estrous cycle and oxytocin-receptor binding. *Endocrinology*, **99**, 1107–1114

159. Sheldrick, E.L. and Flint, A.P.F. (1985). Endocrine control of uterine oxytocin receptors in the ewe. *J. Endocrinol.*, **106**, 249–258

160. Cooke, R.G. and Homeida, A.M. (1982). Plasma concentrations of 13,14-dihydro-15-keto-prostaglandin $F_{2\alpha}$ and progesterone during oxytocin-induced oestrus in the goat. *Theriogenology*, **18**, 453–460

161. Cooke, R.G. and Homeida, A.M. (1985). Suppression of PGF-2α release and delay of

27

luteal regression after active immunization against oxytocin in the goat. *J. Reprod. Fertil.,* **75,** 63–68

162. Wathes, D.C., Swann, R.W., Birkett, S.D., Porter, D.G. and Pickering, B.T. (1983). Characterization of oxytocin, vasopressin and neurophysin from the bovine corpus luteum. *Endocrinology,* **113,** 693–698

163. Rodgers, R.J., O'Shea, J.D., Findlay, J.K., Flint, A.P.F. and Sheldrick, E.L. (1983). Large luteal cells are the source of luteal oxytocin in the sheep. *Endocrinology,* **113,** 2303–2306

164. Flint, A.P.F. and Sheldrick, E.L. (1982). Ovarian secretion of oxytocin is stimulated by prostaglandin. *Nature (Lond.),* **297,** 587–588

165. Schallenberger, E., Schams, D., Bullerman, B. and Walters, D.L. (1984). Pulsatile secretion of gonadotrophins, ovarian steroids and ovarian oxytocin during prostaglandin-induced regression of the corpus luteum in the cow. *J. Reprod. Fertil.,* **71,** 493–501

166. Cooke, R.G. and Homeida, A.M. (1984). Delayed luteolysis and suppression of the pulsatile release of oxytocin after indomethacin treatment in the goat. *Res. Vet. Sci.,* **36,** 48–51

167. Flint, A.P.F. and Sheldrick, E.L. (1983). Evidence for a systemic role for ovarian oxytocin in luteal regression in sheep. *J. Reprod. Fertil.,* **67,** 215–225

168. Sheldrick, E.L. and Flint, A.P.F. (1983). Luteal concentrations of oxytocin decline during early pregnancy in the ewe. *J. Reprod. Fertil.,* **68,** 477–480

169. Schams, D. and Lahloukassi, A. (1984). Circulation concentrations of oxytocin during early pregnancy in ewes. *Acta Endocrinol.,* **106,** 277–281

170. Sheldrick, E.L. and Flint, A.P.F. (1983). Regression of the corpora lutea in sheep in response to cloprostenol is not affected by loss of luteal oxytocin after hysterectomy. *J. Reprod. Fertil.,* **68,** 155–160

171. Rothchild, I. (1981). The regulation of the mammalian corpus luteum. *Rec. Prog. Horm. Res.,* **37,** 183–298

172. Guthrie, H.D. and Rexroad, C.E. Jr. (1980). Blockade of luteal prostaglandin F release *in vitro* during cloprostenol-induced luteolysis in the pig. *Biol. Reprod.,* **23,** 358–362

173. Knobil, E. (1973). On the regulation of the primate corpus luteum. *Biol. Reprod.,* **8,** 246–258

174. Schoonmaker, J.N., Victery, W. and Karsch, F.J. (1981). A receptive period for estradiol-induced luteolysis in the rhesus monkey. *Endocrinology,* **108,** 1874–1877

175. Shaikh, A.A. and Klaiber, E.L. (1974). Effects of sequential treatment with estradiol and $PGF_{2\alpha}$ on the length of the primate menstrual cycle. *Prostaglandins,* **6,** 253–262

176. Auletta, F.J., Kamps, D.L., Pories, S., Bisset, I. and Gibson, M. (1984). An intra-corpus luteum site for the luteolytic action of prostaglandin $F_{2\alpha}$ in the rhesus monkey. *Prostaglandins,* **27,** 285–298

177. Summers, P.M., Wennink, C.J. and Hodges, J.K. (1985). Cloprostenol-induced luteolysis in the marmoset monkey *(Callithrix jacchus). J. Reprod. Fertil.,* **73,** 133–138

178. Sotrel, G., Helvacioglu, A., Dowers, S., Scommegna, A. and Auletta, F.J. (1981). Mechanism of luteolysis — Effect of estradiol and prostaglandin $F_{2\alpha}$ on corpus luteum luteinizing hormone-human chorionic gonadotrophin receptors and cylic nucleotides in the rhesus monkey. *Am. J. Obstet, Gynecol.,* **139,** 134–140

179. Auletta, F.J., Kamps, D.L., Wesley, M. and Gibson, M. (1984). Luteolysis in the rhesus monkey: ovarian venous estrogen, progesterone, and prostaglandin $F_{2\alpha}$-metabolite. *Prostaglandins,* **27,** 299–310

180. Manaugh, L.C. and Novy, M.J. (1976). Effects of indomethacin on corpus luteum function and pregnancy in rhesus monkeys. *Fertil. Steril.,* **27,** 588–598

181. Auletta, F.J., Paradis, D.K., Eesley, M. and Duby, R.T. (1984). Oxytocin is luteolytic in the rhesus monkey. *J. Reprod. Fertil.,* **72,** 401–406

182. Khan-Dawood, F.S., Marat, E.L. and Dawood, M.Y. (1984). Oxytocin in the corpus luteum of the lympomologus monkey *(Macaca fusicularis). Endocrinology,* **115,** 570–574

183. Gore, B.Z., Caldwell, B.V. and Speroff, L. (1973). Estrogen-induced human luteolysis. *J. Clin. Endocrinol. Metab.,* **136,** 615–617

184. Powell, W.S., Hammarstrom, S., Samuelsson, B. and Sjoberg, B. (1974). Prostaglandin $F_{2\alpha}$ receptor in human corpora lutea. *Lancet,* **1,** 1120

185. McNatty, K.P., Henderson, K.M., and Sawers, R.S. (1975). Effects of prostaglandin $F_{2\alpha}$ and E_2 on the production of progesterone by human granulosa cells in tissue culture. *J. Endocrinol.,* **67,** 231–240

186. Hamberger, L., Nilsson, L., Dennefors, B., Khan, I. and Sjogren, A. (1979). Cyclic AMP formation of isolated human corpora lutea in response to HCG—Interference by $PGF_{2\alpha}$. *Prostaglandins*, **17**, 615–621

187. McDougall, A.N.,, Maule Walker, F.M. and Watson, J. (1977). The effect of cloprostenol on human luteal steroid and prostaglandin secretion *in vitro*. *Br. J. Pharmacol.*, **60**, 425–431

188. Korda, A.R., Shutt, D.A., Smith, I.D., Shearman, R.P. and Lyneham, R.C. (1975). Assessment of possible luteolytic effect of intra-ovarian injection of prostaglandin $F_{2\alpha}$ in the human. *Prostaglandins*, **9**, 443–449

189. Lehmann, F., Peters, F., Breckwoldt, M. and Bettendorf, G. (1972). Plasma progesterone levels during infusion of prostaglandin $F_{2\alpha}$ in the human. *Prostaglandins*, **1**, 269–275

190. Shutt, D.A., Clarke, A.H., Fraser, I.S., Goh, P., McMahon, G.R., Saunders, D.M. and Shearman, R.D. (1976). Changes in concentration of prostaglandin F and steroids in relation to growth of the human corpus luteum and luteolysis. *J. Endocrinol.*, **71**, 453–454

191. Swanston, I.A., McNatty, K.P. and Baird, D.T. (1977). Concentration of prostaglandin $F_{2\alpha}$ and steroids in the human corpus luteum. *J. Endocrinol.*, **73**, 115–122

192. Challis, J.R.G., Calder, A.A., Dilley, S., Forster, C.S., Hillier, K., Hunter, D.J.S., McKenzie, I.Z. and Thorburn, G.D. (1976). Production of prostaglandins E and Fα by corpora lutea, corpora albicantes and stroma from the human ovary. *J. Endocrinol.*, **68**, 401–408

193. Patwardhan, V.V. and Lanthier, A. (1985). Luteal phase variations in endogenous concentrations of prostaglandins PGE and PGF and in the capacity for their *in vitro* formation in the human corpus luteum. *Prostaglandins*, **30**, 91–98

194. Askel, S. Schomberg, D.W. and Hammond, C.B. (1977). Prostaglandin $F_{2\alpha}$ production by the human ovary. *Obstet. Gynecol.*, **50**, 347–350

195. Nakano, R., Yamoto, M. and Iwasaki, M. (1981). Effects of oestrogens and prostaglandin $F_{2\alpha}$ on luteinizing hormone receptors in human corpora lutea. *J. Endocrinol.*, **88**, 401–408

196. Wathes, D.C., Swann, R.W., Pickering, B.T., Porter, D.G., Hull, M.G.R. and Drife, J.D. (1982). Neurophyseal hormones in the human ovary. *Lancet*, **2**, 410–412

197. Richardson, M.C. and Masson, G.M. (1985). Lack of direct inhibitory action of oxytocin on progesterone production by dispersed cells from human corpus luteum. *J. Endocrinol.*, **104**, 149–151

198. Leung, P.C.K. (1985). Mechanism of gonadotropin-releasing hormone and prostaglandin action on luteal cells. *Can. J. Physiol. Pharmacol.*, **63**, 249–256

199. Seeley, R.R. (1983). Effect of indomethacin on reproduction under laboratory and field conditions in deermice *(Peromyscus maniculatus)*. *Biol. Reprod.*, **28**, 148–153

2
Eicosanoids, menstruation and menstrual disorders

I. S. Fraser

INTRODUCTION

One of the most exciting recent developments in the understanding of endometrial and myometrial function has been the realization that a range of eicosanoids are synthesized within and have major biological actions on uterine tissues. Evidence is rapidly accumulating to indicate that eicosanoids are responsible for a wide range of physiological uterine functions and pathological disturbances. This is particularly exemplified by their involvement in menstruation and several menstrual disorders.

EICOSANOID SYNTHESIS IN THE UTERUS DURING THE MENSTRUAL CYCLE

The classical prostaglandins E_2 and $F_{2\alpha}$ can be synthesized in substantial amounts by human endometrium, and this varies with the stage of the menstrual cycle. These prostaglandins are not stored in tissues but result from the rapid metabolism of free arachidonic acid. Most of the arachidonic acid in uterine tissues appears to be covalently bound to cell membrane phospholipids[1] and is not directly available for metabolism to prostaglandins. Release of arachidonic acid is catalysed mainly by phospholipase A_2. The uterus also has the capability to synthesize thromboxane A_2 (TXA_2), prostacyclin (PGI_2) and some leukotrienes. The relationships and major synthetic pathways of these eicosanoids are illustrated in simplified form in Figure 2.1. Both cyclo-oxygenase and lipoxygenase pathways appear to be active in different uterine tissues. Prostaglandins E_2 and $F_{2\alpha}$, PGI_2, TXA_2, the cyclic endoperoxides and leukotrienes C_4 and D_4 may all have functional effects on some of the tissues in the uterus.

The first reports of prostaglandins in uterine tissue came from bioassay studies[2,3] and showed a rise in PGE_2 and $PGF_{2\alpha}$ concentration in human

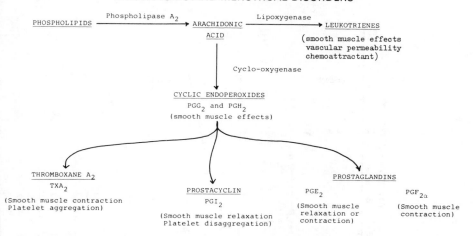

Figure 2.1 Main pathways of synthesis of eicosanoids which have a relevance for uterine function

endometrial curettings in the secretory and especially the premenstrual/menstrual phases of the cycle (Figure 2.2). $PGF_{2\alpha}$ generally increases to a much greater extent than PGE_2. $PGF_{2\alpha}$ may also increase slightly prior to ovulation. Subsequent reports using alternative methodology such as radio-immunoassay for prostaglandin measurement have amply confirmed this pioneering work[4–6], but there have been some disagreements about the cyclical patterns of release[7] and extensive disagreement about absolute concentrations[8]. Endometrial concentrations of $PGF_{2\alpha}$ in the proliferative phase have ranged from 10 to 5790 ng/g, whereas secretory phase concentrations have ranged from 50 to 8280 ng/g. In most studies secretory phase concentrations have been at least double those reported in the proliferative phase.

It now seems clear that assays for endometrial prostaglandins are recording the rapid synthesis of these substances subsequent to trauma during curettage or hysterectomy. These concentrations are therefore the result of a variable, short term incubation of the endometrium at room temperature. In view of the results discussed in the previous paragraph it seems clear that the synthetic capacity of prostaglandins increases substantially towards and at the onset of menses. It seems likely that there is a rapidly synthesizable reserve of prostaglandins present in endometrial cells. This is released within seconds of the initial trauma. However, no matter how standardized the conditions of collection may be, all studies have shown a wide variation in absolute concentrations in specimens collected at the same stage of the cycle.

Several attempts have been made to assess prostaglandin synthesis in endometrium in a more scientific manner using short or long term cultures or perfusions. If these cultures are incubated with excess arachidonic acid the synthesis of PGs should reflect the activity of the cyclo-oxygenase, isomerase and reductase enzymes, which catalyse the metabolism of arachidonic acid[9]. In culture the endogenous secretion of $PGF_{2\alpha}$ and E_2 in normal proliferative endometrium is low and there is reduced capacity to synthesize $PGF_{2\alpha}$ and

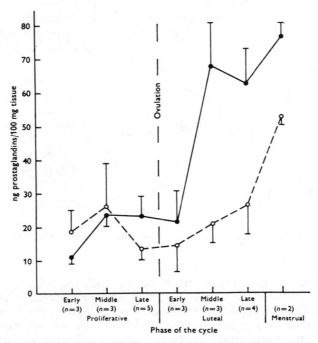

Figure 2.2 Concentrations of PGE_2 (O $--$ O) and $PGF_{2\alpha}$ (● $—$ ●) in endometrium (mean $\pm$ SEM) collected at different stages of the menstrual cycle (from Downie *et al*[3], with permission)

PGE_2 from labelled arachidonic acid when compared with normal secretory endometrium. In secretory endometrium there appears to be increased potential to release arachidonic acid in response to tissue damage or ischaemia.

The prostaglandin synthetase system in endometrium is clearly sensitive to circulating levels of oestrogens and progesterone, although the exact mechanism of action of these hormones is unclear. Throughout the cycle $PGF_{2\alpha}$ levels in the endometrium are linearly related to the log of the concentration of oestradiol in uterine venous blood[6]. However, *in vitro* it has been more difficult to demonstrate a direct stimulatory action of oestradiol on $PGF_{2\alpha}$ production[10,11]. On the other hand a marked and dose dependent stimulation was observed in $PGF_{2\alpha}$ and PGE_2 production using low concentrations of the catechol oestrogen, 2-hydroxyoestradiol[10,11]. The optimal conditions for prostaglandin synthesis in endometrium appear to require progesterone priming followed by oestradiol or a catechol oestrogen. Progesterone inhibits PG synthesis if given simultaneously with oestradiol. It appears that progesterone has an important influence on the activity of the phospholipase A_2 system while oestradiol stimulates later in the prostaglandin synthetase pathway but does not increase arachidonic acid availability.

Several authors have studied prostaglandin release from endometrium during perfusion experiments. The results of these studies are somewhat controversial and tissue damage may occur with perfusion beyond two hours[12]. All these studies have shown a rapid release of prostaglandins E_2 and $F_{2\alpha}$ within the first hour and a plateau is then reached within three to six hours[8,12,13]. These studies have confirmed greater release of $PGF_{2\alpha}$ than PGE_2 from endometrium under most circumstances with particularly high levels in late luteal and menstrual endometrium. This cyclicity of release was not demonstrated for myometrium. These studies have also assessed the release of other prostanoids from endometrium and myometrium. It seems' that thromboxane A_2 and prostacyclin production from endometrium are very low. It is possible that any thromboxane released within the uterus may come entirely from platelets. There is now clear evidence that prostacyclin is produced in larger amounts from myometrium than from endometrium[13,14]. This is particularly obvious when endometrium and myometrium are incubated together allowing cyclic endoperoxide precursors from the endometrium to act as substrate for the myometrial prostacyclin synthetase enzyme system. Since the mass of myometrium in a normal uterus is substantially greater than the endometrial mass the predominant prostaglandin produced by the human uterus *in vivo* in terms of total quantity may be prostacyclin. There is also some evidence for an increase in prostacyclin secretion at the onset of menses.

The prostaglandin cyclo-oxygenase enzyme system appears to be localized in glandular cells of the endometrium[15]. Since the 15-hydroxyprostaglandin dehydrogenase is also found in glandular epithelium[16] it appears that prostaglandins are synthesized and metabolized in similar cell types in endometrium. Although these cells have the capability for metabolizing prostaglandins the concentrations of metabolites such as 13,14-dihydro-15-oxo-$PGF_{2\alpha}$ are very low in endometrium[5].

In passing it should be noted that prostaglandins have also been measured in peripheral venous blood throughout the menstrual cycle and attempts have been made to correlate these levels with changes in uterine function. Unfortunately there are considerable difficulties in measuring eicosanoids in peripheral blood because of their rapid metabolism, especially during passage through the lungs. Measurements of the main metabolite of $PGF_{2\alpha}$ in peripheral venous blood, 13,14-dihydro-15-oxo-$PGF_{2\alpha}$ have usually indicated little change during the normal cycle[17], but one study has shown small pre-ovulatory and pre-menstrual peaks[18]. Although eicosanoids are generally thought to act locally in the tissue where they are generated rather than at a distance, it is possible that precursors from endometrium may be transported through the vascular system over a short distance into myometrium where different actions may be produced[14]. In certain animal species it is well recognized that pulsatile secretion of $PGF_{2\alpha}$ into utero-ovarian venous blood in the late luteal phase is responsible for luteolysis[19]. High levels of $PGF_{2\alpha}$ and PGE_2 have also been measured in menstrual blood[2].

Other factors also have influences on the secretion of eicosanoids from endometrium. For example, oxytocin is capable of enhancing $PGF_{2\alpha}$ release from endometrium via oxytocin receptors, whose availability is stimulated by oestrogen[20]. Adrenaline stimulates the production of all prostaglandins from uterine tissues *in vitro*[10]. $PGF_{2\alpha}$ secretion by endometrium is suppressed in early pregnancy[7] and is thought to be due to an inhibitor of cyclo-oxygenase which is identifiable in amniotic fluid and maternal serum[21]. It has been suggested that this inhibitor might be decidual prolactin or a metabolite[22], since prolactin has been demonstrated to inhibit prostaglandin production in other organs. Secretion of prostaglandins from endometrium *in vitro* can be rapidly suppressed with cyclo-oxygenase inhibitors such as indomethacin[13].

Several studies have demonstrated the effect of contraceptive hormones on endometrial prostaglandins, usually indicating suppression[23] although one study has indicated increased levels of PGE_2[7]. Oestrogen-containing oral contraceptives have been shown to decrease prostacyclin metabolite levels in peripheral plasma, whereas progestogens on their own have no effect[24]. Ethinyl oestradiol on its own may increase the release of thromboxane from endothelial cells *in vitro*[25]. No effect of ethinyl oestradiol, progesterone or testosterone was found on prostacyclin, prostaglandin E or prostaglandin F release from these cultured endothelial cells. Taken together these findings fit in with the clinical evidence for a small increase in venous thromboembolic disease in women using combined oestrogen/progestogen contraceptives.

Finally, mention should be made of the preliminary evidence suggesting an inherent capacity of the human uterus to form lipoxygenase products from arachidonic acid. This has been shown by *in vitro* culture studies of human endometrium exposed to exogenous labelled arachidonic acid with conversion into certain lipoxygenase products[26,27]. It is not known which uterine cell type is responsible for lipoxygenase activity. However, since leukotrienes are actively synthesized by leukocytes, it is possible that the major white cell infiltration which occurs in the later part of the menstrual cycle is predominantly responsible for leukotriene synthesis in endometrium.

PHYSIOLOGICAL AND PHARMACOLOGICAL EFFECTS OF EICOSANOIDS ON THE NON-PREGNANT HUMAN UTERUS

Eicosanoids are synthesized and released to act at a local tissue level rather than as circulating compounds. All of these substances are inactivated rapidly, and sometimes very rapidly, in the peripheral circulation. Different products of the cyclo-oxygenase and lipoxygenase pathways exhibit diverse and sometimes opposing biological actions on uterine tissues. Under certain circumstances the action of the same compound on the same tissue may vary depending on the endocrine milieu. Concentration effects may also be important.

Effects on endometrium

Relatively little is known about the direct effects of eicosanoids on endome-trium. However, it seems probable that various eicosanoids have important actions on endometrial vascular function and menstruation. There is good evidence to suggest that $PGF_{2\alpha}$ and TXA_2 generally act as vasoconstrictors while PGE_2 and PGI_2 act as vasodilators. In addition TXA_2 and PGI_2 have potent and opposing actions on platelet aggregation. Furthermore, leukotrienes have been shown to have potent effects on smooth muscle contraction and small vessel permeability. Leukotriene B_4 appears to be particularly important in eliciting a chemical attractant effect on phagocytic cells, in addition to stimulating lysosomal enzyme release.

Any of these effects may be important in endometrial function throughout the menstrual cycle, at the time of implantation, in early pregnancy and at the time of menstrual breakdown. Very little direct evidence is available for these effects in human endometrium, mainly because *in vivo* models are unsatisfactory. One attempt to look at this problem has been the use of the hamster cheek pouch as a model to study the vascularization and growth of human endometrial explants under direct vision[28]. Preliminary observations using this model have suggested consistent vascular dilatation in the presence of low doses of PGI_2 with vasoconstriction in the presence of higher doses of $PGF_{2\alpha}$. PGE_2 appeared to have little effect on the vasculature of these grafts. Thromboxanes and leukotrienes have not been studied. Little effort has been made to investigate the presence of specific prostaglandin binding sites in human endometrium. However, one study has suggested that $PGF_{2\alpha}$ binding is very low or undetectable at all stages of the menstrual cycle[29]. PGE_2 binding was detected in all specimens and was significantly higher in proliferative than secretory endometrium. The absence of specific $PGF_{2\alpha}$ binding sites suggests that the $PGF_{2\alpha}$ synthesized in relatively large amounts by the endometrium is intended to act on adjacent myometrium.

The possible involvement of eicosanoids in menstruation is considered later in this article.

Effects on myometrium

A considerable amount of information is now available about the major effects of many eicosanoids on myometrial function. There is good evidence for the presence of specific binding sites for PGE_2 and $PGF_{2\alpha}$ in myometrium[30]. Higher concentrations of binding sites are present in the uterine fundus than at the cervical end of the uterine body. In contrast to endometrial PGE_2 binding sites, those in myometrium do not show any cyclical variation. Little evidence is available about binding sites for other eicosanoids.

The first *in vitro* studies of prostaglandins on human myometrium indicated a stimulatory effect of $PGF_{2\alpha}$ and $PGF_{1\alpha}$ and a relaxing effect of PGE_2 and PGI_2[31]. However recent investigations have revealed a complex response of myometrium to different eicosanoids, depending on the localization of the muscle fibers and the phase of the menstrual cycle. The separate effect of different eicosanoids on myometrium has been studied in detail by Wilhelmsson et al.[32,33].

$PGF_{2\alpha}$ stimulates all myometrial layers, and this includes the utero-tubal junction. By contrast PGE_2 inhibits spontaneous contractility in the intermediate and internal muscle layers. However, the subperitoneal myometrial fibers will often show stimulation with low doses of PGE_2 but relaxation with higher doses. The different layers of the utero-tubal junction show complex responses to PGE_2 depending on the phase of the cycle. When PGE_2 and $PGF_{2\alpha}$ are present in equal concentrations myometrial stimulation occurs.

PGE_2 needs to be in considerable excess before it counteracts the effect of $PGF_{2\alpha}$ and produces muscle relaxation.

Prostacyclin produces an inhibitory response in all myometrial fibers including the utero-tubal junction, irrespective of the phase of the menstrual cycle. Thromboxane A_2 is a highly potent stimulator of myometrial contraction including the utero-tubal junction. It is of interest that the cyclic endoperoxides such as PGH_2 are also able to elicit a potent contractile response in the myometrium. Administration of higher doses may initially cause contraction and this is later followed by relaxation.

A small amount of evidence suggests that leukotrienes can affect uterine activity. At low concentrations leukotrienes C_4 and D_4 can elicit contraction of isolated strips of guinea-pig uterus[34]. It has also been demonstrated that an antigen-induced elevation of intrauterine pressure in the guinea-pig is only partially blunted by the cyclo-oxygenase inhibitor, indomethacin. In this model further inhibition of intra-uterine pressure could be produced by infusion of the specific leukotriene receptor antagonist, FPL 55712[35]. This strongly suggests that a leukotriene component had contributed to the induced elevation in intrauterine pressure.

The effects of oestradiol and progesterone on eicosanoid release and effects within the uterus are still far from clear. There are certainly variable changes during the cycle to which ovarian steroids contribute substantially. It has been suggested that these ovarian steroids may help to regulate levels of prostaglandins and leukotrienes by shunting arachidonic acid metabolism from one pathway to another in order to control myometrial function and tone in the uterine vascular bed. Ovarian hormones may also influence the interaction between eicosanoids and such other hormones as oxytocin, vasopressin, relaxin, catecholamines and prolactin. The contractile apparatus of the myometrial smooth muscle cell is based on the interaction of actin and myosin filaments. Enzymatic phosphorylation of the light chains of the myosin molecule activate the contractile mechanism while dephosphorylation inactivates it. The key enzyme, myosin light-chain kinase, requires the presence of the regulatory protein calmodulin, and cyclic AMP. Dephosphorylation by myosin light-chain phosphatase inactivates the contractile apparatus. The relative activity of these two enzymes is also influenced by the presence of calcium ions. The influence of most hormones and drugs on uterine function is explained by their potential effect on the influx and efflux of calcium ions through the cell membrane and their effect on intracellular calcium stores[36]. A direct action of some of these substances may also occur on the contractile proteins. Recently attention has been focussed on the development of gap junctions between myometrial cells[37]. These junctions facilitate the coordination of contractile impulses between myometrial cells and their development appears to be a steroid-dependent phenomenon. The numbers of such junctions appear to increase at the onset of labour and in women with dysmenorrhoea.

Intrauterine pressure studies

The *in vitro* effects of prostaglandins on myometrial strips have, to a great extent, been confirmed by *in vivo* studies. The first studies of the effects of prostaglandin-containing fluids on myometrial activity *in vitro* were carried out with seminal fluid in the early 1930s[38,39]. By contrast the first *in vivo* studies using seminal fluid or purified prostaglandin preparations were carried out in the late 1950s and 1960s[2,40–42]. These and other investigations have demonstrated characteristic myometrial contractility patterns during different phases of the menstrual cycle[43] (Figure 2.3). In the proliferative phase, contractions are usually of small amplitude (10–30 mmHg) with a frequency of 1–3 per minute and a resting tone of 10–25 mmHg. The resting tone increases slightly around the time of ovulation and the frequency increases to 3–5 per minute. At this stage the amplitude usually decreases to 5–20 mmHg. After ovulation the tone again decreases but the amplitude increases up to as much as 80 mmHg. In the late secretory phase increased uterine activity can be recognized. At the onset of menstruation the basal tone may increase to 30–50 mmHg with regular contractions peaking up to 100 mmHg.

Treatment of postmenopausal women with exogenous steroid hormones has demonstrated that oestrogens can cause the proliferative contractile pattern, while the secretory phase pattern is evoked by the addition of progestogens following oestrogen pre-treatment. Therefore it appears likely that ovarian steroids are to a large extent responsible for the different patterns observed during the menstrual cycle.

A number of investigators have studied the response of the human non-pregnant uterus to prostaglandins administered either intravenously or into the uterine cavity through a fine catheter inserted through the cervix[44]. These studies all indicate that PGE_2 and $PGF_{2\alpha}$ generally cause myometrial stimulation with PGE_2 being two to three times more potent. Intrauterine instillations indicate that the myometrium is most sensitive to both PGs in the early proliferative and late secretory phases. At these times as little as 1 μg of PGE_2 or 2–5 μg of $PGF_{2\alpha}$ will elicit a strong response. At ovulation the uterus becomes much less sensitive. At the onset of menstruation $PGF_{2\alpha}$ invariably stimulates uterine contractility although PGE_2 elicits a complex response. Low doses of PGE_2 will stimulate contractions while higher doses cause relaxation. PGE_2 and $PGF_{2\alpha}$ probably have direct effects on uterine blood vessels *in vivo* and there is good evidence to indicate that PGE_2 causes uterine arterial dilatation *in vivo* by a direct relaxation effect as well as by inhibiting sensitivity of the vessels to catecholamines. Prostaglandins probably have a role in regulating uterine blood flow[45].

Although prostacyclin has been shown to cause myometrial relaxation *in vitro*, intravenous injection has no effect on contractility, and intrauterine instillation only elicits a gradual stimulation which may be secondary to its strong vasodilatory effect. Little is known about the *in vivo* effect of other prostaglandins, endoperoxides, thromboxanes and leukotrienes, although it will be surprising if in future they are not shown to have physiological roles.

These basic investigations set the scene for an understanding of the physiology of menstruation, and the pathophysiology and treatment of menstrual disorders such as dysmenorrhoea and dysfunctional uterine bleeding.

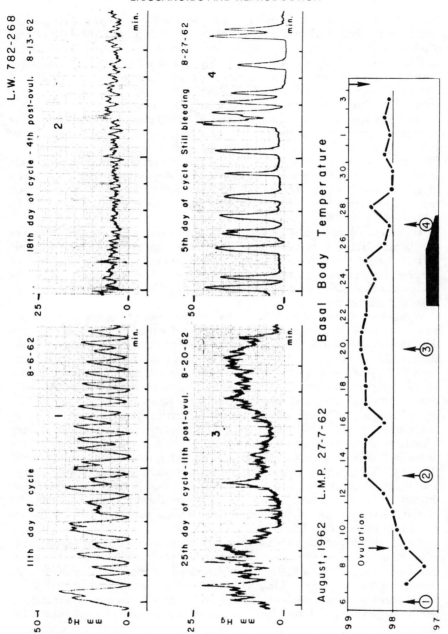

Figure 2.3 Uterine activity as registered by intrauterine pressure recordings at different stages in the menstrual cycle. At the bottom, the basal body temperature chart is marked with circled dates to indicate when pressure records were collected. The solid black area indicates menstrual flow (from Cibils et al.[43], with permission)

THE ROLE OF EICOSANOIDS IN MENSTRUATION

Menstruation is a unique phenomenon which only occurs in primates and is of unknown function. It consists of the loss of blood, endometrial tissue fragments and tissue fluid through the cervix and vagina following the withdrawal of trophic hormone support from the corpus luteum. Until recently homo sapiens lived in an environment where late menarche, early first pregnancy, prolonged lactation and early menopause ensured that regular menstrual cycles were few and far between[46]. Nowadays most women are conditioned to expect a state of regular menstrual bleeding at approximately monthly intervals throughout the major part of their reproductive lives.

The average volume of blood loss per month by women in most Western societies is between 30—40 ml with the upper limit of normal being around 80 ml[47]. It is not widely appreciated that blood only accounts for 30—50 % of the total volume of the menstrual discharge, the remainder probably comprising an endometrial tissue transudate[48]. The amount of endometrial tissue shed at menstruation has been a subject of much controversy over the years and it seems likely that there is wide individual variation[49]. The reason for this tissue breakdown and bleeding in primates is unclear since certain animal species achieve the same degree of endometrial remodelling without actual bleeding.

Our understanding of the sequence of events which occur in the endometrium during menstruation is still relatively poor, and knowledge of the morphological aspects is still based to a great extent on the meticulous observations of Markee[50] who studied intra-ocular endometrial autotransplants in rhesus monkeys. His observations have now been greatly supplemented by corroborative morphological information and new biochemical and hormonal data in women[51].

Endometrial spiral arterioles appear to be essential for the process of menstruation since they are only found in those species in which menstruation has been recorded. Excessive growth and coiling of these vessels occurs during the luteal phase of the cycle and the coiling is greatly accentuated during a period of endometrial regression which occurs immediately prior to endometrial breakdown. This regression is rapid and occurs mainly in the stroma as a result of fluid resorption. Blood flow slows in these excessively coiled arterioles culminating in vascular stasis. This is often followed by a period of vasodilatation accompanied by movement of leukocytes into stroma. This is followed by a period of intense arteriolar constriction which is most obvious at the myometrial—endometrial junction and in the myometrium. This usually lasts between 4—24 hours and precedes the onset of bleeding. Intermittent relaxation of vessels is associated with extravasation of blood into the surrounding stroma and ultimately into the uterine lumen. This accompanies successive shedding of fragments of endometrial glandular and stromal tissue.

The biochemical events which link luteolysis and falling plasma levels of oestradiol and progesterone with actual tissue breakdown are also far from clear. There is reasonable evidence to implicate lysosomes in the initiation of tissue breakdown[52] and these organelles are probably also involved in remodelling of the tissue during and after breakdown. The elegant ultrastructural and histochemical study of Henzl *et al.*[52] demonstrated that acid phosphatase is released from lysosomes into the endometrial cellular cytoplasm and intercellular spaces immediately prior to tissue breakdown. Release of this enzyme appears to follow the fall in plasma levels of oestradiol and progesterone. It has been demonstrated in *in vitro* experiments that hepatic lysosomal membrane stability is influenced by steroid levels, but there is virtually no information on the behaviour of lysosomes of endometrial origin. Little is known about the behaviour of different hydrolase enzymes which could be present in endometrial lysosomes, but it is of some interest that the arachidonic acid mobilising enzyme, phospholipase A_2, is sometimes present in lysosomes. This could provide the link between lysosome activity and the release of eicosanoids at the onset of menstruation.

The exact causes of the endometrial regression, intense vasoconstriction and vascular breakdown, are unknown. In recent years considerable evidence has accumulated to implicate the prostaglandins, especially PGE_2 and $PGF_{2\alpha}$ in the peri-menstrual vascular changes occurring in endometrium, and in the regulation of the volume of blood which is lost. Other eicosanoids may also be involved. Several mechanisms are geared to ensure that increased amounts of $PGF_{2\alpha}$ are secreted by the endometrium just before and at the onset of menstruation. The combined effect of oestradiol and progesterone insures an increased synthetic capacity for $PGF_{2\alpha}$ and this is translated into an increased release of prostaglandin when luteolysis occurs. At the same time there is a decrease in prostaglandin dehydrogenase activity in the endometrium. $PGF_{2\alpha}$ has the ability to induce dose-dependent constriction of human vessels, and infusions of $PGF_{2\alpha}$ into the uterine lumen have been followed within a few hours by menstrual-like bleeding[53]. $PGF_{2\alpha}$ appears to be the major prostaglandin synthesized in secretory endometrium from women with normal ovulatory cycles and a measured menstrual blood loss of less than 50 ml[54]. In this study increased formation of PGE_2 was seen in endometrium from women with heavier bleeding, resulting in a significant inverse correlation between the $PGF_{2\alpha}$ to PGE_2 ratio and blood loss. At the onset of menstruation there is also an increase in uterine contractility which is probably attributable to the increased level of $PGF_{2\alpha}$. These contractions presumably encourage rapid drainage of the uterus.

Haemostatic mechanisms probably also play a central role in control of the volume of blood lost[55,56], and this role is complementary to arteriolar constriction. There is now extensive evidence to indicate that the haemostatic response in endometrium is highly defective compared with other tissues such as skin. This defective response is almost certainly due partly to the highly active fibrinolytic system within the endometrium[57] and possibly also to increased release of PGI_2 and heparin[55]. Morphological studies indicate that bleeding begins when gaps appear in endometrial blood vessel walls. Intravascular haemostatic plugs containing platelets and later some fibrin slowly lead to partial or complete occlusion of vessels. New plugs are formed upstream as tissue fragments are shed but the plugs are always intravascular and typically show an onion skin appearance, suggesting that blood has continued to flow past as they were being formed[58]. In other tissues platelet and fibrin plugs would be seen around the outside as well as inside vessels. The haemostatic response is so defective that in the pre-menstrual phase gaps in vessel walls with exposed collagen may appear without any evidence of platelet plug formation. Platelet plugs only form in the vessel lumina during the first 12–24 hours of menstruation, and fibrin is only detectable in small amounts during the first 48 hours. The haemostatic plugs are shed with the superficial tissue layers into the menstrual fluid. These findings suggest that an imbalance may occur between the pro-aggregatory vasoconstrictor factors and the anti-aggregatory vasodilatory components with a shift in favour of the latter.

Alterations in the intravascular and platelet synthesis of prostacyclin and thromboxane A_2 could contribute to such an imbalance, but there is little evidence to implicate changes in thromboxane A_2 production in the control of blood loss. However the myometrial capacity to synthesise prostacyclin may interact with endometrial $PGF_{2\alpha}$ and PGE_2 to influence bleeding, especially in the first 1–2 days of menstruation. Abnormalities of this interrelationship may be seen in different types of dysfunctional uterine bleeding[59] (Figure 2.4).

Additional evidence to implicate an increase in uterine prostacyclin production at the time of menstruation comes from a study where 6-oxo-$PGF_{1\alpha}$ concentrations were measured in uterine vein and peripheral venous blood in women undergoing abdominal hysterectomy[60]. Concentrations of this metabolite of prostacyclin were found to be significantly higher in uterine venous blood and the highest concentrations were found in three women who were menstruating at the time of surgery. In addition it was found that

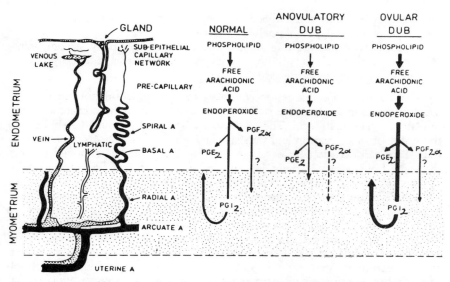

Figure 2.4 Possible involvement of prostaglandins in the vascular control of menstruation and menstrual disorders (from Baird et al.[59], with permission). DUB is dysfunctional uterine bleeding

platelet retention to glass beads was significantly reduced in uterine vein blood. This correlated inversely with the concentrations of 6-oxo-$PGF_{1\alpha}$.

All these mechanisms seem to be aimed at preventing the deposition of significant amounts of fibrin and true blood clot within the uterine cavity. As suggested elsewhere, human pregnancy may only be possible in a uterus which is each month protected from filling with blood clot to reduce the risk of formation of intrauterine adhesions with all their adverse effects on fertility[61]. Thus the poor coagulability of menstrual blood may be important for survival of the species.

Since haemostatic plugs and fibrin are only present in the endometrium during the early stages of menstruation, the mechanism of haemostasis during the remainder of menstruation remains unexplained. It is possible that blood loss after the first twelve hours is limited mainly by vasoconstriction and after forty eight hours by surface regeneration of the epithelium. The major quantity of blood loss occurs during the first two days and then usually tails off rapidly within the next two to three days.

THE ROLE OF EICOSANOIDS IN DYSMENORRHOEA

Dysmenorrhoea is the occurrence of pain in association with menstruation, but in many individuals it may also be accompanied by a symptom-complex which can include nausea, vomiting, diarrhoea, headache, faintness, dizziness, abdominal bloating, back ache and leg pains. Dysmenorrhoea is usually classified into two categories:

(i) primary or spasmodic dysmenorrhoea which typically occurs in the absence of recognizable pelvic disease; and

(ii) secondary or congestive dysmenorrhoea which usually accompanies recognizable pelvic pathology such as endometriosis, adenomyosis or pelvic inflammatory disease.

Most of the following discussion will relate to primary dysmenorrhoea which usually begins in adolescence within a few months after the menarche when ovulatory cycles first occur. The pain usually begins at or immediately before the onset of menstruation and persists through the first 12–48 hours of the flow. Pain can occasionally be so severe that the patient is confined to bed for some hours or even days. Usually there is a constant background pain upon which is superimposed a succession of severe spasmodic cramping pains. Secondary dysmenorrhoea usually has a different symptom pattern with abdominal bloating, pelvic heaviness and dragging pain being prominent.

Primary dysmenorrhoea is a common problem with the maximum incidence in the late teens and twenties[62]. Population surveys indicate that well over half of all menstruating women claim to experience dysmenorrhoea at sometime in their lives, and at least 10% will lose significant time from school or work because of their discomfort. The incidence decreases with increasing age and following child birth. There is a strong association with smoking cigarettes and a strong correlation with mothers and daughters both experiencing dysmenorrhoea. Dysmenorrhoea is clearly influenced by psychological processes and it is still stated that this syndrome seems particularly common in introverted intellectualized neurotic women of obsessive personality[63]. It may well be that these women are more likely to complain about their symptoms than others; however, the converse that all or even most women with dysmenorrhoea have these personality traits is certainly not true. Much of the psychological disturbance may be secondary to the experience of severe recurrent pain which has not responded well to treatment. There is no doubt that there are major socio-economic implications of dysmenorrhoea in all Western societies, since it accounts for a substantial proportion of the total number of hours lost from the female workforce.

Aetiology of primary dysmenorrhoea

There is strong evidence to indicate that the pain of primary dysmenorrhoea is associated with increased uterine muscular activity resulting in increased uterine tone and excessive spasmodic contractions. Baseline intrauterine pressure may easily reach 50 mmHg and pressures up to 100 mmHg have been recorded; superimposed upon this may be spasmodic pressures up to 200 or even 300 mmHg during contractions. This combination of high resting tone and excessive contractions is clearly capable of causing uterine ischaemia. Objective recordings of intrauterine pressure and endometrial blood flow show that flow decreases during contractions and pain is at a maximum when flow is at a minimum[64] (Figure 2.5). It is suggested that pain results from ischaemia by a mechanism analogous to that seen in the heart with myocardial ischaemia and cardiac angina. Treatment resulting in decrease in uterine contractions is usually associated with relief of pain[65] (Figure 2.5). However

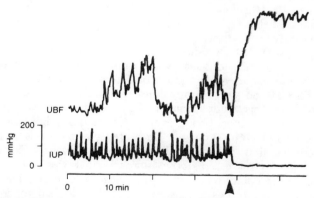

Figure 2.5 High baseline intrauterine pressure (IUP) and extremely high pressure contractions in a patient with dysmenorrhoea on day 1 of her menstrual period. Endometrial blood flow (UBF) was initially low and fluctuating but rose markedly after an injection of terbutaline (arrow). This injection also abolished contractions and greatly reduced baseline tone (from Akerlund *et al.*[64], with permission)

on occasions high amplitude peaks may occur in the absence of pain[66]. Also, in experimental situations pain may sometimes be induced without an obvious increase in contractions. This suggests that there may be other mechanisms resulting in pain which are not directly associated with uterine spasm. This is supported by the fact that dysmenorrhoeic pain can be produced by autologous transfusion of plasma from dysmenorrhoeic women[67]. In this experiment venous plasma was removed from women at the time of severe dysmenorrhoea and, when transfused back into the women some weeks later, produced typical abdominal pain and sometimes associated symptoms in eight out of twelve women. Plasma withdrawn at symptom-free periods did not cause pain when retransfused. A fascinating feature was that the pain could be reproduced in some eight women at a later stage after hysterectomy had been carried out. This phenomenon may be related to the hyperaesthetic effects of prostaglandins, although direct evidence for this in the uterus has not yet been sought[68].

There is now substantial evidence to implicate an excessive endometrial release of $PGF_{2\alpha}$ in the mechanism of primary dysmenorrhoea. The perimenstrual increase in $PGF_{2\alpha}$ in normal cycles has been discussed above. The work of several investigators has demonstrated increased amounts of $PGF_{2\alpha}$ or its main metabolite in endometrium, menstrual fluid and peripheral venous blood from women complaining of dysmenorrhoea, on the first day of the menstrual cycle[2,69,70]. It has recently been demonstrated that $PGF_{2\alpha}$ concentrations in menstrual fluid correlate with uterine work[71], indicating that $PGF_{2\alpha}$ may contribute to the pain of dysmenorrhoea by increasing overall uterine activity.

When $PGF_{2\alpha}$ is infused into the uterus it produces an increase in uterine contractility and dysmenorrhoea-like pain[72], and can also mimic the associated symptoms of nausea, vomiting, diarrhoea and headaches. It is not clear whether other substances which are capable of causing uterine contraction may also sometimes contribute. Possible candidates for this role include the cyclic endoperoxides, thromboxane A_2 and the leukotrienes. There is scanty evidence to suggest that leukotrienes may have an aetiological role in some cases of primary dysmenorrhoea[73].

If indeed excessive $PGF_{2\alpha}$ production is the main mechanism for primary dysmenorrhoea it is still not clear what causes this excessive secretion. Abnormalities of ovarian secretion of oestradiol or progesterone could certainly play a part and such abnormalities have indeed been demonstrated in one study[74]. In this study women with dysmenorrhoea exhibited a significantly higher late-luteal phase level of plasma oestradiol than controls (163 pg/ml compared with 93 pg/ml). Decreased plasma levels of prolactin were also demonstrated, a finding of uncertain significance. Extrapolation from *in vitro* studies discussed above suggests that this abnormality of oestrogen secretion could have an aetiological role in dysmenorrhoea. Abnormalities of catechol oestrogens have not been looked for in women with dysmenorrhoea, but since they are even more potent stimulants of prostaglandin synthesis than oestradiol the possibility exists that they could also have a role.

It has been known for several years that plasma levels of vasopressin are elevated at the time of menstruation and are higher in women with dysmenorrhoea. Recent work now indicates that plasma vasopressin levels remain excessively high in women whose dysmenorrhoea is successfully controlled with prostaglandin inhibitors[75]. This suggests that vasopressin could have an aetiological role mediated through uterine prostaglandin synthesis. Recent studies in rat uterine tissues indicate that vasopressin-induced contractions can be inhibited by nordihydroguaretic acid, a chemical inhibitor of lipoxygenase activity[73]. These contractions were not affected by indomethacin. These observations may suggest a role for lipoxygenase products in vasopressin-induced uterine contractions. The extent of involvement of catecholamines and the autonomic nervous system in the mechanism of dysmenorrhoea is unknown. Dysmenorrhoea can be abolished by presacral neurectomy, but it is also suggested that the decrease in dysmenorrhoea following pregnancy may be related to a marked decrease in autonomic nerve fibers in the uterus at that time[76].

It has long been recognized that intrauterine devices increase the incidence of both dysmenorrhoea and menorrhagia. The reason for this is not clear but one study has demonstrated a clear and statistically significant increase in the PGE content of endometrium from women following insertion of an intrauterine device[77]. In this study there was no evidence for an increase in the PGF content but it is quite possible that elevated PGE levels could stimulate abnormal uterine contractions as well as causing vasodilatation.

Finally, gap junctions between adjacent muscle cells facilitate transmission of contractile impulses, and appear with greater frequency in myometrium at the time of menstruation. They appear to be more frequent than usual in women with dysmenorrhoea[37]. Gap junctions appear to be a steroid dependent phenomenon and may also be influenced by the presence of $PGF_{2\alpha}$.

Management of primary dysmenorrhoea

A vast range of medications and procedures have at various times been proposed for the management of this condition[62]. Severity of the pain and individual tolerance clearly influence the approach to management, and counselling and an explanation of physiology are an integral part of all management approaches. Many women experiencing dysmenorrhoea are also susceptible to the temporary power of suggestion known as the placebo effect. However this effect usually wears off within a few cycles. It does mean that assessment of the efficacy of any new method of treatment requires careful comparison either against placebo or some standard mode of therapy, preferably on a double-blind and cross-over basis. Mild analgesics are often recommended but there is little good evidence to indicate that agents such as paracetamol or aspirin are superior to placebo[70,78].

Many of the drugs which are most effective result in the suppression of endometrial prostaglandin concentrations. These include the combined oral contraceptive pill which produces almost complete relief of menstrual pain in up to 50% of women, with a further 30–40% experiencing marked relief[79]. The constant dose formulations with a more progestogenic balance seem most effective. These agents suppress ovulation, produce suppressed secretory changes in endometrial histology and substantially alter uterine contractility patterns. It seems likely that the altered pattern of circulating oestrogen and progestogen levels act on the endometrium to reduce capacity for prostaglandin synthesis[23] (Table 2.1). The lower levels of $PGF_{2\alpha}$ secretion presumably mean lower intrauterine pressures and therefore less pain. This is clearly the approach of choice if the subject wishes contraceptive cover.

For those who do not wish oral contraceptive cover the medication of choice nowadays is probably the use of a prostaglandin inhibitor administered only for the duration of symptoms. These have recently become extremely popular because of their relatively high degree of efficacy, the simplicity of administration and the relatively low incidence of side effects. Most studies have reported major benefits in 60–90 % of subjects and several different agents have proven very significantly superior to placebo. The clinical value of a prostaglandin inhibitor in women with severe dysmenorrhoea was first convincingly demonstrated in 1974 using flufenamic acid[80]. The fenamates appear to be particularly valuable agents, and benefits of mefenamic acid have been convincingly demonstrated with excellent relief in up to 89 % of women when less than 15 % responded to placebo[81,82]. A chemically different type of prostaglandin inhibitor which has been extensively tested and provides excellent benefit is naproxen and its sodium salt[83,84]. Other agents which may have a similar level of efficacy include ibuprofen, ketoprofen, tolfenamic acid, sulindac and indomethacin.

All of these clinically useful prostaglandin inhibitors are inhibitors of the cyclo-oxygenase enzyme system (Figure 2.1), and are therefore inhibitors of the synthesis of PGE_2, $PGF_{2\alpha}$, PGI_2 and thromboxane A_2. The chemistry and the individual biological half-lives of these drugs are different and therefore recommended dosage schedules vary. Some of these drugs require a loading dose and thereafter individual response usually dictates the frequency of subsequent administration. It is of interest that some women seem to obtain a good response with one agent and less satisfactory results with another. These prostaglandin inhibitors clearly suppress endometrial prostaglandin secretion[23,69,70,85] (Table 2.1), and this leads to the substantial decrease in uterine tone and contractions which accompany the clinical benefits[65,83] (Figure

Table 2.1 Effects of ibuprofen, combined oral contraceptives and placebo on menstrual fluid prostaglandin content. (Adapted from Chan et al.[23])

	Number of patients	Number of cycles	Total menstrual prostaglandin content per cycle (mean ± SEM; μg $PGF_{2\alpha}$ equivalents)
Control cycles	6	6	59.8 ± 7.2
Placebo	6	11	54.4 ± 5.8
Ibuprofen	6	11	16.8 ± 2.3
Control cycles	2	5	60.3 ± 4.1
Combined pill	2	5	12.3 ± 2.4

2.6). Although these agents act predominantly by cyclo-oxygenase inhibition, there is also some controversial evidence for a weak end-organ effect by some of them. All of these drugs should be taken in appropriate dosage at the very first sign of pain or bleeding, whichever comes first, and continued every four to eight hours according to the recurrence of pain. The first onset of action is usually within thirty to forty minutes of ingestion and treatment need only be continued for the normal duration of symptoms, that is to say for no more than 1–3 days per month. The occasional patient obtains added benefit by starting medication just before the onset of menstruation if this is predictable. Side effects are generally uncommon and minor when taken in such short term dosage. Minor gastrointestinal effects such as dyspepsia, nausea or diarrhoea may be noted in up to 5% of subjects and this incidence is reduced if the drug is taken with food. Central nervous system effects such as headache, dizziness and drowsiness are very uncommon. In fact the cyclo-oxygenase inhibitors usually produce very substantial benefit in the symptom complex which often accompanies primary dysmenorrhoea.

There has been a suggestion that selective inhibitors of $PGF_{2\alpha}$ synthesis may be more appropriate than general cyclo-oxygenase inhibitors. However, no such agents are currently available and they could theoretically result in increased PGE_2 or PGI_2 synthesis and an abnormal increase in menstrual blood loss (see below). There seems little clinical reason to make an effort to develop such agents. For this reason a more productive line of research may be to develop drugs which specifically block the action of different prostaglandins at the receptor level[86]. There remain concerns about the 10–40% of dysmenorrhoea patients who do not respond well to the usual agents. The reason for treatment failures with cyclo-oxygenase inhibiting drugs is unknown. This may reflect the fact that the aetiology of primary dysmenorrhoea is still not well understood, and may not always be due to excessive $PGF_{2\alpha}$ secretion. It is possible that in some cases there may be excessive production of leukotrienes C_4 and D_4[73]. Unfortunately, as yet there are no clinically available specific leukotriene antagonists, or inhibitors of the 5-lipoxygenase pathway which leads to leukotriene synthesis. It is possible that a combination of specific lipoxygenase and cyclo-oxygenase inhibitors

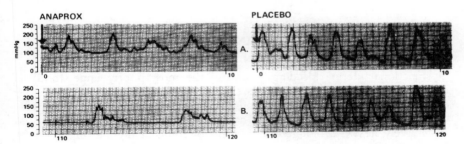

Figure 2.6 Intrauterine pressure tracings in two patients with dysmenorrhoea. One received oral naproxen sodium (Anaprox), with rapid marked reduction in uterine contractions and baseline tone. The other subject showed no reduction in intrauterine pressure following placebo (from Henzl et al.[83], with permission)

may be required to produce the best therapeutic response.

It is worth noting that in many countries some of the cyclo-oxygenase inhibitors are now registered for over-the-counter sale, which means that pharmacists are a very important first line of management. This means that the medical profession is only likely to see the treatment failures, and knowledge about other approaches to treatment is very important. These approaches include the β-adrenergic receptor agonists such as terbutaline[64]. Terbutaline is given in a dosage of 5 mg three times daily for the duration of symptoms in the same way as the prostaglandin inhibitors. Drugs of this type are probably almost as effective as prostaglandin inhibitors, although they appear to have slightly greater incidence of side effects such as tachycardia. A further approach is the research use of calcium channel blocking agents such as nifedipine[87]. These agents probably act at one step beyond prostaglandin and leukotriene involvement in the biochemistry of uterine contractions. There is some hope for the future development of calcium channel blockers specific for uterine smooth muscle, which will hopefully avoid the side effects which sometimes limit their current use. Adjuncts to drug therapy such as relaxation training, acupuncture, behavioural modification therapy, osteopathy and hypnosis may have a role in any patient with troublesome dysmenorrhoea.

Management of secondary dysmenorrhoea

The therapy of secondary dysmenorrhoea is really the management of the underlying diseases and is too extensive for discussion here. However it is worth emphasizing that at least in patients with endometriosis there is evidence for prostaglandin release within the peritoneal cavity and this might contribute to the mechanism of pain. There is also evidence that cyclo-oxygenase inhibitors such as tolfenamic acid may produce relief of secondary dysmenorrhoea in some patients with endometriosis[88], but this relief is not nearly so dramatic as seen with primary dysmenorrhoea sufferers. It should not be forgotten that women with dysmenorrhoea which is secondary to an intrauterine device will usually respond well to antiprostaglandin agents[89].

THE ROLE OF EICOSANOIDS IN DYSFUNCTIONAL UTERINE BLEEDING

Dysfunctional uterine bleeding is one of the most poorly understood of common gynaecological conditions. This is partly due to great confusion over definitions and terminology, and few authorities can agree on consistent criteria to delineate the condition. The definition which this author prefers is 'excessively heavy, prolonged or frequent bleeding of uterine origin which is not due to recognizable pelvic or generalized medical disease, or to pregnancy'. Therefore this is a diagnosis of exclusion — a useful 'working diagnosis'. The commonest complaint is of excessively heavy bleeding (menorrhagia) and it is this symptom which is mainly considered in the following review.

There is little doubt that whatever definition is used the aetiology is multifactorial and only a few categories can be defined clearly. Perception of symptoms by the patient can be quite misleading but clearly forms a crucial part of the initial presentation and the clinical assessment. It is convenient to group the women into those with acute or chronic symptoms and ideally also those who are predominantly ovulatory or predominantly anovulatory[62].

Menorrhagia is a common diagnosis but the actual incidence is very difficult to determine. It is calculated that between 5–25% of women will complain of menorrhagia at some time and that it is particularly common in the ten years leading up to the menopause. Population studies of menstrual blood loss indicate that menorrhagia with measured loss over 80 ml per cycle is relatively infrequent[47,90]. These studies are subject to many biases but give an indication that perhaps 5–10% of menstruating women in a general population will exhibit objective menorrhagia at any one time. This is very different from the subjective complaint of 'menorrhagia' as made by the patient which is probably much commoner. Many women lose their menstrual discharge in small gushes which lead to 'accidents', soiling or soaking of underclothes, and there are considerable individual variations in perception and tolerance of this menstrual loss[62]. It should also be remembered that blood itself accounts only for about one third of the total menstrual fluid discharge[48], the remainder probably being made up mainly by an endometrial transudate.

Increasing evidence points to abnormalities of arachidonic acid metabolism in the uterus of women in whom excessive menstrual bleeding is not obviously secondary to organic pelvic disease.

Aetiology of anovulatory dysfunctional uterine bleeding

In these women a range of hypothalamic and ovarian mechanisms may contribute to the failure of ovulation[62]. The erratic, prolonged and excessively heavy bleeding which is typical of anovulatory DUB is clearly associated with prolonged unopposed stimulation of the endometrium by fluctuating and sometimes excessively high levels of follicular oestradiol[91]. Heavy menstrual bleeding usually occurs when oestrogen levels are falling but occasionally when levels are steady and rarely even when oestrogen levels are rising. The exact mechanism of abnormal breakdown of the endometrium under these circumstances has not been elucidated. The histological findings have been well described[92]. Orderly development of the endometrial vasculature does not occur and there is usually poor spiral arterial development with exaggerated venous vascularity and the development of venous sinusoids[93].

The relative importance of different biochemical mechanisms in the initiation and maintenance of abnormal bleeding has not been defined. There is increasing evidence to implicate the prostaglandins and several abnormalities have been reported. Willman et al.[94] reported an increased endometrial concentration of prostaglandin E_2 while Smith et al.[95] demonstrated that basal amounts of $PGF_{2\alpha}$ and PGE_2 in persistent proliferative endometrium were similar to those obtained from normal proliferative endometrium. However these levels of $PGF_{2\alpha}$ were significantly less than those found in normal secretory endometrium. Therefore the PGE_2 to $PGF_{2\alpha}$ ratio is greater at the time of bleeding than in the normal cycle. Persistent proliferative endometrium appears to lack the capacity to synthesize normal amounts of $PGF_{2\alpha}$ *in vivo* because it lacks the endogenous precursor, arachidonic acid. When incubated in the presence of exogenous arichidonic acid its capacity to synthesize prostaglandins is similar to that of normal secretory endometrium. In this study a highly significant inverse correlation was found between the ratio of the endogenous concentrations of $PGF_{2\alpha}$ and PGE_2 and the measured menstrual blood loss[95].

Abnormal intrauterine haemostasis due to excessive fibrinolysis or to excessive heparin production by endometrial mast cells may also contribute in some women[55,57]. It is not known whether there is any abnormality of endometrial lysosome function although it could be expected that lysosome membrane stability would be reduced in the presence of unopposed oestrogen. Unopposed oestrogen may also lead to endometrial vasodilatation and an excessive rate of endometrial blood flow at the time of endometrial breakdown. All these factors could be expected to be translated into an excessive blood loss.

Aetiology of ovulatory dysfunctional uterine bleeding

Most of these women have ovulatory hormone levels and secretory endometrium which are indistinguishable from those of normal women.

Increasing evidence once again implicates abnormalities of prostaglandin metabolism in the mechanism of bleeding. Willman *et al.*[94] found increased endometrial concentrations of PGE_2 and $PGF_{2\alpha}$ throughout the menstrual cycle in women complaining of heavy periods. Smith *et al.*[54] found that heavy menstrual blood loss in ovulating women was associated with a shift in the endometrial synthetic capacity in favour of PGE_2 over $PGF_{2\alpha}$. There is also evidence to indicate that endometria from ovulatory patients with DUB have an increased capacity to enhance the production of prostacyclin by myometrium and endometria from women with normal menstrual blood loss[96]. The factors responsible for such a shift in the endometrial conversion of cyclic endoperoxides towards PGE_2 and PGI_2 (Figure 2.4) are unknown. It will be of interest to look for an abnormality of catechol oestrogen metabolism in these patients. The abnormalities described above could not be confirmed by Rees *et al.*[97] although limited data from three menstrual specimens suggested a possible relationship between menstrual blood loss and $PGF_{2\alpha}$, PGE_2 and prostacyclin production in both endometrium and myometrium.

Little is known about prostaglandin receptors in target tissues in women with bleeding disorders. However one study has demonstrated that proliferative phase endometrium from women with a diagnosis of abnormal uterine bleeding is associated with significantly higher prostaglandin E_2 binding than women with other gynaecological diagnoses[98]. No abnormality of $PGF_{2\alpha}$ binding was demonstrated. It must also be remembered that the endometrium is a highly active endocrine organ[22] and there may well also be abnormalities of fibrinolysis, heparin secretion, lysosome activity, prolactin secretion or even relaxin or renin secretion. Nothing is known about the possible involvement of leukotrienes in abnormal bleeding.

Management of dysfunctional uterine bleeding

Medical management usually first includes the establishment of a correct diagnosis, and the exclusion of diseases such as coagulation disorders, systemic lupus erythematosus, hypothyroidism and pelvic conditions such as leiomyomata, adenomyosis, endometriosis, endometrial polyps, chronic pelvic inflammatory disease, polycystic ovarian disease and a few other rare conditions which may need to be managed surgically or in some specific medical manner. The remaining women with ovulatory or anovulatory dysfunctional uterine bleeding have been treated over the years with a wide range of different agents, and several of these have been shown to have considerable efficacy. This review will concentrate on the effects of agents which influence prostaglandin release but it must be borne in mind that other treatments of value in women with dysfunctional bleeding include steroidal hormone preparations such as combined oral contraceptives, progestogens alone or Danazol and such other varied drugs as fibrinolytic inhibitors, ethamsylate and a long acting vasopressin analogue.

In the last ten years increasing interest has been focussed on a number of the cyclo-oxygenase inhibitors and their ability to reduce menstrual blood loss[99-101]. The most intensively investigated preparation is mefenamic acid used in the same manner as for dysmenorrhoea. This results in a mean reduction in measured blood loss of 28%, but is usually proportionally greater in those with more excessive loss[102] (Figure 2.7). The benefit is usually maintained with repeated treatment over long periods of time[101], and interestingly may also be seen in women with menorrhagia due to an IUCD, fibroids, endometriosis, adenomyosis and occasionally other conditions[100,103,104]. Women with DUB treated with mefenamic acid also experience a significant long term reduction in other menstrually associated symptoms such as secondary dysmenorrhoea, nausea, vomiting, diarrhoea, headache, depression and a decrease in duration of bleeding. Limited published information suggests that flufenamic acid, indomethacin and naproxen may also have some effects on the reduction of excessive menstrual blood loss[99,105,106]. The rather mysterious drug, Ethamsylate, may also significantly reduce menstrual blood loss by a series of mechanisms including reduction in capillary fragility, anti-hyaluronidase and anti-prostaglandin activity[107,108].

Women with anovulatory DUB do not respond as effectively to anti-prostaglandin agents as women who are ovulatory. It is generally recommended that anovulatory women should first of all be treated with hormonal preparations. On the other hand at least 20% of ovulatory DUB sufferers will not experience any reduction in blood loss with mefenamic acid, and some will even exhibit an increase. It is probable that these women have other, as yet undefined, abnormalities of uterine arachidonic acid metabolism.

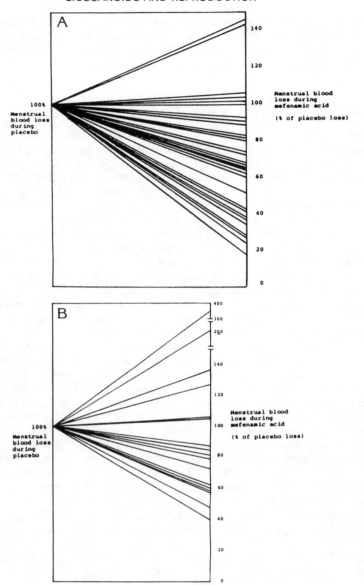

Figure 2.7 Percentage change in menstrual blood loss in 69 women with a convincing clinical complaint of menorrhagia during treatment with mefenamic acid by comparison with their loss during placebo treatment (100%). A: group of women with placebo blood loss greater than 60 ml per cycle. B: group of women with placebo blood loss less than 40 ml per cycle (from Fraser[102], with permission)

It should also be appreciated that many women with DUB, perhaps the majority, will need long-term medical therapy. When this consideration is added to the significant number of treatment failures it is not difficult to understand the popularity of hysterectomy as a treatment for women with these disorders who have already completed their families.

THE ROLE OF EICOSANOIDS IN OTHER MENSTRUALLY-RELATED DISORDERS

There are a number of other conditions which occur cyclically with some relationship to the menstrual cycle which may involve abnormalities of eicosanoid metabolism. Several of these will be briefly discussed.

Premenstrual syndrome

This disorder is a highly variable symptom-complex which is probably not a single entity, but due to a range of different biochemical, endocrine or neurotransmitter–neuromodulator abnormalities. Symptoms occur in a regular and cyclical fashion during the 1–2 weeks prior to menstruation and usually disappear during menstruation. Typically they occur in women who are ovulating but rarely similar cyclical symptoms have been described during the premenarchal and postmenopausal years and even after bilateral oophorectomy.

Mood and behavioural changes are common and may be accompanied by muddled thinking, poor memory, indecisiveness, clumsiness, headaches, back ache, faintness, altered appetite, cravings and a range of physical symptoms such as abdominal bloating and breast tenderness and swelling. In a small proportion of women these changes have such an influence on personality that accidents, crimes, suicides etc. occur more commonly during this phase of the cycle.

The aetiology of the premenstrual syndrome is unknown and many theories have been proposed[109]. Only the evidence relating to eicosanoids will be discussed here.

Prostaglandins of several different types produce multiple effects in the central nervous system, some of which could easily cause symptoms of the type reported in premenstrual syndrome[110,111]. Most of the evidence for central actions of various prostaglandins comes from animal studies. There is good evidence that several prostaglandins interact with various neurotransmitters, neuromodulators and central nervous system hormones. In particular they may modify concentrations of biogenic amines and may block dopaminergic receptors in the central nervous system[112]. Prostaglandins of the E series have a substantial depressant action on behaviour, resulting in sedation, reduction in spontaneous motor activity, loss of interest in surroundings, motor incoordination, disturbances of posture, inhibition of conditioned avoidance and escape responses and decreased skeletal muscle tone. Most prostaglandins also cause anorexia and inhibition of food intake although PGE_1 may produce an increase in food intake through certain hypothalamic regions[113]. There may also be effects on thirst, sexual behaviour and sensitization of pain receptors. Prostaglandin E_1 is particularly potent in facilitating pain[114].

All of this evidence is very theoretical in relation to pre-menstrual symptom aetiology. However there is evidence for improvement of certain symptoms associated with the pre-menstrual syndrome in women using cyclo-oxygenase inhibitors. Four separate therapeutic studies have been reported which have bearing on this aetiology. Three involve the use of mefenamic acid taken from early in the luteal phase by women with a medically confirmed diagnosis of pre-menstrual syndrome[115-117]. A short-term, double-blind placebo comparison confirmed a significantly better response of a range of PMS symptoms with mefenamic acid in 60–80 % of patients. Tension, irritability, depression, pain and headaches were helped but breast symptoms were not[116]. A recent study with a more thorough methodology has confirmed beneficial effects of this drug in women with carefully defined PMS[117]. These results appear to suggest that excessive secretion of one or more prostaglandins in some tissue constitutes an integral part of PMS. The fourth study utilized evening primrose oil, which contains the dietary prostaglandin precursors, linoleic and dihomogamma linolenic acid[118]. This study was not placebo controlled but did improve all symptoms. This combination of essential fatty acids should promote the synthesis of some prostaglandins, and may imply an imbalance of certain prostaglandins in PMS rather than an abnormality of absolute level. Ultimately, it is probable that certain prostaglandins will be found to play a role in the aetiology of the pre-menstrual syndrome in some women but it is likely that they are only part of a cascade of factors which all have a small part to play.

Endometriosis

Endometriosis is a unique and highly variable condition in which endometrium-like tissue is present in extra-uterine sites. On histological examination the deposits often have considerable similarities to normal endometrium but may exhibit significant differences. The deposits respond to oestrogens and progesterone in a rather similar manner to the endometrium although the response is frequently not identical to true endometrium. There is also evidence that oestrogen and progesterone receptors in endometriosis vary in different ways to those seen in true endometrium.

Endometriotic tissue almost certainly has similar endocrine properties to endometrium, which means that it may have the capacity to produce a range of biologically active substances. These substances may be normal for the intrauterine milieu but they may not be normal for the intraperitoneal environment. This means that the substances could have unexpected effects on ovulation, ovum release, tubal function including ovum pick-up, fertilization, implantation and perhaps other genital tract functions. The deposits of endometriosis show cyclical variations and will frequently break down and bleed at the time of menstruation. This may result in local inflammation and a number of associated symptoms. Typical clinical symptoms are those of secondary dysmenorrhoea, uterine tenderness and deep dyspareunia, menorrhagia, pre-menstrual spotting and infertility.

It would not be surprising if abnormalities of arachidonic acid metabolism were responsible for some of the symptoms or functional disturbances with endometriosis. In 1981 evidence was presented which suggested that prostaglandin F concentrations in endometriotic lesions ($2.72 \pm 0.14 \, ng/mg$ of protein) were significantly higher than levels in uterine endometrium collected from the same women at the same time ($0.54 \pm 0.03 \, ng/mg$). Levels were also higher in endometriotic cyst fluid than in follicular fluid and endometriotic tissue in culture secreted more PGF than ovarian stroma or true endometrium[119]. Since that first report there has been considerable controversy about the involvement of arachidonic acid abnormalities in patients with endometriosis. Published results have been inconsistent. It has been suggested that the concentration of thromboxane and prostacyclin metabolites are increased in peritoneal fluid of women with endometriosis[120]. The same investigators found an increase in peritoneal fluid volume in endometriosis which meant that both the concentration and total amount of thromboxane and prostacyclin metabolites was increased compared with normal controls. This finding could not be confirmed in another similar and much larger study[121]. Yet another study found no elevation of the concentrations of PGE_2, $PGF_{2\alpha}$, $PGF_{2\alpha}$ metabolite and thromboxane B_2 in peritoneal fluid of women with endometriosis[122].

There seems little doubt that eicosanoids can be produced from endometriotic tissue. However the controversy centres on the possibility that abnormalities of eicosanoid levels in peritoneal fluid might influence the function of adjacent reproductive structures. The fact that differing results have been reported suggests any genuine involvement of eicosanoids will only be confirmed by more subtle studies. There are a number of problems with the published studies which mainly centre around the difficulty of excluding occult or microscopic endometriotic deposits in so called 'controls'. There is no question that eicosanoids have the capability to contribute to many of the symptoms experienced by women with endometriosis and could cause infertility by subtle effects on reproductive physiology.

The use of cyclo-oxygenase inhibitors may produce significant relief of secondary dysmenorrhoea in women with endometriosis[88]. Unfortunately these agents are not nearly so effective in treating the pain associated with this condition as they are in primary dysmenorrhoea. This also tends to suggest that other mechanisms are involved in endometriosis.

Menstrual migraine

Cyclical pre-menstrual or menstrual headaches typically of the migraine type are a relatively common occurrence. They are often associated with visual disturbances or other systemic symptoms. Some of these symptoms can be reproduced by intravenous infusions of PGE_1[123] or prostacyclin[124]. Most if not all drugs effective in headache and migraine therapy oppose prostaglandin synthesis or antagonise its actions[125], and some cyclo-oxygenase inhibitors are widely used in the therapy of migraine. Menstrual and pre-menstrual migraine is usually related in some way to sensitivity to oestrogen or oestrogen withdrawal and it is suggested that certain prostaglandins may help to mediate this action.

Other menstrual disorders

Some women complain of troublesome mid-cycle (peri-ovulatory) pain or bleeding/spotting. Ultrasound scanning suggests that mid-cycle pain occurs during the immediate pre-ovulatory hours and anecdotal reports suggest substantial benefit from cyclo-oxygenase inhibitor therapy. Mid-cycle bleeding is probably associated with a temporary instability of the endometrium as oestrogen levels fall during the early stages of formation of the corpus luteum. Suggestions of benefit from prostaglandin inhibitor therapy in such patients with persistent mid-cycle bleeding are also anecdotal but could have a realistic theoretical basis. More careful studies need to be designed to evaluate cyclo-oxygenase inhibitor therapy in these conditions.

CONCLUSION

A range of eicosanoids are important in the physiology of the endometrium and myometrium during the normal menstrual cycle and in pregnancy. Disturbances of their synthesis, secretion and metabolism may be important in a number of gynaecological conditions and in particular those related to menstruation.

There is now excellent evidence that several cyclo-oxygenase inhibitors have excellent therapeutic value in some of these conditions. Nevertheless there are a reasonable number of therapeutic failures and future research needs to concentrate closely on the basic involvement of eicosanoids in these conditions and on the reasons for therapeutic failure. There is little doubt that a vast amount of information on leukotrienes will become available over the next few years and it would be surprising if they are not shown to have important roles. There is a considerable need to study therapy in detail and for the pharmaceutical industry to develop specific inhibitors, and perhaps receptor blockers, for individual eicosanoids. These would provide us with very valuable physiological, pharmacological and therapeutic information.

REFERENCES

1. Leaver, H.A. and Poyser, N.L. (1983). Arachidonic acid in guinea-pig uterus and plasma. In Samuelsson, B., Ramwell, P.W. and Paoletti, R. (eds.) *Advances in Prostaglandin and Thromboxane Research*, **8**, pp. 1361–1363 (New York: Raven Press)
2. Pickles, V.R., Hall, W.J., Best, F.A. and Smith G.N. (1965). Prostaglandins in endometrium and menstrual fluid from normal and dysmenorrhoeic women. *J. Obstet. Gynaecol. Br. Commonw.*, **72**, 185–192
3. Downie, J., Poyser, N.L. and Wunderlich, N. (1974). Levels of prostaglandins in human endometrium during the normal menstrual cycle. *J. Physiol.*, **236**, 465–469
4. Singh, E.J., Baccarini, I.M. and Zuspan, F.P. (1975). Levels of prostaglandins $F_{2\alpha}$ and E_2 in

human endometrium during the menstrual cycle. *Am. J. Obstet. Gynecol.*, **121**, 1003–1006

5. Gréen, K. and Hagenfeldt, K. (1975). Prostaglandins in the human endometrium. Gas chromatographic–mass spectrometric quantitation before and after IUD insertion. *Am. J. Obstet. Gynecol.*, **122**, 611–614

6. Jordan, V.C. and Pokoly, T.V. (1977). Steroid and prostaglandin relations during the menstrual cycle. *Obstet. Gynecol.*, **49**, 449–453

7. Maathuis, J.V. and Kelly, R.W. (1978). Concentration of prostaglandins $F_{2\alpha}$ and E_2 in endometrium throughout the human menstrual cycle, after the administration of Clomiphene or an oestrogen/progestogen pill, and in early pregnancy. *J. Endocrinol.*, **77**, 361–376

8. Liggins, G.C., Campos, G.A., Roberts, C.N. and Skinner, S.J. (1980). Production rates of prostaglandin F, 6-keto-$PGF_{1\alpha}$ and thromboxane B_2 by perifused human endometrium. *Prostaglandins*, **19**, 461–477

9. Yamanoto, S., Ohki, S., Ogino, N., Shimizu, T., Yoshimoto, T., Watanabe, K. and Hayaishi, O. (1980). Enzymes involved in the formation and further transformations of prostaglandin endoperoxides. In Samuelsson, B., Ramwell, P.W. and Paoletti, R. (eds.) *Advances in Prostaglandin and Thromboxane Research*, pp. 27–33. (New York: Raven Press)

10. Kelly, R.W. and Abel, M.H. (1980). Catechol oestrogens stimulate and direct prostaglandin synthesis. *Prostaglandins*, **20**, 613–626

11. Abel, M.H. and Baird, D.T. (1980). The effect of 17-β oestradiol and progesterone on prostaglandin production by human endometrium maintained in organ culture. *Endocrinology*, **106**, 1599–1605

12. Peek, M.J., Fraser, I.S., Phillips, C.A., Resta, T.M., Blackwell, P.M. and Markham, R. (1985). The measurement of human endometrial prostaglandin production: a comparison of two in vitro methods. *Prostaglandins*, **29**, 3–18

13. Rees, M.C.P., Anderson, A.B.M., Demers, L.M. and Turnbull, A.C. (1984). Endometrial and myometrial prostaglandin release during the menstrual cycle in relation to menstrual blood loss. *J. Clin. Endocrinol. Metab.*, **58**, 813–818

14. Abel, M.H. and Kelly, R.W. (1979). Differential production of prostaglandin within the human uterus. *Prostaglandins*, **18**, 821–834

15. Rees, M.C.P. (1982). Uterine prostaglandins and menstrual blood loss. *Res. Clin. Forums*, **4**, 19–22

16. Casey, M.L., Hensell, D.L., MacDonald, P.C. and Johnston, J.M. (1980). NAD + dependent 15-hydroxyprostaglandin dehydrogenase activity in human endometrium. *Prostaglandins*, **19**, 115–127

17. Ghodgaonkar, R.V., Dubin, N.H. and Blake, D.A. (1979). 13, 14-dihydro-15-keto-prostaglandin $F_{2\alpha}$ concentrations in human plasma and amniotic fluid. *Am. J. Obstet. Gynecol.*, **134**, 265–272

18. Koullapis, E.N. and Collins, W.P. (1980). The concentration of 13, 14-dihydro-15-oxo-prostaglandin $F_{2\alpha}$ in peripheral venous plasma throughout the normal ovarian and menstrual cycle. *Acta Endocrinol.*, **93**, 123–138

19. Thorburn, G.D., Cox, R.I., Currie, W.B., Restall, B.J. and Schneider, W. (1973). Prostaglandin F and progesterone concentrations in the utero-ovarian venous plasma of the ewe during the oestrus cycle and early pregnancy. *J. Reprod. Fertil.*, Supplement 18, 151–158

20. Roberts, J.S., McCracken, J.A., Gavagan, J.E. and Soloff, M.S. (1976). Oxytocin stimulated release of prostaglandin $F_{2\alpha}$ from ovine endometrium in vitro: correlation with oestrus cycle and oxytocin-receptor binding. *Endocrinology*, **99**, 1107–1114

21. Saaed, S.A., Strickland, D.M., Young, D.C., Dang, A. and Mitchell, M.D. (1982). Inhibition of prostaglandin synthesis by human amniotic fluid: acute reduction in inhibitory activity of amniotic fluid obtained during labour. *J. Clin. Endocrinol. Metab.*, **55**, 801–811

22. Healy, D.L. and Hodgen, G.D. (1983). The endocrinology of human endometrium. *Obstet. Gynecol. Survey*, **38**, 509–530

23. Chan, W.Y., Dawood, M.Y. and Fuchs, F. (1981). Prostaglandins in primary dysmenorrhoea: comparison of prophylactic and non-prophylactic treatment with Ibuprofen and use of oral contraceptives. *Am. J. Med.*, **70**, 535–539

24. Ylikorkala, O., Puolakka, J. and Viinikka, L. (1981). Oestrogen containing oral contraceptives decrease prostacyclin production. *Lancet*, **1**, 42

25. Witter, F.R. and Di Blasi, M.C. (1984). Effect of steroid hormones on arachidonic acid metabolites of endothelial cells. *Obstet. Gynecol.*, **63**, 747–751
26. Saeed, S.A. and Mitchell, M.D. (1982). Formation of arachidonate lipoxygenase metabolites by human foetal membranes, uterine decidua vera and placenta. *Prostagl., Leukotr. and Med.*, **8**, 635–642
27. Demers, L.M., Rees, M.C.P. and Turnbull, A.C. (1984). The metabolism of arachidonic acid by the non-pregnant human uterus. *Prostagl., Leukotr. and Med.*, **14**, 175–181
28. Abel, M.H., Zhu, C. and Baird, D.T. (1982). An animal model to study menstrual bleeding. *Res. Clin. Forums*, **4**, 25–34
29. Hofmann, G.E., Rao, C.V., De Leon, F.D., Toledo, A.A. and San Filippo, J.S. (1985). Human endometrial prostaglandin E_2 binding sites and their profiles during the menstrual cycle and in pathologic states. *Am. J. Obstet. Gynecol.*, **151**, 269–375
30. Hofmann, G.E., Rao, C.V., Barrows, G.H. and San Fillipo, J.S. (1983). Topography of human uterine prostaglandin E and $F_{2\alpha}$ receptors and their profiles during pathological states. *J. Clin. Endocrinol. Metab.*, **57**, 360–368
31. Bygdeman, M. (1964). The effect of different prostaglandins on human myometrium in vitro. *Acta Physiol. Scand.*, **63**, (supplement) 1–15
32. Wilhelmsson, L., Lindblom, D. and Wiqvist, N. (1979). The human utero-tubal junction: contractile patterns of different smooth muscle layers and the influence of prostaglandin E_2, prostaglandin $F_{2\alpha}$ and prostaglandin I_2 in vitro. *Fertil. Steril.*, **32**, 303–307
33. Wilhelmsson, L., Wikland, M. and Wiqvist, N. (1981). PGH_2, TXA_2 and PGI_2 have potent and differentiated actions on human uterine contractility. *Prostaglandins*, **21**, 277–286
34. Weichman, B.M. and Tucker, S.S. (1982). Contraction of the guinea pig uterus by synthetic leukotrienes. *Prostaglandins*, **24**, 245–256
35. Carraher, R., Hahn, D.W., Ritchie, D.M. and McGuire, J.L. (1983). Involvement of lipoxygenase products in myometrial contractions. *Prostaglandins*, **26**, 23–34
36. Huszar, G. (1981). Biology and biochemistry of myometrial contractility and cervical maturation. *Semin. Perinatol.*, **3**, 216–221
37. Garfield, R.E. and Hayashi, R.H. (1980). Presence of gap junctions in the myometrium of women during various stages of menstruation. *Am. J. Obstet. Gynecol.*, **138**, 569–574
38. Goldblatt, M.W. (1933). A depressor substance in seminal fluid. *J. Soc. Chem. Ind.*, **52**, 1056–1060
39. Von Euler, U.S. (1934). Zur kenntnis der pharmakologischen wirkungen von nativsekreten und extrakten männlicher accessorischer geschlechtsdrüsen. *Naunyn Schmiedeberg Arch. Pharm. Exp. Pathol.*, **175**, 78–84
40. Karlson, S. (1959). The influence of seminal fluid on the motility of the non-pregnant human uterus. *Acta Obstet. Gynecol. Scand.*, **38**, 503–511
41. Eliasson, R. and Posse, N. (1960). The effect of prostaglandin on the non-pregnant human uterus in vivo. *Acta Obstet. Gynecol. Scand.*, **39**, 112–119
42. Roth-Brandel, U., Bygdeman, M. and Wiqvist, N. (1970). Effect of intravenous administration of prostaglandin E_1 and $F_{2\alpha}$ on the contractility of the non-pregnant human uterus in vivo. *Acta Obstet. Gynecol. Scand.*, **49**, supplement 5, 19–25
43. Cibils, L.A. (1967). Contractility of the non-pregnant human uterus. *Obstet. Gynecol.*, **30**, 441–461
44. Borell, U., Bygdeman, M., Gréen, K. and Lundström, V. (1985). Physiology and pharmacology of prostacyclins and prostaglandins. In Shearman, R.P. (ed.) *Clinical Reproductive Endocrinology*, pp. 249–263. (Edinburgh: Churchill Livingstone)
45. Clark, K.E., Farley, D.B., Van Orden, D.E. and Brodie, M.J. (1977). Role of endogenous prostaglandins in regulation of uterine blood flow and adrenergic neurotransmission. *Am. J. Obstet. Gynecol.*, **127**, 455–461
46. Short, R.V. (1976). The evolution of human reproduction. *Proc. R. Soc. London*, **B195**, 3–24
47. Hallberg, L., Hogdahl, A.M., Nilson, L. and Rybo, G. (1966). Menstrual blood loss – a population study. *Acta Obstet. Gynecol. Scand.*, **45**, 320–351
48. Fraser, I.S., McCarron, G., Markham, R. and Resta, T. Blood and total fluid content of menstrual discharge. *Obstet. Gynecol.*, **65**, 194–198
49. Flowers, C.E. and Willborn, W.H. (1978). New observations on the physiology of menstruation. *Obstet. Gynecol.*, **51**, 16–24

50. Markee, J.E. (1940). Menstruation in intraocular endometrial transplants in the rhesus monkey. *Contrib. Embryol.*, (Carnegie Inst. of Washington), **28**, 219–308
51. Abel, M.H. (1985). Prostaglandins and leukotrienes in menstruation. *Prostagl. Perspect.*, **1**, 1–4
52. Henzl, M.R., Smith, R.C., Boost, G. and Tyler, E.T. (1972). Lysosomal concept of menstrual bleeding in humans. *J. Clin. Endocrinol. Metab.*, **34**, 860–875
53. Wiqvist, N., Bygdeman, M. and Kirton, K. (1971). Non-steroidal infertility agents in the female. In Diczfalusy, E. and Borell, U. (eds.) *Control of Human Fertility, Nobel Symposium*, **15**, 137–148
54. Smith, S.K., Abel, M.H., Kelly, R.W. and Baird, D.T. (1981). Prostaglandin synthesis in the endometrium of women with ovular dysfunctional uterine bleeding. *Br. J. Obstet. Gynaecol.*, **88**, 434–439
55. Paton, R.C., Tindall, H., Zuzel, M. and McNicol, G.P. (1980). Haemostatic mechanisms in the normal endometrium and endometrium exposed to contraceptive steroids. In Diczfalusy, E., Fraser, I.S. and Webb, F.T.G. (eds.) *Endometrial Bleeding and Steroidal Contraception*, pp. 325–341. (Bath: Pitman Press)
56. Sixma, J.J., Christiaens, G.C.M.L. and Haspels, A.A. (1980). The sequence of haemostatic events in the endometrium during normal menstruation. In Diczfalusy, E, Fraser, I.S., Webb, F.T.G. (eds.) *Endometrial Bleeding and Steroidal Contraception*, pp. 86–96. (Bath: Pitman Press)
57. Rybo, G. (1966). Plasminogen activator in the endometrium. *Acta Obstet. Gynecol. Scand.*, **45**, 411–450
58. Christiaens, G.C.M.L., Sixma, J.J. and Haspels, A.A. (1980). Morphology of haemostasis in menstrual endometrium. *Br. J. Obstet. Gynaecol.*, **87**, 425–439
59. Baird, D.T., Abel, M.H., Kelly, R.W. and Smith, S.K. (1981). Endocrinology of dysfunctional uterine bleeding: the role of endometrial prostaglandins. In Crosignani, P.G. and Rubin, B. (eds.) *Endocrinology of Human Infertility : New Aspects*, pp. 399–417. Proceedings of the Serono clinical colloquia on reproduction 2, September 1980. (Oxford: Academic Press)
60. Goodfellow, C.F., Paton, R.C., Salmon, J.A., Moncada, S., Clayton, J.K., Davies, J.A. and McNicol, G.P. (1982). 6-oxo-prostaglandin $F_{1\alpha}$ and thromboxane B_2 in uterine vein blood – a possible role in menstrual bleeding. *Thromb. Haemostas.*, **48**, 9–12
61. Fraser, I.S. (1982). Quoted by Turnbull, A.C. Aspects of dysfunctional uterine bleeding; summary and conclusion. *Res. Clin. Forums*, **4**, 143
62. Fraser, I.S. (1985). The 'dysfunctional' uterus: dysmenorrhoea and dysfunctional uterine bleeding. In Shearman, R.P. (ed.) *Clinical Reproductive Endocrinology*, pp. 579–598 (Edinburgh: Churchill Livingstone)
63. Carney, M.W. (1981). Menstrual disturbance: a psychogenic disorder? *Clin. Obstet. Gynaecol.*, **8**, 103–109
64. Åkerlund, M., Anderssen, K.-E., Ingermarsson, I. (1976). Effects of terbutaline on myometrial activity, uterine blood flow and lower abdominal pain in women with primary dysmenorrhoea. *Br. J. Obstet. Gynaecol.*, **83**, 673–681
65. Smith, R.P. and Powell, J.R. (1980). The objective evaluation of dysmenorrhoea therapy. *Am. J. Obstet. Gynecol.*, **137**, 314–319
66. Lumsden, M.A. and Baird, D.T. (1985). Intrauterine pressure in dysmenorrhoea. *Acta Obstet. Gynecol. Scand.*, **64**, 183–186
67. Irwin, J., Morse, E. and Riddick, D. (1981). Dysmenorrhoea induced by autologous transfusion. *Obstet. Gynecol.*, **58**, 286–294
68. Ferreira, S.H. (1981). Inflammatory pain, prostaglandin hyperalgesia and the development of peripheral analgesic trends. *Pharmacol. Sci.*, **2**, 183–186
69. Lundström, V. and Gréen, K. (1978). Endogenous levels of $PGF_{2\alpha}$ and its main metabolites in plasma and endometrium of normal and dysmenorrheic women. *Am. J. Obstet. Gynecol.*, **130**, 640–649
70. Rosenwaks, Z., Jones, G.S., Henzl, M.R., Dubin, N.H., Ghodgoankar, R.B. and Hofmann, S. (1981). Naproxen sodium, aspirin and placebo in primary dysmenorrhoea. *Am. J. Obstet. Gynecol.*, **140**, 592–599
71. Lumsden, M.A., Kelly, R.W. and Baird, D.T. (1983). Is prostaglandin $F_{2\alpha}$ involved in the increased myometrial contractility of primary dysmenorrhoea. *Prostaglandins*, **25**, 683–691

72. Lundström, V. (1977). The myometrial response to intrauterine administration of $PGF_{2\alpha}$ and PGE_2 in dysmenorrhoeic women. *Acta Obstet. Gynecol. Scand.*, **56**, 167–173

73. Demers, L.M., Hahn, D.W. and McGuire, J.L. (1984). Newer concepts in dysmenorrhoea research. In Dawood, M.Y., McGuire, J.L. and Demers, L.M. (eds.) *Premenstrual Syndrome and Dysmenorrhoea*, pp. 205–220. (Baltimore: Urban and Schwarzenburg)

74. Ylikorkala, O., Puolakka, J. and Kauppila, A. (1979). Serum gonadotrophins, prolactin and ovarian steroids in primary dysmenorrhoea. *Br. J. Obstet. Gynecol.*, **86**, 648–653

75. Stromberg, P., Forsling, M.L. and Akerlund, M. (1981). Effects of prostaglandin inhibition on vasopressin levels in women with primary dysmenorrhoea. *Obstet. Gynecol.*, **58**, 206–208

76. Sjoberg, N.-O. (1979). Dysmenorrhoea and uterine neurotransmitters. *Acta. Obstet. Gynecol. Scand.*, **87**, (supplement) 57–60

77. Hillier, A. and Kasonde, J.M. (1976). Prostaglandin E and F concentrations in human endometrium after insertion of an intrauterine contraceptive device. *Lancet*, **1**, 15–16

78. Janbu, T., Lokken, P. and Neshein, B.-I. (1979). Effect of acetyl salicyclic acid, paracetamol and placebo on pain and blood loss in dysmenorrhoeic woman. *Acta Obstet. Gynecol. Scand.*, **87**, (supplement) 81–86

79. Kremser, E. and Mitchell, G.M. (1971). Treatment of primary dysmenorrhoea with a combined-type oral contraceptive: a double blind study. *J. Am. Coll. Health Assoc.*, **19**, 195–199

80. Schwarz, A., Zor, U., Lindner, H.R. and Naor, S. (1974). Primary dysmenorrhoea: alleviation by an inhibitor of prostaglandin synthesis and action. *Obstet. Gynecol.*, **44**, 709–714

81. Anderson, A.B.M., Fraser, I.S., Haynes, P.J. and Turnbull, A.C. (1978). Trial of prostaglandin synthetase inhibitors in primary dysmenorrhoea. *Lancet*, **1**, 345–348

82. Kintis, G.A. and Contifaris, B. (1980). The treatment of primary dysmenorrhoea with mefenamic acid. *Int. J. Gynecol. Obstet.*, **18**, 172–175

83. Henzl, M.R., Ortega-Herrera, E., Rodriguez, C. and Izu, A. (1979). Anaprox in dysmenorrhoea; reduction of pain and intrauterine pressure. *Am. J. Obstet. Gynecol.*, **135**, 455–460

84. Henzl, M.R., Massey, S. and Hanson, F.W. (1980). Primary dysmenorrhoea: the therapeutic challenge. *J. Reprod. Med.*, **25**, (supplement) 226–234

85. Pulkkinen, M.O. and Csapo, A.I. (1978). Effect of ibuprofen on menstrual blood prostaglandin levels in dysmenorrhoeic women. *Prostaglandins*, **18**, 137–142

86. Poyser, N.L. (1985). Prostaglandin pharmacology: five differential inhibitors of prostanoid synthesis. *Prostagl. Perspect.*, **2**, 10–11

87. Andersson, K.-E. and Ulmsten, U. (1978). Effects of nifedipine on myometrial activity and lower abdominal pain in patients with primary dysmenorrhoea. *Br. J. Obstet. Gynaecol.*, **85**, 142–149

88. Kauppila, A., Puolakka, J. and Ylikorkala, O. (1979). Prostaglandin biosynthesis inhibitors and endometriosis. *Prostaglandins*, **18**, 655–661

89. Buttram, V., Izu, A. and Henzl, M.R. (1979). Naproxen sodium in uterine pain following intrauterine contraceptive device insertion. *Am. J.. Obstet. Gynecol.*, **134**, 575–580

90. Cole, S.K., Billewicz, W.Z. and Thomson, A.M. (1971). Sources of variation in menstrual blood loss. *J. Obstet. Gynecol. Br. Commonw.*, **78**, 933–939

91. Brown, J.B., Kellar, R.J. and Matthew, G.D. (1959). Preliminary observations on urinary oestrogen excretion in certain gynaecological disorders. *J. Obstet. Gynaecol. Br. Emp.*, **66**, 177–211

92. Sutherland, A.M. (1949). The Histology of the endometrium in functional uterine haemorrhage. *Glasgow Med. J.*, **30**, 1–28

93. Beilby, J.O.W., Farrer-Brown, G. and Tarbit, M.H. (1971). The microvasculature of common uterine abnormalities excluding fibroids. *J. Obstet. Gynaecol. Br. Commonw.*, **78**, 361–368

94. Willman, E.A., Collins, W.P. and Clayton, S.G. (1976). Studies in the involvement of prostaglandins in uterine symptomatology and pathology. *Br. J. Obstet. Gynaecol.*, **83**, 337–345

95. Smith, S.K., Abel, M.H., Kelly, R.W. and Baird, D.T. (1982). The synthesis of prostaglandins from persistent proliferative endometrium. *J. Clin. Endocrinol. Metab.*, **55**, 284–289

96. Smith, S.K., Abel, M.H., Kelly, R.W. and Baird, D.T. (1981). A role for prostacyclin (PGI_2) in excessive menstrual bleeding. *Lancet*, **1**, 522–524

97. Rees, M.C.P., Anderson, A.B.M., Demers, L.M. and Turnbull, A.C. (1984). Endometrial and myometrial prostaglandin release during the menstrual cycle in relation to menstrual blood loss. *J. Clin. Endocrinol. Metab.*, **58**, 813–818

98. Hoffman, G.E., Rao, C.V., De Leon, F.D., Toledo, A.A. and San Filippo, J.S. (1985). Human endometrial prostaglandin E_2 binding sites and their profiles during the menstrual cycle and in pathologic states. *Am. J. Obstet. Gynecol.*, **151**, 369–375

99. Anderson, A.B.M., Haynes, E.J., Guillebaud, J. and Turnbull, A.C. (1976). Reduction of menstrual blood loss by prostaglandin synthetase inhibitors. *Lancet*, **1**, 774–776

100. Fraser, I.S., Pearse, C., Shearman, R.P., Elliott, P.M., McIlveen, J. and Markham, R. (1981). Efficacy of mefenamic acid in patients with a complaint of menorrhagia. *Obstet. Gynecol.*, **58**, 543–551

101. Fraser, I.S., McCarron, G., Markham, R., Robinson, M. and Smyth, E. (1983). Long term treatment of menorrhagia with mefenamic acid. *Obstet. Gynecol.*, **61**, 109–112

102. Fraser, I.S. (1983). The treatment of menorrhagia with mefenamic acid. *Res. Clin. Forums*, **5**, No. 3, 93–99

103. Guillebaud, J., Anderson, A.B.M. and Turnbull, A.C. (1978). Reduction by mefenamic acid of increased menstrual blood loss associated with intrauterine contraception. *Br. J. Obstet. Gynaecol.*, **85**, 53–62

104. Fraser, I.S., McCarron, G., Markham, R., Resta, T. and Watts, A. (1986). Measured menstrual blood loss in women with menorrhagia associated with pelvic disease or coagulation disorder. *Obstet. Gynecol.*, (in press)

105. Damarawy, H. and Toppozada, M. (1976). Control of bleeding due to I.U.D.'s by a prostaglandin biosynthesis inhibitor. *IRCS Med. Sci., Reprod., Obstet. Gynecol.*, **4**, 5–7

106. Davies, A.J., Anderson, A.B.M. and Turnbull, A.C. (1981). Reduction by Naproxen of excessive menstrual bleeding in women using intrauterine devices. *Obstet. Gynecol.*, **57**, 74–78

107. Harrison, R.F. and Campbell, S. (1976). Double-blind trial of Ethamsylate in the treatment of primary and intrauterine device menorrhagia. *Lancet*, **2**, 283–285

108. Kovacs, L. and Annus, J. (1978). Effectiveness of Ethamsylate in intrauterine device menorrhagia. *Gynecol. Invest.*, **9**, 161–165

109. Reid, R. (1985). Premenstrual syndrome. *Curr. Probl. Obstet. and Gynecol.*, **8**, No. 2, 1–57

110. Craig, G. (1980). The premenstrual syndrome and prostaglandin metabolism. *Br. J. Fam. Plann.*, **6**, 74–77

111. Jakubowicz, D.L. (1983). The significance of prostaglandins in the premenstrual syndrome. *Res. Clin Forums*, **5**, No. 3, 59–66

112. Poddubiuk, Z. (1976). A comparison of the central actions of prostaglandins A_1 E_1 $F_{1\alpha}$ and $F_{2\alpha}$ in the rat. 1. Behavioural, antinociceptive and anticonvulsant actions of intraventricular prostaglandins in the rat. *Psychol. Pharmacol.*, **50**, 89–94

113. Baile, C.A. and Martin, F.H. (1973). Relationship between prostaglandin E_1 polyphloretin phosphate and β-adrenoreceptor bound feeding loci in the hypothalamus of sheep. *Pharmacol. Biochem. Behav.*, **1**, 530–545

114. Juan, H. (1978). Prostaglandins as modulators of pain. *Gen. Pharmacol.*, **9**, 403–409

115. Wood, C. and Jakubowicz, D.L. (1980). The treatment of premenstrual symptoms with mefenamic acid. *Br. J. Obstet. Gynaecol.*, **87**, 627–630

116. Jakubowicz, D.L., Wood, C. and Dewhurst, C.J. (1982). The treatment of premenstrual tension. *Res. Clin. Forums*, **4**, 119–124

117. Mira, M., McNeil, D., Fraser, I.S., Vizzard, J. and Abraham, S. (1986). The use of mefenamic acid in the treatment of premenstrual tension sufferers. *Obstet. Gynecol.*, **68**, 395–398

118. Brush, M.G. (1981). Efamol in the treatment of premenstrual syndrome. Proceedings of the 1st symposium on the clinical uses of Efamol and essential fatty acids. St Thomas' Hospital, London

119. Moon, Y.S., Leung, T.C.S., Yuen, B.H. and Gomel, V. (1981). Prostaglandin F. in human endometriotic tissue. *Am. J. Obstet. Gynecol.*, **141**, 344–345

120. Drake, T.S., O'Brien, W.F., Ramwell, P.W. and Metz, S.A. (1981). Peritoneal fluid thromboxane B_2 and 6-keto $PGF_{1\alpha}$ in endometriosis. *Am. J. Obstet. Gynecol.*, **140**, 401–406

121. Mudge, T.J., James, M.J., Jones, W.R. and Walsh, J.A. (1985). Peritoneal fluid 6-keto $PGF_{1\alpha}$ levels in women with endometriosis. *Am. J. Obstet. Gynecol.*, **152**, 901–904

122. Rock, J.A., Dubin, N.H., Ghodgaonkar, R.B., Bergquist, C.A., Erozan, Y.S. and Kimball,

A.W. (1982). Cul-de-sac fluid in women with endometriosis: fluid volume and prostanoid concentration during the proliferative phase of the cycle. *Fertil. Steril.*, **37**, 747–758
123. Carlson, L.A., Ekelund, L.G. and Oro, L. (1968). Clinical and metabolic effects of prostaglandin E_1 in man. *Acta Med. Scand.*, **183**, 423–430
124. Peatfield, R.C., Gawell, M.J. and Clifford-Rose, F. (1981). The effect of infused prostacyclin in migraine and cluster headache. *Headache*, **21**, 190–195
125. Horrobin, D.F. (1977). Hypothesis: prostaglandins and migraine. *Headache*, **17**, 113–117

3
Menstrual regulation

M. Bygdeman

INTRODUCTION

The most prevalent technique for first trimester abortion is suction curettage and was developed to minimize the complications of infection and blood loss encountered with dilatation and sharp curettage. A desire to further reduce these risks coupled with the development of highly sensitive pregnancy tests led to the development of the early suction abortion, which has been variously termed menstrual regulation, menstrual extraction and mini-abortion. Later experience demonstrated that in at least some patients local anaesthesia to minimize vasovagal symptoms and mechanical cervical dilatation could not be avoided. In addition, even with local anaesthesia, 4% had developed endometritis when seen at follow-up, and another 4% required a repeat extraction or suction curettage for incomplete abortion[1]. In a multicentre study the frequency of pregnancy continuation and incomplete abortion was 4.9% and 3.7% respectively[2].

The development of the prostaglandins offered the hope of an effective pharmacological alternative to surgical interruption of early first trimester pregnancy that would avoid the potential problems associated with anaesthesia, mechanical dilatation of the cervix and uterine instrumentation.

The prostaglandins have the ability to stimulate uterine activity and to interrupt pregnancy throughout all stages of gestation. The present review will, however, be restricted to the first three weeks following the first missed menstrual period, or more precisely, up to 49 days of amenorrhoea.

NATURAL PROSTAGLANDINS

In the early 1970s Bygdeman and Wiqvist[3-5] and Karim and Filshie[6,7] independently demonstrated the ability of intravenous infusions of the naturally occurring prostaglandins (PG), PGE_2 and $PGF_{2\alpha}$, to terminate first trimester pregnancy. It soon became obvious that treatment with both intravenous infusion[8,9] and vaginal[10] administration of these prostaglandins was associated with too high a frequency of mainly gastrointestinal side-effects, precluding the routine application of these techniques for early pregnancy interruption.

Administration of the prostaglandins directly to the target organ, the myometrium, is one way to enhance the myometrial effect and reduce the systemic absorption of prostaglandins and therefore minimize side-effects. The first study showing that extra-amniotic administration of $PGF_{2\alpha}$ and PGE_2 gave an acceptable success rate and that side-effects were considerably reduced was published in 1970[11]. These preliminary findings were confirmed in later studies in which large numbers of patients were treated[12,13]. Csapo and co-workers treated a total of 542 patients with either 5 mg $PGF_{2\alpha}$ or 1.5 mg PGE_2 by the intrauterine route. Both treatments were equally effective, 95 % of the patients had a complete evacuation of the uterus[12]. However, it was necessary to pre-treat the patients with analgesic and sedative drugs to reduce side-effects to an acceptable level. If the prostaglandin dose was reduced to a level which did not cause side-effects, the efficacy was also decreased[14].

These early studies were of importance since they clearly demonstrated that PGE_2 and $PGF_{2\alpha}$ were effective as abortifacients during very early pregnancy. However, it was equally obvious that the procedures had no, or very limited, clinical usefulness due to side-effects and, with regard to intrauterine administration, the need for premedication and the use of a catheter which was not adaptable to self-administration.

PROSTAGLANDIN ANALOGUES

The results of clinical studies of natural prostaglandins for termination of both first and second trimester pregnancy initiated the search for analogues with a more specific effect on the myometrium and a greater resistance to enzymatic degradation by prostaglandin 15-dehydrogenase. A number of such analogues have been developed. Among the first of these to be tested clinically were 15-methyl-$PGF_{2\alpha}$ methyl ester and 16,16-dimethyl-PGE_2, both administered by the vaginal route. Satisfactory results with regard to frequency of complete abortion (91–97 %) was reported for the F-analogue, both following repeated, 0.5–1.5 mg, and single, 3.0 mg, vaginal administration. The frequency of gastrointestinal side-effects, although lower than for classical prostaglandins was, however, still too high to encourage more widespread clinical use[15–18] (Table 3.1). The E-analogue in a dose of 0.8–1.0 mg repeated two to four times was equally effective but the treatment was associated with a significantly lower frequency of gastrointestinal side-effects than encountered with 15-methyl-$PGF_{2\alpha}$ methyl ester[19,20]. A problem with 16,16-dimethyl-PGE_2 was that the compound was not stable in the suppository base and therefore not suitable for more routine clinical use.

More recently, E-analogues which are sufficiently stable for routine clinical use have been developed. The efficacy and safety of three such analogues for

Table 3.1 Termination of very early pregnancy by prostaglandin analogues administered by the vaginal route. Results from selected studies

Type of analogue Reference	Route of administration	No. of patients	Frequency of complete abortion (%)	Side-effects	(%)
15-methyl PGF$_{2\alpha}$ methyl ester					
Bygdeman et al.[15]	repeated vaginal	63	97	vomiting } diarrhoea }	58
				endometritis	0
Hamberger et al.[16]	repeated vaginal	42	93	vomiting } diarrhoea }	50
Gréen et al.[17]	single vaginal	128	94.5	vomiting	54
				diarrhoea	59
				endometritis	0.8
Mandelin[18]	single vaginal	104	91	vomiting	24
				diarrhoea	37
				endometritis	1.0
16,16-dimethyl PGE$_2$					
Mackenzie et al.[19]	repeated vaginal	34	100	vomiting	26.5
				diarrhoea	35.3
				endometritis	0
Lundström et al.[20]	repeated vaginal	88	94	vomiting	12.5
				diarrhoea	13.6
				endometritis	1.1
16,16-dimethyl PGE$_1$					
Karim et al.[21]	repeated vaginal	50	92	vomiting	4
				diarrhoea	6
				endometritis	0
Tagaki et al.[22]	repeated vaginal	63	86	vomiting	1.6
				diarrhoea	4.8
				endometritis	0
9-methylene PGE$_2$					
Bygdeman et al.[25]	repeated vaginal	101	94	vomiting } diarrhoea }	40
				endometritis	3

termination of early pregnancy has been evaluated. The analogues are 16-phenoxy-tetranor PGE$_2$ methyl sulphonylamide (16-phenoxy PGE$_2$), 16,16-dimethyl-trans-Δ^2 PGE$_1$ methyl ester (16,16-dimethyl PGE$_1$) and 9-deoxo-16,16-dimethyl-9-methylene PGE$_2$ (9-methylene PGE$_2$). The first analogue is administered by the intramuscular route, the other two vaginally.

Vaginal administration of 1.0 mg 16,16-dimethyl PGE$_1$ in triglyceride base five times at four-hourly intervals resulted in complete abortion in 46 out of 50 women with a delay in menstruation of up to 14 days. Uterine cramps were experienced by most patients but these were mild and only seven resorted to mild analgesics for pain relief. Gastrointestinal side-effects were very infrequent[21]. Tagaki et al.[22], using a lower total dose, also found a very low frequency of gastrointestinal side-effects following repeated vaginal administration of this analogue. The frequency of incomplete abortion was, however, higher (Table 3.1). Repeated intramuscular injection of 16-phenoxy PGE$_2$ (0.5 mg) has also proved an effective first trimester abortifacient with a success rate of 95 % and an incidence of gastrointestinal side-effects around 30 %[23,24]. A similarly high success rate was found also for repeated vaginal administration of 9-methylene PGE$_2$[25].

In a study which included 198 early pregnant patients (duration of amenorrhoea of up to 49 days) these PGE analogues were compared[25]. The patients received one of the following treatments: three intramuscular injections of 0.5 mg 16-phenoxy PGE$_2$ administered at three-hourly intervals; five suppositories containing 1.0 mg 16,16-dimethy PGE$_1$ at three-hourly intervals; or two suppositories containing 75 and 30 mg or 60 and 45 mg respectively, of 9-methylene PGE$_2$ at six-hourly intervals. All three treatments were highly effective in terminating early pregnancy. The frequency of complete abortion varied between 92 and 94 % whilst the frequency of patients in whom pregnancy continued despite treatment was 4 % or less in all three groups. Side-effects were limited to occasional vomiting and diarrhoea in approximately 40–50 % of the patients. One group of patients was allowed self-treatment at home. This group has been expanded to include 100 patients in a new study[26]. Selection criteria for home treatment were the same as for the other patients except that at least one previous pregnancy was a prerequisite. The patients received a total amount of 100–120 mg of 9-methylene PGE$_2$ divided into two doses administered with a six-hour interval. In 94 % of the patients the therapy was regarded as successful, resulting in complete abortion. The only problem was uterine pain. Four patients out of 100 experienced strong uterine pain necessitating hospital visit and an analgesic injection for alleviation of pain.

COMPARISON BETWEEN PROSTAGLANDIN ANALOGUES AND VACUUM ASPIRATION

Randomized studies comparing vacuum aspiration and treatment with prosta-glandin analogues are few. In two studies vaginal administration of a PGE analogue was used. In the first, 16,16-dimethyl PGE$_2$ and in the second 9-methylene PGE$_2$ was administered[20,27]. In a third multicentre study including 486 women repeated intramuscular injections of 16-phenoxy PGE$_2$ was used[28].

Efficacy of treatment

Prostaglandin administration results in an increase in uterine contractility followed by bleeding, which generally starts three to six hours after the initiation of therapy and lasts for one to two weeks. Visual observation of the patients, ultrasound examination of the uterus and the decreased level of plasma hCG indicate that most patients abort during the first 24 hours. Minor residues of the conceptus without clinical importance may, however, remain in the cavity for several weeks[18]. The efficacy of the surgical and non-surgical procedure in the randomized studies was equal. The frequency of complete abortion for vacuum aspiration was 95–100 % and for the PGE analogues 92–97.5 % (Table 3.2).

Table 3.2 Randomized comparison between prostaglandin analogues and vacuum aspiration for termination of early pregnancy

Reference	Treatment	Complete abortion (%)	Vomiting and/or diarrhoea (%)	Analgesic injections (%)	Duration of bleeding (days)
Rosén et al.[27]	9-methylene PGE$_2$ home treatment	94.4	50	5.6	10.5
	9-methylene PGE$_2$ hospital treatment	100	60	39	9.9
	vacuum aspiration	100	0	0*	4.4
Lundström et al.[20]	16,16-dimethyl PGE$_1$	93	26	30	11.9
	vacuum aspiration	95	0	0*	9.3
WHO[28]	16-phenoxy- PGE$_2$	92.1	35	10	10.8
	vacuum aspiration	94.7	2	0	5.3

*except at surgery

Bleeding

The mean duration of bleeding was significantly longer in the patients treated with prostaglandins (9.9–11.9 days) than with vacuum aspiration (4.4–9.3 days) in the three studies. In 20 patients treated with 9-methylene PGE$_2$, the amount of bleeding was measured[25]. The mean blood loss from the start of treatment to the end of the whole bleeding period was 61.7 ml with a range of 21 to 150 ml. These figures are somewhat higher than those normally reported for vacuum aspiration, but no significant changes in haemoglobin values were found following either of the two treatments. That heavy bleeding is a rare phenomenon in association with prostaglandin treatment for termination of early pregnancy was also shown in a large multicentre study in which repeated vaginal administration of 16,16-dimethyl PGE$_1$ was used. Only one out of the 358 patients included in the study experienced heavy bleeding requiring blood transfusion[29].

Complications

Clinical evidence of pelvic infection was occasionally observed but did not seem to be more common following prostaglandin treatment than following vacuum aspiration. In the large multicentre study mentioned above the frequency of endometritis was 2%[29]. The frequency of gastrointestinal side-effects was significantly higher with prostaglandin treatment than after vacuum aspiration but was not severe enough to interrupt therapy. To evaluate which procedure is the more painful is not possible since the analgesic treatment was different. All patients treated with vacuum aspiration received analgesic injections together with paracervical block at operation. Only occasionally additional injections during the post-operative period was needed. In the prostaglandin treated patients, the pain resulted from stimulation of uterine contractility and occurred during the first six to eight hours. In the different studies between 15 and 40% of the patients treated in the hospital and 4%

of the patients treated at home required injection of meperidine chloride for the alleviation of pain. From these data it is obvious that patients treated with prostaglandins experience more pain than if vacuum aspiration is used. If the patients are treated at home however, the pain seems more acceptable.

Acceptability

In two studies the acceptability of both the surgical and non-surgical procedures has been evaluated[27,30]. Acceptability to the individual user is important and may eventually become the crucial factor for the success of a new method related to fertility regulation. Both the surgical and non-surgical procedures were evaluated positively but were perceived to have very different characteristics. The patients' preference for the method they received increased in both groups after abortion. With either method approximately two out of three patients found their treatment so satisfactory that they indicated a preference for the same procedure in the case of a repeated abortion. The drawbacks of prostaglandin treatment were the pain experienced and/or the amount or length of bleeding and, in a few patients, the waiting time from the insertion of a suppository to the onset of bleeding and abortion. The advantages of prostaglandin therapy were mainly a more 'natural' abortion, no intrauterine manipulations and no routine hospital admission and treatment.

COMBINATION OF ANTIPROGESTIN AND PROSTAGLANDIN

It has long been accepted that progesterone is essential for the maintenance of an early pregnancy. Inhibition of progesterone production or blocking the effect of progesterone may thus be possible methods of terminating early pregnancy. Recently, both possibilities have been evaluated clinically with epostane and RU 486. Epostane is a competitive inhibitor of the 3β-hydroxy steroid dehydrogenase enzyme system[31] and RU 486 a progesterone antagonist which acts at the receptor level[32]. Clinical studies have shown that oral administration of RU 486 resulted in termination of an early pregnancy in the majority of cases. However, the frequency of incomplete abortion was too high for the treatment to compete with vacuum aspiration[33,34]. In the study by Kovacs et al.[34] different amounts of RU 486, from 50 to 200 mg daily for four days, were used. Within this dose range the frequency of complete abortion was the same, about 60 %. Even when the dose was further increased[35] or the duration of treatment was prolonged to seven days[36] the success rate did not increase significantly. Most of the patients experienced only minor side-effects in terms of mild uterine pain and nausea. However, some patients suffered heavy bleeding requiring blood transfusion and curettage (Table 3.3).

As shown by Bygdeman and Swahn[37] pre-treatment with RU 486 in early pregnant patients will result in the appearance of co-ordinated uterine contractions which were in sharp contrast to the almost silent contractility pattern observed in non-treated patients of the same gestational age (Fig.

Table 3.3 Comparison of treatment with RU 486 or prostaglandin analogues alone or in combination for termination of early pregnancy. To avoid influence of different definitions of success rate and side-effects only results from one centre are included

Treatment Reference	Dose (mg)	Frequency of complete abortion (%)	Vomiting and/or diarrhoea (%)	Uterine pain Frequency of analgesic injections (%)
RU 486 alone Kovacs et al.[34]	50–200 daily for 4 days	61	0	0
9-methylene PGE$_2$ Bygdeman et al.[25]	75 and 30 or 60 and 45 with 6 h interval between doses	94	40	34
16-phenoxy PGE$_2$ Bygdeman et al.[25]	0.5 at 3 h interval 3 times	94	55	56
RU 486 Bygdeman and Swahn[37]	50 daily for 4 days plus 16-phenoxy PGE$_2$ 0.25 single dose	94	0	8.8

3.1). Also the sensitivity to prostaglandin was markedly increased. It is likely that the increase in spontaneous contractility and in sensitivity to prostaglandin was due to the local withdrawal of progesterone suppression.

In a recent study, treatment with RU 486 was thus supplemented with a small dose, 0.25 mg, of the PGE analogue 16-phenoxy PGE$_2$, administered as an intramuscular injection on the last day of RU 486 therapy to increase efficacy and reduce the risk for bleeding of RU 486 alone. The dose of RU 486 was 25 mg twice or four times daily for four days. The study included 34 early pregnant women admitted to the hospital for termination of the pregnancy. The combined treatment resulted in complete abortion in 32 patients (94%). One patient experienced an incomplete abortion and in another the pregnancy continued unaffected. The patients started to bleed on the third or fourth day of treatment. The bleeding resembled a heavy menstruation with a duration of one to two weeks. Side-effects were few, 20% of the patients complained of some nausea and three patients (8.8%) of strong uterine pain shortly after the prostaglandin injection[37].

Similar results have been published for the progesterone enzyme inhibitor epostane. Epostane alone was not sufficiently effective to terminate early pregnancy even in high doses. However, if combined with three 10 mg PGE$_2$ suppositories administered at two-hour intervals the success rate increased significantly[38]. It thus seems that a combination of a compound inhibiting progesterone production or progesterone effect with a prostaglandin analogue may be developed into a highly effective, non-surgical method to terminate early pregnancy without many of the drawbacks of each type of compound if used alone.

CONCLUSIONS

The most widely used method for termination of early first trimester pregnancy, often called menstrual regulation, is vacuum aspiration. It is a

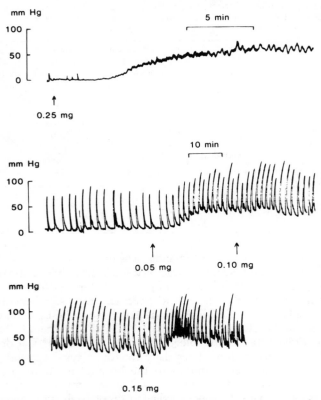

Figure 3.1 The figure shows uterine contractility and response to intramuscular 16-phenoxy PGE$_2$ in one control patient not pre-treated with RU 486 (upper tracing) and in one patient in the morning of the fourth day of treatment with RU 486 25 mg twice daily (lower tracings). Both patients were in the 7th week of pregnancy. Administration of 16-phenoxy PGE$_2$ is indicated by arrows (From Bygdeman and Swahn[37])

highly effective procedure and the overall complication rate is low. The prostaglandins offer a non-surgical alternative for menstrual regulation. Both vaginal and intramuscular administration of the latest generation of PGE analogues have been shown in several studies to be equally effective as vacuum aspiration if the treatment is restricted to the first three weeks following the first missed menstrual period. Preliminary studies in which one of these PGE analogues was administered by the vaginal route indicate that self-administration at home starts to be a reality in selected patients. Gastrointestinal side-effects and uterine pain are still problems although of significantly less importance than if natural prostaglandins are used. It seems possible that with a combination of an antiprogesterone and a prostaglandin analogue these problems can be further reduced. The prospects for the development of a non-surgical, self-administered method for menstrual regulation which can gain widespread acceptability seem bright.

ACKNOWLEDGEMENTS

Most of the studies performed at the Department of Obstetrics and Gynecology, Karolinska Hospital, included in this review were supported by grants from the World Health Organization, Special Programme of Research, Development and Research Training in Human Reproduction. The skilful assistance of Astrid Häggblad is gratefully acknowledged.

REFERENCES

1. Landesman, R., Kay, R.E. and Wilson, K.H. (1973). Menstrual extraction: a review of 400 procedures at Women's Services, New York, N.Y. *Contraception*, **8**, 527–39
2. Annual Report, WHO Special Programme of Research, Development and Research Training in Human Reproduction (1979). pp. 60–61
3. Roth-Brandel, U., Bygdeman, M., Wiqvist, N. and Bergström, S. (1970). Prostaglandins for induction of therapeutic abortion. *Lancet*, **1**, 190
4. Wiqvist, N. and Bygdeman, M. (1970). Induction of therapeutic abortion with intravenous prostaglandin $F_{2\alpha}$. *Lancet*, **2**, 889
5. Bygdeman, M. and Wiqvist, N. (1971). Early abortion in the human. *Ann. N.Y. Acad. Sci.*, **180**, 473–82
6. Karim, S.M.M. and Filshie, G.M. (1970). Therapeutic abortion using prostaglandin $F_{2\alpha}$. *Lancet*, **1**, 157–9
7. Karim, S.M.M. (1971). Prostaglandins as abortifacients. *N. Engl. J. Med.*, **285**, 1534–5
8. Kinoshita, K., Wagatsuma, T., Hogaki, M. and Sakamoto, S. (1971). The induction of abortion by prostaglandin $F_{2\alpha}$. *Am. J. Obstet. Gynecol.*, **111**, 855–8
9. Wentz, A.C. and Jones, G.S. (1973). Intravenous prostaglandin $F_{2\alpha}$ for induction of menses. *Fertil. Steril.*, **24**, 569–77
10. Treadway, D. and Mishell, D.R. Jr. (1973). Therapeutic abortion of early human gestation with vaginal suppositories of prostaglandin $F_{2\alpha}$. *Am. J. Obstet. Gynecol.*, **116**, 795–98
11. Wiqvist, N. and Bygdeman, M. (1970). Therapeutic abortion by local administration of prostaglandin. *Lancet*, **2**, 716–17
12. Mocsary, P. and Csapo, A.I. (1975). Menstrual induction with $PGF_{2\alpha}$ and PGE_2. *Prostaglandins*, **10**, 545–47
13. Ragab, M.I. and Edelman, D.A. (1976). Early termination of pregnancy. A comparative study of intrauterine prostaglandin $F_{2\alpha}$ and vacuum aspiration. *Prostaglandins*, **11**, 275
14. Mackenzie, I.Z., Hillier, K. and Embrey, M.P. (1976). Intrauterine prostaglandin E_2 as an early postconceptional abortifacient. In Samuelsson, B. and Paoletti, R. (eds.) *Advances in Prostaglandin and Thromboxane Research*. Vol. II., pp. 687–91. (New York: Raven Press)
15. Bygdeman, M., Martin, J.N. Jr., Leader, A., Lundström, V., Ramadan, M., Eneroth, P. and Gréen, K. (1976). Early pregnancy interruption by 15(S)15-methyl prostaglandin $F_{2\alpha}$ methyl ester. *Obstet. Gynecol.*, **48**, 221–4
16. Hamberger, L., Nilsson, L., Björn-Rasmussen, E., Atterfelt, P. and Wiqvist, N. (1978). Early abortion by vaginal prostaglandin suppositories: blood loss in relation to elimination of serum chorionic gonadotrophin, progesterone and estradiol-17β. *Contraception*, **17**, 183–94
17. Gréen, K., Bygdeman, M. and Bremme, K. (1978). Interruption of early first trimester pregnancy by single vaginal administration of 15-methyl-$PGF_{2\alpha}$ methyl ester. *Contraception*, **18**, 551–60
18. Mandelin, M. (1978). Termination of early pregnancy by a single dose 3 mg 15-methyl $PGF_{2\alpha}$ methyl ester vaginal suppository. *Prostaglandins*, **16**, 143–52
19. Mackenzie, I.Z., Embrey, M.P., Davies, A.J. and Guillebaud, J. (1978). Very early abortion by prostaglandins. *Lancet*, **1**, 1223–6
20. Lundström, V., Bygdeman, M., Fotiou, S., Gréen, K. and Kinoshita, K. (1977). Abortion in early pregnancy by vaginal administration of 16,16-dimethyl-PGE_2 in comparison with vacuum aspiration. *Contraception*, **16**, 167–73
21. Karim, S.M.M., Ratnam, S.S. and Ilancheran, A. (1977). Menstrual induction with vaginal administration of 16,16-dimethyl trans Δ^2-PGE_1 methyl ester (ONO-802). *Prostaglandins*, **14**, 615–16

22. Takagi, S., Sakata, H., Yoshida, T., Den, K., Fujii, T.K., Amenyia, H. and Tomita, M. (1978). Termination of early pregnancy by ONO-802 suppositories (16,16-dimethyl-trans-Δ^2-PGE$_1$ methyl ester). *Prostaglandins*, **15**, 913–19

23. Karim, S.M.M., Rao, B., Ratnam, S.S., Prasad, R.N.V., Wong, Y.M. and Ilancheran, A. (1977). Termination of early pregnancy (menstrual induction) with 16-phenoxy-ω-tetranor-PGE$_2$ methyl-sulfonylamide. *Contraception*, **16**, 377–81

24. Fleischer, A., Schulman, H., Blattner, P., Jagani, N. and Fayemi, A. (1982). Early pregnancy-abortion model using sulprostone. *Prostaglandins*, **23**, 643–55

25. Bygdeman, M., Christensen, N.J., Gréen, K., Zheng, S. and Lundström, V. (1983). Termination of early pregnancy: future development. *Acta Obstet. Gynecol. Scand. Suppl.*, **113**, 125–9

26. Bygdeman, M., Christensen, N.J., Gréen, K. and Vesterqvist, O. (1984). Self-administration at home of prostaglandin for termination of early pregnancy. In Toppozada, M., Bygdeman, M. and Hafez, E.S.E. (eds.) *Advances in Reproductive Health Care*, pp. 83–90. (Lancaster: MTP)

27. Rosén, A.S., von Knorring, K., Bygdeman, M. and Christensen, N. (1984). Randomized comparison of prostaglandin treatment in hospital or at home with vacuum aspiration for termination of early pregnancy. *Contraception*, **29**, 423–35

28. WHO Task Force on Post-ovulatory Methods for Fertility Regulation (1986). Menstrual regulation by intramuscular injections of 16-phenoxy-tetranor-PGE$_2$ methyl sulfonylamide or vacuum aspiration. *Br. J. Obstet. Gynaecol.* (in press).

29. WHO Prostaglandin Task Force (1982). Termination of early first trimester pregnancy by vaginal administration of 16,16-dimethyl-trans-Δ^2 PGE$_1$ methyl ester. *Asia Oceania J. Obstet. Gynaecol.*, **8**, 263–68

30. Rosén, A.S., Nystedt, L., Bygdeman, M. and Lundström, V. (1979). Acceptability of a non-surgical method to terminate very early pregnancy in comparison with vacuum aspiration. *Contraception*, **19**, 107–17

31. Pattison, N.S., Webster, M.A., Phipps, S.L., Anderson, A.B.M. and Gillmer, M.D.G. (1985). Inhibition of 3β-hydroxy steroid dehydrogenase activity in first and second trimester pregnancy and in the luteal phase using Epostane. *Fertil. Steril.*, **42**, 875–81

32. Baulieu, E.E. (1985). RU 486: an antiprogestin steroid with contragestive activity in women. In Baulieu, E.E. and Segal, S.J. (eds.) *The Antiprogestin RU 486 and Human Fertility Control*, pp. 1–26. (New York: Plenum Press)

33. Herrmann, W., Wyss, R., Riondel, A., Philibert, D., Teutsch, G., Sakiz, E. and Baulieu, E.E. (1982). Effet d'un steroide antiprogesterone chez la femme: interruption du cycle menstruel et de la grossesse au début. *C.R. Acad. Sci. Paris*, **294**, 933–38

34. Kovacs, L., Sas, M., Resch, B.A., Ugocsai, G., Swahn, M.L., Bygdeman, M. and Rowe, P.J. (1984). Termination of very early pregnancy by RU 486 – An anti-progestational compound. *Contraception*, **24**, 399–410

35. Sitruk-Ware, R., Billaud, L., Mowszowicz, I., Yaneva, H., Mauvais-Jarvis, P., Bardin, C.W. and Spitz, I.M. (1985). The use of RU 486 as an abortifacient in early pregnancy. In Baulieu, E.E. and Segal, S.J. (eds.) *The Antiprogestin Steroid RU 486 and Human Fertility Control*, pp. 243–48. (New York: Plenum Press)

36. Birgersson, L., Odlind, V. and Johansson, E. (1985). Clinical effects of RU 486 administered for seven days in early pregnancy. In Baulieu, E.E. and Segal, S.J. (eds.) *The Antiprogestin Steroid RU 486 and Human Fertility Control*, pp. 235–42. (New York: Plenum Press)

37. Bygdeman, M. and Swahn, M.L. (1985). Progesterone receptor blockage. Effect on uterine contractility and early pregnancy. *Contraception*, **32**, 45–51

38. Webster, M.A., Phipps, S.L. and Gillmer, M.D.G. (1985). Interruption of first trimester human pregnancy following Epostane therapy. Effect of prostaglandin E$_2$ pessaries. *Br. J. Obstet. Gynaecol.*, **92**, 963–68

4
Interactions of eicosanoids and other factors in blastocyst implantation

T.G. Kennedy

INTRODUCTION

Implantation involves a series of reactions between the embryo and uterus which result in the embryo becoming fixed in position within the uterus in physical contact with the maternal organism[1]. There are considerable species differences in these reactions, most notably in the extent of trophoblastic invasion of the endometrium[2-4]. In all species, however, the embryo–endometrial interactions can only be initiated when the embryo and endometrium have reached a precise stage of maturity; the embryo must be at the blastocyst stage of development, and hormone-dependent changes leading to the development of a 'receptive' (or 'sensitized') endometrium must have occurred. Lack of synchronization in the development of the embryo and the endometrium results in the failure, or less commonly the postponement, of implantation and largely explains why implantation is such a critical period for the establishment of pregnancy.

For a number of reasons, research into implantation has been stimulated in recent years. First, the recognition that implantation is such a critical event has led to the suggestion that at least some unexplained infertility in man is caused by implantation failure. Secondly, a better understanding of implantation might lead to the development of improved contraceptive techniques, and finally, it has become apparent that implantation is the least efficient step in *in vitro* fertilization programmes for the treatment of human infertility.

In virtually all species investigated, the earliest macroscopically-identifiable sign of blastocyst implantation is an increase in endometrial vascular permeability which is localized to the areas adjacent to the blastocysts[4]. This increase in permeability is usually taken as defining the beginning of implantation, and is thought to be an essential prerequisite for implantation[4]. The increase in permeability precedes trophoblastic invasion of the endometrium in those species in which invasion occurs. In species in which endometrial

73

stromal cells differentiate into decidual cells (decidualization, or the decidual cell reaction) in response to artificial stimuli, an increase in endometrial vascular permeability precedes the differentiation of decidual cells[4].

The localized nature of the permeability increase at implantation in most species suggests that it occurs in response to a signal from the blastocyst. In women, however, there is no need to invoke a locally acting embryonic signal since there is a generalized increase in endometrial vascular permeability, as well as stromal differentiation of pre-decidual cells, during each menstrual cycle, presumably as a consequence of a systemic stimulus[4]. Where an embryonic signal seems to be involved, its nature is uncertain[5] but there is now considerable evidence that eicosanoids, particularly prostaglandins, have an obligatory role in endometrial vascular permeability changes and decidualization in a number of species. The eicosanoids probably do not act alone, but rather interact with other vasoactive compounds.

This chapter will review the evidence for the involvement of eicosanoids in implantation and decidualization. Little work has been done in our own species or in primates; hence most of the data reviewed are from non-primate species. Since the decidual cell reaction has been widely used as a model for implantation, particularly in rodents, the involvement of eicosanoids in this reaction will also be reviewed.

PROSTAGLANDINS AND IMPLANTATION – DECIDUALIZATION

Evidence

There is now considerable experimental evidence that prostaglandins have an obligatory role in the endometrial vascular permeability changes and decidualization in a number of species. With hindsight, it is possible to attribute the first indications of the involvement of prostaglandins in this process to Rozenkranz[6] and Horan[7] who reported effects of non-steroidal anti-inflammatory drugs on implantation at a time when the mechanism of action of this class of drugs was unknown.

More recently, in pregnant animals indomethacin, a potent inhibitor of prostaglandin biosynthesis[8], has been shown to delay or inhibit the localized increase in endometrial vascular permeability in rats[9,10], mice[11], hamsters[12], and rabbits[13], and implantation in rats[14,15], mice[16–18], rabbits[19,20], and pigs[21]. The only exception reported to date appears to be the ewe in which treatment from day 7 to 22 after mating with either indomethacin or acetylsalicylic acid at doses which substantially reduced endometrial prostaglandin concentrations had no apparent effect on the establishment of pregnancy[22].

Consistent with the notion that prostaglandins are involved in implantation are the observations that intrauterine administration of prostaglandin antagonists at the expected time of implantation reduces the number of implantation sites[23]. In addition, the concentrations of prostaglandins are elevated in the areas of increased endometrial vascular permeability[5,12,24,25], and exogenous prostaglandins can reverse, at least partially, the effects of indomethacin on implantation[17,18,15,26].

In non-pregnant animals with uteri sensitized for the decidual cell reaction, decidualization in response to artificial stimuli is reduced by indomethacin administration[27–34], as is the increase in endometrial vascular permeability which preceeds decidualization[35]. Uterine concentrations are elevated by artificial deciduogenic stimuli[33,35–39] before there are detectable changes in permeability; the time-course is consistent with the proposal that prostaglandin levels are elevated as a cause, rather than a consequence, of the increased permeability. Prostaglandins administered into the uterine lumen of animals in which endogenous prostaglandin production has been inhibited can increase endometrial vascular permeability[31,35–37] and bring about decidualization[31,32,40]. There is evidence that prostaglandins are involved not only in the initiation of the endometrial vascular changes, but also throughout the growth and differentiation of decidual cells[32].

Taken together, these data strongly suggest that prostaglandins are involved in implantation and decidualization.

Source of prostaglandins

In considering the potential sources of the prostaglandins which are involved in implantation, the two most likely sources are the blastocysts and the endometrium.

The blastocysts as a source of prostaglandins could readily explain the localized nature of the permeability response. There are reports of blastocyst biosynthesis of prostaglandins for a number of species[22,41–47], in all of which the blastocysts undergo marked expansion prior to implantation. In contrast, attempts to demonstrate prostaglandin biosynthesis by rat[48] or mouse[49] blastocysts, which remain small prior to implantation, have been unsuccessful; this lack of success may have been the result of a combination of the limited amount of tissue available, lack of sensitivity of the techniques employed and/or inappropriate culture conditions. There is indirect evidence for prostaglandin production by mouse blastocysts: inhibitors of prostaglandin biosynthesis prevent the hatching of mouse blastocysts in vitro[50–52]. However, it should be emphasized that the demonstration of blastocyst prostaglandin production by itself is insufficient to implicate the blastocyst as the source of prostaglandins in implantation; it will be necessary to demonstrate that the blastocyst-produced prostaglandins act on the endometrium. Blastocyst-produced prostaglandins may have functions within the blastocyst[50].

Based on the results of embryo transfer studies in which blastocysts recovered from control or indomethacin-treated donor rabbits were transferred to control or indomethacin-treated recipients, Snabes and Harper[53] suggested that the prostaglandins involved in implantation are produced in the endometrium. The endometrium as the source of prostaglandins regulating endometrial vascular permeability and decidualization is potentially capable of explaining the increase in permeability brought about by both blastocysts and artificial stimuli. It is possible that blastocysts, as a result of their interaction with the luminal epithelium, and artificial stimuli have the common property of 'traumatizing' the endometrium thereby stimulating prostaglandin production. Ultrastructural studies of the early stages of implantation suggest the possibility of physical interactions between trophoblastic cells and endometrial luminal epithelial cells. The endometrial vascular permeability changes are preceded by interdigitation of microvilli on trophoblastic and epithelial cells, followed by broad areas of apposition of cell membranes[54-56]. This intimate contact between trophoblastic and epithelial cells may be sufficient to stimulate the production of prostaglandins by the epithelial cells. In addition, the blastocyst may play a more active role in physically perturbing the luminal epithelium than indicated by morphological studies. When cultured *in vitro*, rat and mouse blastocysts undergo repetitive contractions and dilatations[52,57,58] which, if they also occur *in vivo*, may augment the physical signal attributable to the close contact between the blastocyst and uterine luminal epithelium.

Artificial deciduogenic stimuli cause tissue damage[59,60] and in other tissues, injury is known to stimulate prostaglandin synthesis[61,62].

If the signal from the blastocyst is not physical in nature, then it is presumably a chemical. The chemical signal, if not a prostaglandin, would presumably stimulate prostaglandin production within the endometrium. If during the initiation of implantation, the endometrium produces prostaglandins in response to a physical or chemical signal from the blastocysts, which endometrial cells produce the prostaglandins? If the luminal epithelium is not the source of the prostaglandins, it would be necessary for the physical or chemical signal from the blastocyst to be transferred across the epithelium to act on the underlying stromal cells; for a physical signal this would require the transformation of the original signal to a chemical signal capable of stimulating stromal cell prostaglandin production. Possibly of relevance to these considerations is the localized depletion of neutral lipids which occurs in the epithelium surrounding rat blastocysts[63]. These neutral lipids are mainly triacylglycerols[64] and, if they contain arachidonic acid, their depletion may represent mobilization of stored precursor for prostaglandin biosynthesis. There is evidence for luminal epithelial cell production of prostaglandins[65]; *in vitro*, epithelial cell enriched preparations produce more prostaglandins than do corresponding endometrial stromal cell preparations (E.J. Psenicka and T.G. Kennedy, unpublished). As indicated by histochemistry, prostaglandin synthetase activity in the sensitized rat uterus is confined to the luminal and glandular epithelial cells of the endometrium[66]. Thus the prostaglandins may be produced within the luminal epithelium in response to a physical or chemical signal from the blastocyst, and then diffuse into the endometrial stroma to bring about their effects. Alternatively they may be produced within the stroma in response to a chemical signal which arises either from the epithelium (as a result of its interaction with the blastocyst) or from the blastocyst.

Which prostaglandins?

In attempting to identify the prostaglandin(s) involved in mediating the endometrial vascular permeability response at implantation and following the application of an artificial deciduogenic stimulus, use has been made of uterine prostaglandin measurements and/or production, and uterine responses to exogenously administered prostaglandins.

The measurements of prostaglandins have not identified a single prostaglandin as the mediator of the endometrial vascular changes. The concentrations of prostaglandins E, F and I_2 (measured as 6-oxo-prostaglandin $F_{1\alpha}$) are elevated at implantation sites[9,24,25,67] and in the uterus following the application of an artificial deciduogenic stimulus[33,35-37,68]. Not all reports are consistent; in the hamster, prostaglandins E but not F, are elevated at implantation sites[12], while in the mouse, uterine concentrations of prostaglandins F, but not E or I_2 are elevated in response to a deciduogenic stimulus[39]. Homogenates of pregnant and pseudopregnant uteri produce prostaglandins E_2, $F_{2\alpha}$ and 6-oxo-prostaglandin $F_{1\alpha}$, with the latter being produced in the greatest amounts[10,69].

The uterine responses to exogenously administered prostaglandins have been no more enlightening than their measurements. Indirect evidence that prostaglandin $F_{2\alpha}$ may be involved has come from reports that this prostaglandin can induce implantation in rats and mice when given systemically[17,26]. However, when applied locally into the uterine lumen, prostaglandin $F_{2\alpha}$ was found to be less effective than prostaglandin E_2 at inducing implantation in mice[18]. Intrauterine administration of prostaglandin $F_{2\alpha}$ results in decidualization in rats[29] and rabbits[70], although in the latter study prostaglandin E_2 was more effective than prostaglandin $F_{2\alpha}$. However, in these studies no inhibitors of endogenous prostaglandin production were used and consequently the reported responses may have been due to the exogenous prostaglandin, endogenously produced prostaglandins, or an interaction between exogenous and endogenous prostaglandins. It is of interest in this regard to note that while prostaglandin $F_{2\alpha}$ induced decidualization when given to animals not treated with indomethacin, it was ineffective when given to indomethacin-treated animals[30]. To circumvent these problems of interpretation of results, prostaglandins have been infused into the uterine lumen of rats treated with indomethacin. Prostaglandins E_2 and $F_{2\alpha}$, alone or combined, were effective in bringing about an increase in endometrial vascular permeability and decidualization and, in terms of the latter response, were equally potent[31,32].

Based on the observation that tranylcypromine, purportedly a selective inhibitor of prostaglandin I_2 synthesis[71], inhibits decidualization, Jonsson et al.[68] have suggested that prostaglandin I_2 may be a mediator of decidualization in mice. However the specificity of this inhibitory action of tranylcypromine has been questioned[34,72] and the inhibition has not been overriden with prostaglandin I_2. Because of the chemical instability of prostaglandin I_2 in aqueous solutions, it is difficult to determine its biological activity. Neither prostaglandin I_2 (in Tris–saline buffer, pH9) nor a stable analogue of prostaglandin I_2, ZK 36374 (Schering), increased endometrial vascular permeability or caused decidualization when infused into the uterine lumen of indomethacin-treated rats; under the same conditions, prostaglandin E_2 was effective (T.G. Kennedy, unpublished).

Recently, 6-oxo-prostaglandin E_1 has been identified as a biological product[73,74]; at present it is not known if its precursor is prostaglandin I_2 or 6-oxo-prostaglandin $F_{1\alpha}$[75]. When infused into the uterine lumen of indomethacin-treated rats, 6-oxo-prostaglandin E_1 is equally as potent as prostaglandin E_2

in producing decidualization[76]. However, a deciduogenic stimulus did not increase uterine concentrations of 6-oxo-prostaglandin E_1, suggesting that uterine production of this prostaglandin, if it occurs at all, was not stimulated. Hence it seems unlikely that 6-oxo-prostaglandin E_1 has a role in decidualization.

Thus there is considerable uncertainty about the identity of the prostaglandins involved in the initiation of implantation and decidualization. In this regard it is of interest to note that while endometrial binding sites for E-series prostaglandins have been reported in rats[77,78], humans[79] and pigs[80], binding sites for prostaglandins $F_{2\alpha}$ have not been found[79,81].

Prostaglandins and control of uterine sensitization

There is a very limited time in pregnancy during which mature blastocysts can interact with the endometrium and implant successfully; at other times, the uterus is incapable of responding appropriately to the signal(s) from the blastocysts[4]. Likewise, decidualization in response to artificial stimuli can only be obtained during a limited period of pregnancy, pseudopregnancy, or when the uterus has been prepared by an appropriate regimen of hormone treatments[3,4]. In addition, oestrogens in low dosages act synergistically with progesterone to sensitize the rat and mouse uterus for the decidual cell reaction[3,82,83]. That these temporal and endocrine changes in uterine sensitization might be related to the ability of the uterus to produce prostaglandins is suggested first, by reports[10,69] that the production of prostaglandins by uterine homogenates from pregnant and pseudopregnant rats is maximal on day five, corresponding to the timing of maximal uterine sensitization for the decidual cell reaction[84], and secondly by the observations that oestrogens affect uterine prostaglandin production[85,86]. However, the results of investigations of temporal and endocrine changes in uterine sensitization indicate that uterine prostaglandin levels in response to standardized artificial stimuli do not provide a ready explanation for the changes in sensitization[36,37,39]. Rather, maximal uterine sensitization corresponded with the maximal ability of the endometrium to respond to intrauterine-injected prostaglandin E_2 with increased endometrial vascular permeability.

Of the many possible explanations for the changes in responsiveness to prostaglandins, one is that in the non-sensitized uterus the exogenous prostaglandins are cleared rapidly, either by metabolism or translocation across the uterus. In the rabbit, the rates of translocation of prostaglandins across the uterine wall varies throughout early pregnancy and pseudopregnancy[87]. In an attempt to expose the endometrium to elevated prostaglandin levels over an extended time, prostaglandins have been infused into the uterine lumen of differentially sensitized rat uteri, and decidualization subsequently assessed[88]. Temporal and endocrine changes in uterine sensitization were only partially circumvented by the intrauterine infusions of prostaglandins, suggesting that the reduced responsiveness of the non-sensitized uteri is probably not due solely to more rapid clearance of prostaglandins.

An alternative explanation for changes in sensitization is the possibility that mediators in addition to prostaglandins are involved and it is the production, release or action of these other mediators which determines maximal uterine sensitization. It has been suggested that the vascular permeability changes during the early inflammatory response, which are similar to those occurring at implantation, involve mediators in addition to prostaglandins[89,90]. An unsuccessful attempt has been made to override oestrogen-induced non-sensitization by the intrauterine injection of prostaglandin E_2 combined with either histamine or bradykinin[91]. The interpretation of these negative data are limited, however, by the assumption that bradykinin and histamine were able to move out of the uterine lumen to reach their presumed site of action, the endothelial cells within the endometrium. There is good evidence for a barrier which restricts the free movement of some compounds, depending on molecular size and lipid solubility, from blood to the uterine lumen[92,93]; this barrier is probably located at the level of the uterine luminal epithelium[94]. If this barrier also impedes the movement of substances in the opposite direction, then histamine and bradykinin, because of their molecular size and hydrophilic nature, may not readily enter the endometrium from the uterine lumen.

Endometrial responsiveness to prostaglandins may be related to the properties of endometrial receptors for prostaglandins. Endometrial membrane preparations from sensitized rat uteri and from pig and human uteri have specific, saturable, high-affinity binding sites for E-series prostaglandins[77-80], but not for prostaglandin $F_{2\alpha}$[79,81]. In the rat, the endometrial concentrations of prostaglandin E binding sites are controlled primarily by progesterone and seem to be located in the stroma but not the luminal epithelium[78]. Endocrine regulation and localization of the binding sites in human and pig endometrium have been less well investigated. Although in the rat the onset of uterine sensitization is temporally correlated with the appearance of detectable concentrations of these binding sites[77], no simple relationship exists between their endometrial concentrations and uterine sensitization for the decidual cell reaction[78].

In the rat, there is an excellent correlation between the proportion of endometrial stromal capillaries which are sheathed by pericytes and uterine receptivity for implantation and sensitization for the decidual cell reaction[92]. On day five of pregnancy, the day of uterine receptivity, there is a transient but substantial increase (to 74 % compared to < 15 % on days four and six) in the percentage of capillaries sheathed by pericytes[95]. A sequence of treatment with progesterone and oestrogen which sensitizes the uterus for the decidual cell reaction also results in a high proportion of capillaries with associated pericytes[95]. At present the function of pericytes is unknown but it is conceivable that these cells may regulate the responsiveness of capillaries to prostaglandins and it is their low numbers in the non-sensitized uteri which renders the endometrial vasculature unresponsive to prostaglandins. It would be of great interest to know if pericytes have receptors for prostaglandins.

Mode of action of prostaglandins

Little is known about the mechanisms by which prostaglandins bring about increased endometrial vascular permeability and the subsequent decidualization. Experimental evidence suggests that prostaglandins are involved not only in the permeability response but also throughout the transformation of stromal cells to decidual cells[28,31,32]. Inhibition of prostaglandin biosynthesis by the administration of indomethacin 12 h[28] or even up to 48 h[31] after the application of a deciduogenic stimulus suppresses the decidual cell reaction. The mechanism of action as well as the types of prostaglandins may differ in the two processes.

Arguing by analogy with the inflammatory response, Kennedy and Armstrong[48] have suggested that there may be two mediators of the endometrial vascular permeability response; one, a prostaglandin of the E or I series, may cause vasodilatation; the other, possibly histamine, may increase vascular permeability. In support of this suggestion is the observation that vasodilatation accompanies the endometrial permeability response to an artificial stimulus[96]. The evidence for the involvement of histamine is indirect. Rabbit and mouse blastocysts are capable of histamine synthesis[97,98] and in rabbits the injection into the uterine lumen of an inhibitor of histidine decarboxylase, the enzyme which converts histidine to histamine, interrupts implantation[97,99]. Implantation in rabbits is also adversely affected by the intrauterine instillation of disodium cromoglycate, an inhibitor of histamine release from mast cells[100]. Rabbit blastocysts and endometrium have histamine H_2- and H_1-receptors, respectively[101]. However, in rats the initiation of implantation was not affected when the animals were treated with both histamine H_1- and H_2-receptor antagonists[102]. Thus the possibility that prostaglandins interact with other vasoactive substances, particularly histamine, remains uncertain, and requires further investigation.

The mode of action of prostaglandins at the cellular level within the endometrium is poorly understood. In a number of cell types, c-AMP acts as a second messenger for prostaglandins of the E series[86,103,104]. Some, but by no means all, of the available evidence suggests that c-AMP may be involved in implantation and decidualization. The uterine concentrations of c-AMP are elevated at the areas of increased endometrial vascular permeability on day six of pregnancy in the rat[105], and in ovariectomized progesterone-treated mice, blastocysts implant following the intraluminal injection of c-AMP[106] or its dibutyryl analogue[107]. However the specificity of this implantation response has been questioned since AMP (non-cyclic) will also induce implantation in these animals[108]. Other evidence for the involvement of c-AMP in the initiation of implantation is the report that the intrauterine administration of an inhibitor of adenylate cyclase reduced the implantation rate in rabbits[109]. In animals sensitized for the decidual cell reaction, artificial deciduogenic stimuli cause a rapid increase in uterine c-AMP concentrations[33,110–112]; this increase is inhibited by indomethacin, suggesting that the response is prostaglandin-mediated[33,112]. The intraluminal injection of prostaglandin E_2 into the uteri of rats pretreated with indomethacin increases uterine c-AMP concentrations[113]. Cholera toxin, a stimulator of adenylate cyclase, is a potent inducer of endometrial vascular permeability changes in rats[112,114], and of decidualization in rats[112] and mice[33]. However, the mechanism of action of cholera toxin in these circumstances is uncertain; whereas Rankin et al.[33] reported a 10-fold increase in uterine c-AMP concentrations after intrauterine administration of cholera toxin to mice, Johnston and Kennedy[113,114] were unable to detect any increase in rats. Other observations which raise doubts about the role of c-AMP in the endometrial permeability response and decidualization are the reports that in rats in which endogenous prostaglandin synthesis has been inhibited with indomethacin, analogues of c-AMP, with or without inhibitors of phosphodiesterase, when given into the uterine lumen do not increase endometrial vascular permeability above that produced by the vehicle[112–114]. In addition, in mice, rats and rabbits, the intrauterine administration of c-AMP or its analogues does not induce decidualization[70,110,111,115]. It is possible, therefore, that prostaglandins have their effects within the endometrium by mechanisms not involving c-AMP as a second messenger.

The endometrial cells which respond to prostaglandins are not known. If E-series prostaglandins are the important mediators, then presumably the responding cells are within the endometrial stroma since high-affinity binding sites for E-series prostaglandins have been detected in the stroma but not epithelium[78]. Endometrial stroma is not a homogenous tissue; it consists of stromal cells, vascular endothelial cells, pericytes and other cells. Prostaglandin E_2 can act directly on stromal cells; stromal cell alkaline phosphatase activity in vitro is maintained at a higher level in the presence of PGE_2 than its absence[116]. Whether PGE_2 can also act directly on endothelial cells or on pericytes is at present unknown.

OTHER EICOSANOIDS

At present, little is known about the role, if any, of eicosanoids other than the prostaglandins in blastocyst implantation. To date, the only investigations which have any relevance to implantation–decidualization have been restricted to defining the metabolism of arachidonic acid by lipoxygenase pathways in the uterus; the physiological significance of the products of these pathways has not been determined.

As indicated by the production of hydroxyeicosatetraenoic (HETE) acids, lipoxygenase activities are present in human[117], rat[118], and rabbit[119,120] endometrium. Endometrium from the non-pregnant human uterus produces predominantly 12-HETE, with 5-HETE[117] indicating the presence of 12- and 5-lipoxygenase activities, respectively. Rat endometrium also produces 12-HETE, with possibly 15-HETE but no 5-HETE[118]. In rabbits, Pakrasi and Dey[119] and Pakrasi et al.[120] have reported the synthesis of 5-HETE by endometrium, and also by day five blastocysts.

In all the studies utilizing endometrium, the cellular source of the lipoxygenase products has not been definitively established; they may be produced by the white cells present in the endometrium, rather than by the endometrial cells themselves.

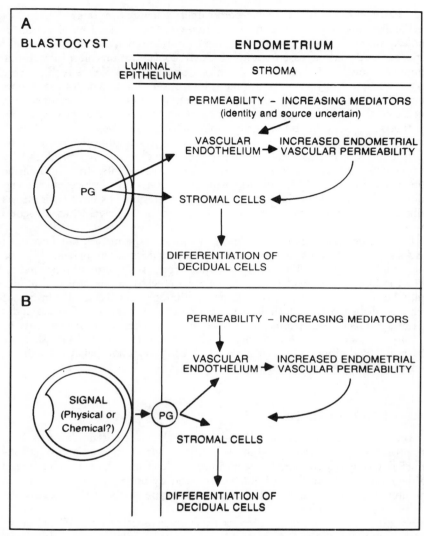

Figure 4.1 Schematic representation of possible interactions between the blastocyst and endometrium which result in the initiation of implantation and decidualization. In scheme A, the blastocyst is the source of prostaglandins; in B, the prostaglandins are produced in the endometrium (luminal epithelium and/or stroma) in response to a signal from the blastocyst. (Modified from Kennedy[123], reproduced from *Prostaglandin Perspectives* with permission of Media Medica)

Since the leukotrienes are potent vasoactive compounds[121], they may be involved in mediating the endometrial vascular changes which occur at implantation. No data on this are presently available. That leukotrienes may have a role in the uterine vasculature is suggested by the observation that

FPL 55712, a selective leukotriene antagonist, potentiated oestrogen-induced hyperaemia in rabbits[122], thereby suggesting that leukotrienes inhibit the uterine vascular responses to oestrogen. From this observation, it would be expected that leukotriene synthesis should be inhibited at the implantation site in order to allow the increase in vascular permeability to occur.

CONCLUSIONS

While considerable experimental evidence suggests that prostaglandins have an obligatory role in the initiation of implantation as well as decidualization in a number of species, other eicosanoids have not been investigated to any extent. Little is known about the types of prostaglandins involved in implantation–decidualization, their site of production or mode of action. It is likely that the prostaglandins do not act alone, but interact with other vasoactive substances. Some of the possible relationships are presented in Figure 4.1. A question which remains to be answered is whether these findings in animals are relevant to our own species.

REFERENCES

1. McLaren, A. (1972). The embryo. In Austin, C.R. and Short, R.V. (eds.) *Reproduction in Mammals*. Book 2: *Embryonic and Fetal Development*, pp. 1–42 (London: Cambridge University Press)
2. Amoroso, E.C. (1952). Placentation. In Parkes, A.S. (ed.) *Marshall's Physiology of Reproduction*, Vol. II pp. 127–311. (London: Longmans, Green and Co.)
3. Finn, C.A. and Porter, D.G. (1975). *The Uterus*. (Action: Publishing Sciences Group)
4. Psychoyos, A. (1973). Endocrine control of egg implantation. In Greep, R.O., Astwood, E.B. and Geiger, S.R. (eds.) *Handbook of Physiology*. Section 7, Vol. II, Part 2, pp. 187–215. (Bethesda: American Physiological Society)
5. Kennedy, T.G. (1983). Embryonic signals and the initiation of blastocyst implantation. *Aust. J. Biol. Sci.*, **36**, 531–543
6. Rosenkranz, V.W. (1955–56). Über hemmung der deciduombildung durch butazolidin. *Z. Biol.*, **108**, 53–57
7. Horan, A.H. (1971). The suppression of inflammatory edema at the nidation site by sodium salicylate and nitrogen mustard in the rat. *Fertil. Steril.*, **22**, 392–397
8. Vane, J.R. (1971). Inhibition of prostaglandin synthesis as a mechanism of action of aspirin-like drugs. *Nature (London) New Biol.*, **231**, 232–235
9. Kennedy, T.G. (1977). Evidence for a role for prostaglandins in the initiation of blastocyst implantation in the rat. *Biol. Reprod.*, **16**, 286–91
10. Phillips, C.A. and Poyser, N.L. (1981). Studies on the involvement of prostaglandins in implantation in the rat. *J. Reprod. Fertil.*, **62**, 73–81
11. Lundkvist, Ö. and Nilsson, B.O. (1980). Ultrastructural changes of the trophoblast-epithelial complex in mice subjected to implantation blocking treatment with indomethacin. *Biol. Reprod.*, **22**, 719–26
12. Evans, C.A. and Kennedy, T.G. (1978). The importance of prostaglandin synthesis for the initiation of blastocyst implantation in the hamster. *J. Reprod. Fertil.*, **54**, 255–261
13. Hoffman, L.H., DiPietro, D.L. and McKenna, T.J. (1978). Effects of indomethacin on uterine capillary permeability and blastocyst development in rabbits. *Prostaglandins*, **15**, 823–828
14. Gavin, M.A., Dominguez Fernandez-Tejerina, J.C., Montanes de las Heras, M.F. and Vijil Maeso, E. (1974). Efectos de un inhibidos de la biosíntesis de las prostaglandinas (Indometacina) sobre la implantación en le rata. *Reproduccion*, **1**, 177–183

15. Garg, S.K. and Chandhury, R.R. (1983). Evidence for a possible role of prostaglandins in implantation in rats. *Arch. Int. Pharmacodyn.*, **262**, 299–307
16. Lau, I.F., Saksena, S.K. and Chang, M.C. (1973). Pregnancy blockade by indomethacin, an inhibitor of prostaglandin synthesis: its reversal by prostaglandins and progesterone in mice. *Prostaglandins*, **4**, 795–803
17. Saksena, S.K., Lau, I.F. and Chang, M.C. (1976). Relationship between oestrogen, prostaglandin $F_{2\alpha}$ and histamine in delayed implantation in the mouse. *Acta Endocrinol.*, **81**, 801–807
18. Holmes, P.V. and Gordashko, B.J. (1980). Evidence for prostaglandin involvement in blastocyst implantation. *J. Embryol. Exp. Morphol.*, **55**, 109–122
19. El-Banna, A.A. (1980). The degenerative effect on rabbit implantation sites by indomethacin. I. Timing of indomethacin action, possible effect on uterine proteins and the effect of replacement doses of $PGF_{2\alpha}$. *Prostaglandins*, **20**, 587–599
20. Cao, Z.-D., Jones, M.A. and Harper, M.J.K. (1985). Progesterone and oestradiol receptor concentration and translocation in uterine tissue of rabbits treated with indomethacin. *J. Endocrinol.*, **107**, 197–203
21. Kraeling, R.R., Rampacek, G.B. and Fiorello, N.A. (1985). Inhibition of pregnancy with indomethacin in mature gilts and prepuberal gilts induced to ovulate. *Biol. Reprod.*, **32**, 105–110
22. Lacroix, M.C. and Kann, G. (1982). Comparative studies of prostaglandins $F_{2\alpha}$ and E_2 in late cyclic and early pregnant sheep: in vitro synthesis by endometrium and conceptus-effects of in vivo indomethacin treatment on establishment of pregnancy. *Prostaglandins*, **23**, 507–526
23. Biggers, J.D., Baskar, J.F. and Torchiana, D.F. (1981). Reduction of fertility of mice by the intrauterine injection of prostaglandin antagonists. *J. Reprod. Fertil.*, **63**, 365–372
24. Kennedy, T.G. and Zamecnik, J. (1978). The concentration of 6-keto-prostaglandin $F_{1\alpha}$ is markedly elevated at the site of blastocyst implantation in the rat. *Prostaglandins*, **16**, 599–605
25. Sharma, S.C. (1979). Temporal changes in PGE, PGF_α oestradiol 17β and progesterone in uterine venous plasma and endometrium of rabbits during early pregnancy. *INSERM Symp.*, **91**, 243–264
26. Oettel, M., Koch, M., Kurischko, A. and Schubert, K. (1979). A direct evidence for the involvement of prostaglandin $F_{2\alpha}$ in the first step of estrone-induced blastocyst implantation in the spayed rat. *Steroids*, **33**, 1–8
27. Castracane, V.D., Saksena, S.K. and Shaikh, A.A. (1974). Effect of IUD's prostaglandins and indomethacin on decidual cell reaction in the rat. *Prostaglandins*, **6**, 387–404
28. Tobert, J.A. (1976). A study of the possible role of prostaglandins in decidualization using a nonsurgical method for the instillation of fluids into the rat uterine lumen. *J. Reprod. Fertil.*, **47**, 391–393
29. Sananès, N., Baulieu, E.-E. and Le Goascogne, C. (1976). Prostaglandin(s) as inductive factor of decidualization in the rat uterus. *Mol. Cell. Endocrinol.*, **6**, 153–158
30. Sananès, N., Baulieu, E.-E. and Le Goascogne, C. (1981). A role for prostaglandins in decidualization of the rat uterus. *J. Endocrinol.*, **89**, 25–33
31. Kennedy, T.G. and Lukash, L.A. (1982). Induction of decidualization in rats by the intrauterine infusion of prostaglandins. *Biol. Reprod.*, **27**, 253–260
32. Kennedy, T.G. (1985). Evidence for the involvement of prostaglandins throughout the decidual cell reaction in the rat. *Biol. Reprod.*, **33**, 140–146
33. Rankin, J.C., Ledford, B.E., Jonsson, H.T. and Baggett, B. (1979). Prostaglandins, indomethacin and the decidual cell reaction in the mouse uterus. *Biol. Reprod.*, **20**, 399–404
34. Buxton, L.E. and Murdoch, R.N. (1982). Lectins, calcium ionophore A23187 and peanut oil as deciduogenic agents in the uterus of pseudopregnant mice : effects of tranylcypromine, indomethacin, iproniazid and propanolol. *Aust. J. Biol. Sci.*, **35**, 63–72
35. Kennedy, T.G. (1979). Prostaglandins and increased endometrial vascular permeability resulting from the application of an artificial stimulus to the uterus of the rat sensitized for the decidual cell reaction. *Biol. Reprod.*, **20**, 560–566
36. Kennedy, T.G. (1980). Timing of uterine sensitivity for the decidual cell reaction: role of prostaglandins. *Biol. Reprod.*, **22**, 519–525
37. Kennedy, T.G. (1980). Estrogen and uterine sensitization for the decidual cell reaction: role of prostaglandins. *Biol. Reprod.*, **23**, 955–962

38. Kennedy, T.G., Barbe, G.J. and Evans, C.A. (1980). Prostaglandin I_2 and increased endometrial vascular permeability preceding the decidual cell reaction. In Kimball, F.A. (ed.) *The Endometrium*, pp. 331–341. (New York: Spectrum Publications, Inc.)

39. Milligan, S.R. and Lytton, F.D.C. (1983). Changes in prostaglandin levels in the sensitized and non-sensitized uterus of the mouse after the intrauterine instillation of oil or saline. *J. Reprod. Fertil.*, **67**, 373–377

40. Miller, M.M. and O'Morchoe, C.C.C. (1982). Inhibition of artificially induced decidual cell reaction by indomethacin in the mature oophorectomized rat. *Anat. Rec.*, **204**, 223–230

41. Shemesh, M., Milaguir, F., Ayalon, N. and Hansel, W. (1979). Steroidogenesis and prostaglandin synthesis by cultured bovine blastocysts. *J. Reprod. Fertil.*, **56**, 181–185

42. Watson, J. and Patek, C.E. (1979). Steroid and prostaglandin secretion by the corpus luteum, endometrium and embryos of cyclic and pregnant pigs. *J. Endocrinol.*, **82**, 425–428

43. Dey, S.K., Chien, S.M., Cox, C.L. and Crist, R.D. (1980). Prostaglandin synthesis in the rabbit blastocyst. *Prostaglandins*, **19**, 449–453

44. Marcus, G.J. (1981). Prostaglandin formation by the sheep embryo and endometrium as an indication of maternal recognition of pregnancy. *Biol. Reprod.*, **25**, 56–64

45. Lewis, G.S., Thatcher, W.W., Bazer, F.W. and Curl, J.S. (1982). Metabolism of arachidonic acid in vitro by bovine blastocysts and endometrium. *Biol. Reprod.*, **27**, 431–439

46. Hyland, J.H., Manns, J.G. and Humphrey, W.D. (1982). Prostaglandin production by ovine embryos and endometrium *in vitro*. *J. Reprod. Fertil.*, **65**, 299–304

47. Harper, M.J.K., Norris, C.J. and Rajkumar, K. (1983). Prostaglandin release by zygotes and endometria of pregnant rabbits. *Biol. Reprod.*, **28**, 350–362

48. Kennedy, T.G. and Armstrong, D.T. (1981). The role of prostaglandins in endometrial vascular changes at implantation. In Glasser, S.R. and Bullock, D.W. (eds.) *Cellular and Molecular Aspects of Implantation*, pp. 349–363. (New York: Plenum Press)

49. Racowsky, C. and Biggers, J.D. (1983). Are blastocyst prostaglandins produced endogenously? *Biol. Reprod.*, **29**, 379–388

50. Biggers, J.D., Leonov, B.V., Baskar, J.F. and Fried, J. (1978). Inhibition of hatching of mouse blastocysts in vitro by prostaglandin antagonists. *Biol. Reprod.*, **19**, 519–533

51. Baskar, J.F., Torchiana, D.F., Biggers, J.D., Corey, E.J., Andersen, N.H. and Subramanian, N. (1981). Inhibition of hatching of mouse blastocysts *in vitro* by various prostaglandin antagonists. *J. Reprod. Fertil.*, **63**, 359–363

52. Hurst, P.R. and MacFarlane, D.W. (1981). Further effects of nonsteroidal anti-inflammatory compounds on blastocyst hatching in vitro and implantation rates in the mouse. *Biol. Reprod.*, **25**, 777–784

53. Snabes, M.C. and Harper, M.J.K. (1984). Site of action of indomethacin on implantation in the rabbit. *J. Reprod. Fertil.*, **71**, 559–565

54. Parkening, T.A. (1976). An ultrastructural study of implantation in the golden hamster. I. Loss of the zona pellucida and initial attachment to the uterine epithelium. *J. Anat.*, **121**, 161–184

55. Enders, A.C. and Schlafke, S. (1979). Comparative aspects of blastocyst-endometrial interactions at implantation. *Ciba Found. Symp.*, **64**, 3–32

56. Segalen, J. and Chambon, Y. (1983). Ultrastructural aspects of the antimesometrial implantation in the rabbit. *Acta Anat.*, **115**, 1–7

57. Cole, R.J. (1967). Cinemicrographic observations on the trophoblast and zona pellucida of the mouse blastocyst. *J. Embryol. Exp. Morphol.*, **17**, 481–490

58. Bitton-Casimiri, V., Brun, J.L., and Psychoyos, A. (1970). Comportement *in vitro* des blastocysts du 5e jour de la gestation chez la ratte. Étude micro-cinematographique. *C.R. Seances Acad. Sci. {III}*, **270**, 2979-2982

59. Finn, C.A. (1977). The implantation reaction. In Wynn, R.M. (ed.) *Biology of the Uterus*, pp. 245-308. (New York: Plenum Press)

60. Lundkvist, Ö., Ljungkvist, I. and Nilsson, Ö. (1977). Early effects of oil on rat uterine epithelium sensitized for decidual induction. *J. Reprod. Fertil.*, **51**, 507–509

61. Ramwell, P.W. and Shaw, J.E. (1970). Biological significance of the prostaglandins. *Rec. Progr. Horm. Res.*, **26**, 139–173

62. Piper, P. and Vane, J. (1971). The release of prostaglandins from lung and other tissues. *Ann. N.Y. Acad. Sci.*, **180**, 363–385

63. Boshier, D.P. (1976). Effects of the rat blastocyst on neutral lipids and non-specific esterases in the uterine luminal epithelium at the implantation area. *J. Reprod. Fertil.*, **46**, 245–247

64. Boshier, D.P., Holloway, H. and Millener, N.M. (1981). Triacylglycerols in the rat uterine epithelium during the oestrous cycle and early pregnancy. *J. Reprod. Fertil.*, **62**, 441–446

65. Moulton, B.C. (1984). Epithelial cell function during blastocyst implantation. *J. Biosci.*, **6**, Suppl. 2, 11–21

66. Ohta, Y. (1985). Histochemical localization of prostaglandin synthetase in the rat endometrium with reference to decidual cell reaction. *Proc. Jpn. Acad.*, **61**, Ser. B, 467–470

67. Pakrasi, P.L. and Dey, S.K. (1982). Blastocyst is the source of prostaglandins in the implantation site in the rabbit. *Prostaglandins*, **24**, 73–77

68. Jonsson, H.T., Rankin, J.C., Ledford, B.E. and Baggett, B. (1979). Uterine prostaglandin levels following stimulation of the decidual cell reaction: effect of indomethacin and tranylcypromine. *Prostaglandins*, **18**, 847–857

69. Fenwick, L., Jones, R.L., Naylor, B., Poyser, N.L. and Wilson, N.H. (1977). Production of prostaglandins by the pseudopregnant rat uterus, *in vitro*, and the effect of tamoxifen with the identification of 6-keto-prostaglandin F_1 as a major product. *Br. J. Pharmacol.*, **59**, 191–199

70. Hoffman, L.H., Strong, G.B., Davenport, G.R. and Frolich, J.C. (1977). Deciduogenic effect of prostaglandins in the pseudopregnant rabbit. *J. Reprod. Fertil.*, **50**, 231–237

71. Gryglewski, R.J., Bunting, S., Moncada, S., Flower, R.J. and Vane, J.R. (1976). Arterial walls are protected against deposition of platelet thrombi by a substance (prostaglandin X) which they make from prostaglandin endoperoxides. *Prostaglandins*, **12**, 685–713

72. Rajtar, G. and de Gaetano, G. (1979). Tranylcypromine is not a selective inhibitor of prostacyclin in rats. *Thromb. Res.*, **14**, 245–248

73. Wong, P.Y.-K., Malik, K.U., Desiderio, D.M., McGiff, J.C. and Sun, F.F. (1980). Hepatic metabolism of prostacyclin (PGI$_2$) in the rabbit: formation of a potent novel inhibitor of platelet aggregation. *Biochem. Biophys. Res. Commun.*, **93**, 486–494

74. Quilley, C.P., McGiff, J.C., Lee, W.H., Sun, F.F. and Wong, P.Y.-K. (1980). 6-keto PGE$_1$: a possible metabolite of prostacyclin having platelet antiaggregatory effects. *Hypertension*, **2**, 524–528

75. Lewis, R., Scholkens, B.A. and Beck, G. (1984). Biological activities of 6-keto-prostaglandin E$_1$. *Prostagl. Leukotr. Med.*, **16**, 303–324

76. Doktorcik, P.E. and Kennedy, T.G. (1986). 6-Keto-prostaglandin E$_1$ and the decidual cell reaction in rats – *Prostaglandins*, **32**, 679–689

77. Kennedy, T.G., Martel, D. and Psychoyos, A. (1983). Endometrial prostaglandin E$_2$ binding: characterization in rats sensitized for the decidual cell reaction and changes during pseudopregnancy. *Biol. Reprod.*, **29**, 556–564

78. Kennedy, T.G., Martel, D. and Psychoyos, A. (1983). Endometrial prostaglandin E$_2$ binding during the estrous cycle and its hormonal control in ovariectomized rats. *Biol. Reprod.*, **29**, 565–571

79. Hofmann, G.E., Rao, Ch.V., De Leon, F.D., Toledo, A.A. and Sanfilippo, J.S. (1985). Human endometrial prostaglandin E$_2$ binding sites and their profiles during the menstrual cycle and in pathologic states. *Am. J. Obstet. Gynecol.*, **151**, 369–375

80. Kennedy, T.G., Keys, J.L. and King, G.J. (1986). Endometrial prostaglandin E$_2$-binding sites in the pig: characterization and changes during the estrous cycle and early pregnancy. *Biol. Reprod.*, **35**, 624–632.

81. Martel, D., Kennedy, T.G., Monier, M.N. and Psychoyos, A. (1985). Failure to detect specific binding sites for prostaglandin F-2α in membrane preparations from rat endometrium. *J. Reprod. Fertil.*, **75**, 265–274

82. Yochim, J.M. and De Feo, V.J. (1963). Hormonal control of the onset, magnitude and duration of uterine sensitivity in the rat by steroid hormones of the ovary. *Endocrinology*, **72**, 317–326

83. Armstrong, D.T. and King, E.R. (1971). Uterine progesterone metabolism and progestational response: effects of estrogens and prolactin. *Endocrinology*, **89**, 191–197

84. De Feo, V.J. (1967). Decidualization. In Wynn, R.M. (ed.) *Cellular Biology of the Uterus*, pp. 191–290. (New York: Meredith Publishing Co.)

85. Castracane, V.D. and Jordan, V.C. (1975). The effect of estrogen and progesterone on uterine prostaglandin biosynthesis in the ovariectomized rat. *Biol. Reprod.*, **13**, 587–596
86. Kuehl, F.S., Cirillo, V.J., Zanetti, M.E., Beveridge, G.C. and Ham, E.A. (1976). The effect of estrogen upon cyclic nucleotide and prostaglandin levels in the rat uterus. *Adv. Prostagl. Thromb. Res.*, **1**, 313–323
87. Cao, Z.-D., Jones, M.A. and Harper, M.J.K. (1984). Prostaglandin translocation from the lumen of the rabbit uterus in vitro in relation to day of pregnancy or pseudopregnancy. *Biol. Reprod.*, **31**, 505–519
88. Kennedy, T.G. (1986). Intrauterine infusion of prostaglandins and decidualization in rats with uteri differentially sensitized for the decidual cell reaction. *Biol. Reprod.*, **34**, 327–335
89. Williams, T.J. (1977). Chemical mediators of vascular responses in inflammation: a two mediator hypothesis. *Br. J. Pharmacol.*, **61**, 447–448
90. Williams, T.J. and Peck, M.J. (1977). Role of prostaglandin-mediated vasodilation in inflammation. *Nature*, **270**, 530–532
91. Power, S.G.A. and Kennedy, T.G. (1982). Estrogen-induced changes in uterine sensitivity for the decidual cell reaction: interactions between prostaglandin E_2 and histamine or bradykinin. *Prostaglandins*, **23**, 219–226
92. McRae, A.C. and Kennedy, T.G. (1983). Selective permeability of the blood-uterine lumen barrier in rats: importance of molecular size. *Biol. Reprod.*, **29**, 879–885
93. McRae, A.C. and Kennedy, T.G. (1983). Selective permeability of the blood-uterine lumen barrier in rats: importance of lipid solubility. *Biol. Reprod.*, **29**, 886–894
94. McRae, A.C. (1984). The blood-uterine lumen barrier and its possible significance in early embryo development. *Oxf. Rev. Reprod. Biol.*, **6**, 129–173
95. Lunam, C. and Rogers, A.W. (1981). Pericytes in the stroma of the rat uterus. *J. Reprod. Fertil.*, **63**, 267–270
96. Bitton, V., Vassent, G. and Psychoyos, A. (1965). Réponse vasculaire de l'utérus au traumatisme, au cours de la pseudogestation chez la ratte. *C.R. Seances Acad. Sci. {III}*, **261**, 3474–3477
97. Dey, S.K., Johnson, D.C. and Santos, J.G. (1979). Is histamine production by the blastocyst required for implantation in the rabbit? *Biol. Reprod.*, **21**, 1169–1173
98. Dey, S.K. and Johnson, D.C. (1980). Histamine formation by mouse preimplantation embryos. *J. Reprod. Fertil.*, **60**, 457–460
99. Dey, S.K. (1981). Role of histamine in implantation: inhibition of histidine decarboxylase induces delayed implantation in the rabbit. *Biol. Reprod.*, **24**, 867–869
100. Dey, S.K., Villanueva, C., Chien, S.M. and Crist, R.D. (1978). The role of histamine in implantation in the rabbit. *J. Reprod. Fertil.*, **53**, 23–26
101. Dey, S.K., Villanueva, C. and Abdou, N.I. (1979). Histamine receptors on rabbit blastocyst and endometrial cell membranes. *Nature*, **278**, 648–649
102. Brandon, J.M. and Raval, P.J. (1979). Interaction of estrogen and histamine during ovum implantation in the rat. *Eur. J. Pharmacol.*, **57**, 171–177
103. Biddulph, D.M., Sawyer, L.M. and Smales, W.P. (1984). Chondrogenesis of chick limb mesenchyme in vitro. Effects of prostaglandins on cyclic AMP. *Exp. Cell Res.*, **153**, 270–274
104. Lazarus, S.C., Basbaum, C.B. and Gold, W.M. (1984). Prostaglandins and intracellular cyclic AMP in respiratory secretory cells. *Am. Rev. Respir. Dis.*, **130**, 262–266
105. Vilar-Rojas, C., Castro-Osuna, G. and Hicks, J.J. (1982). Cyclic AMP and cyclic GMP in the implantation site of the rat. *Int. J. Fertil.*, **27**, 56–59
106. Holmes, P.V. and Bergstrom, S. (1975). Induction of blastocyst implantation in mice by cyclic AMP. *J. Reprod. Fertil.*, **43**, 329–332
107. Webb, F.T.B. (1975). Implantation in ovariectomized mice treated with dibutyryl adenosine 3′,5′-monophosphate (dibutyryl cyclic AMP). *J. Reprod. Fertil.*, **42**, 511–517
108. Fernandez-Noval, A. and Leroy, F. (1978). Induction of implantation in the mouse by intrauterine injection of adenosine monophosphate. *J. Reprod. Fertil.*, **53**, 7–8
109. Dey, S.K. and Hubbard, C.J. (1981). Role of histamine and cyclic nucleotides in implantation in the rabbit. *Cell Tissue Res.*, **220**, 549–554
110. Leroy, F., Vansande, J., Shetgen, G. and Brasseur, D. (1974). Cyclic AMP and the triggering of the decidual reaction. *J. Reprod. Fertil.*, **39**, 207–211
111. Rankin, J.C., Ledford, B.E. and Baggett, B. (1977). Early involvement of cyclic nucleotides

in the artificially stimulated decidual cell reaction of the mouse uterus. *Biol. Reprod.*, **17**, 549–554

112. Kennedy, T.G. (1983). Prostaglandin E$_2$, adenosine 3':5'-cyclic monophosphate and changes in endometrial vascular permeability in rat uteri sensitized for the decidual cell reaction. *Biol. Reprod.*, **29**, 1069–1076

113. Johnston, M.E.A. and Kennedy, T.G. (1984). Estrogen and uterine sensitization for the decidual cell reaction in the rat: role of prostaglandin E$_2$ and adenosine 3':5'-cyclic monophosphate. *Biol. Reprod.*, **31**, 959–966

114. Johnston, M.E.A. and Kennedy, T.G. (1985). Temporal desensitization of rat uteri for the decidual cell reaction is abolished by cholera toxin acting by a mechanism apparently not involving adenosine 3':5'-cyclic monophosphate. *Can. J. Physiol. Pharmacol.*, **63**, 1052–1056

115. Webb, F.T.G. (1975). The inability of dibutyryl adenosine 3':5'-monophosphate to induce the decidual reaction in intact pseudopregnant mice. *J. Reprod. Fertil.*, **42**, 187–188

116. Daniel, S.A.J. and Kennedy, T.G. (1985). Prostaglandin E$_2$ stimulates uterine stromal cell alkaline phosphatase activity *in vitro*. *Can. J. Physiol. Pharmacol.*, **63**, Ax.

117. Demers, L.M., Rees, M.C.P. and Turnbull, A.C. (1984). Arachidonic acid metabolism by the non-pregnant human uterus. *Prostagl. Leukotr. Med.*, **14**, 175–180

118. Vesin, M.F., Bourgoin, S., Leiber, D. and Harbon, S. (1984). Lipoxygenase and cyclooxygenase products of arachidonic acid in uterus. Selective interaction with the cGMP and cAMP systems. *Prostagl. Leukotr. Med.*, **13**, 75–78

119. Pakrasi, P.L. and Dey, S.K. (1985). Evidence for an inverse relationship between cyclooxygenase and lipoxygenase pathways in the pregnant rabbit endometrium. *Prostagl. Leukotr. Med.*, **18**, 347–352

120. Pakrasi, P.L., Becka, R. and Dey, S.K. (1985). Cyclooxygenase and lipoxygenase pathways in the preimplantation rabbit uterus and blastocyst. *Prostaglandins*, **29**, 481–495

121. Samuelsson, B. (1983). Leukotrienes: mediators of immediate hypersensitivity reactions and inflammation. *Science*, **220**, 568–575

122. Parisi, V.M., Rankin, J.H.G., Phernetton, T.M. and Makowski, E.L. (1984). The effect of a leukotriene receptor antagonist, FPL 55712, on estrogen-induced uterine hyperemia in the nonpregnant rabbit. *Am. J. Obstet. Gynecol.*, **148**, 365–369

123. Kennedy, T.G. (1985). Prostaglandins and blastocyst implantation. *Prostagl. Persp.*, **1**, 1–3

5
Occurrence and measurement of eicosanoids during pregnancy and parturition

M.D. Mitchell

INTRODUCTION

Prostaglandins play important roles in pregnancy and the mechanisms of parturition in all mammalian species that have been studied. There is evidence that these products of arachidonic acid metabolism not only play a part in cervical ripening and uterine contractions but also may be of significance in the regulation of uterine and feto-placental haemodynamics. In this review, I shall attempt to provide an outline of current knowledge on the concentrations of prostaglandins in a variety of biological fluids throughout gestation and the changes that occur during labour. Moreover, potential uterine sources of prostaglandins will be indicated together with information on alterations in rates of production by tissues in association with the onset and progression of labour.

It is now well established that products of arachidonic acid metabolism by way of lipoxygenase pathways have potent biological activities, and are more important than products of the cyclo-oxygenase pathway in many biological mechanisms. Hence, whenever possible, information will be presented on the production of arachidonate lipoxygenase metabolites by uterine tissues and concentrations of such metabolites in biological fluids as they pertain to pregnancy and parturition. Finally, it is necessary to limit the scope of this review since the literature relating products of arachidonic acid (eicosanoids) to pregnancy and parturition is overwhelming. I will therefore concentrate attention mainly, but not exclusively, on information related to human pregnancy and parturition. The reader is directed to other reviews that are available on this topic[1-5].

EICOSANOIDS IN AMNIOTIC FLUID

The presence of prostaglandins in amniotic fluid was reported first by Sultan Karim[6] and shortly thereafter he also observed that labour was associated with greatly increased concentrations of prostaglandins in amniotic fluid of women at term of pregnancy[7]. Although the identity of the specific prostaglandins in amniotic fluid has been questioned (e.g. by Keirse[2]) the general precept that concentrations of prostaglandins in amniotic fluid are elevated greatly during labour has been amply confirmed. Amniotic fluid has proven to be a popular fluid in which to measure prostaglandins since there is essentially no biosynthesis or metabolism of prostaglandins in this fluid[8]. Indeed, in numerous studies[2] it has been shown that concentrations of prostaglandin E_2 (PGE$_2$), and of prostaglandin $F_{2\alpha}$ (PGF$_{2\alpha}$) increase slowly from mid-pregnancy until term and then increase sharply with the onset of labour and continue to increase in parallel with cervical dilatation (Figure 5.1). Since, during labour, amniotic fluid levels of 13,14-dihydro-15-keto-prostaglandin $F_{2\alpha}$ (PGFM; a major metabolite of PGF$_{2\alpha}$) exhibit changes similar to those of PGF$_{2\alpha}$[9], it is assumed that the increased PGF$_{2\alpha}$ (and PGE$_2$) concentrations reflect enhanced rates of prostaglandin biosynthesis rather than reduced rates of catabolism. This assumption has been proved correct since it has been demonstrated that the activities of prostaglandin catabolizing enzymes within intrauterine tissues do not change with labour[2].

Both 6-keto-prostaglandin $F_{1\alpha}$ (6-keto-PGF$_{1\alpha}$) and thromboxane B_2 (TxB$_2$), the major hydrolysis products of prostacyclin (PGI$_2$) and thromboxane A_2 (TxA$_2$) respectively, have been detected in amniotic fluid[10,11]. Although the concentrations of these products are elevated in labour, there is no trend for levels to rise further as labour progresses. Hence, it has been suggested that in labour there is a redistribution in the flow through different prostanoid

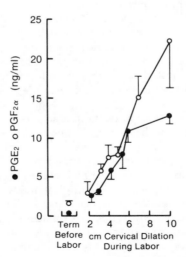

Figure 5.1 Concentrations (mean ± SEM) of prostaglandin E_2 and prostaglandin $F_{2\alpha}$ in amniotic fluid during late pregnancy and labour at term (from 2, with permission)

pathways that favour PGE_2 and $PGF_{2\alpha}$[4]. A similar suggestion has been made on the basis of detailed investigations in pregnant sheep[12]. Hence, labour is characterized by an increasing ratio in the rates of formation of prostaglandins that contract the uterus versus those that are inhibitory or have no action on uterine contractility.

The mechanism(s) responsible for increased prostaglandin concentrations in amniotic fluid during labour are functional prior to term since preterm labour and therapeutic abortions are associated with elevated levels of amniotic fluid prostaglandins[13,14]. Such mechanisms are highly responsive since prostaglandin concentrations in amniotic fluid can increase within minutes. For instance, vaginal and cervical manipulation can raise amniotic fluid prostaglandin levels within five minutes[8]. It is interesting to note also that a significant fraction of PGE_2 applied to the vagina can reach the amniotic sac after a lag period of a few hours without being degraded[15]. This finding was quite unexpected since it was considered highly unlikely that PGE_2 could diffuse so far without being metabolized or cleared. Thus, some degree of caution is warranted whenever prostaglandins are applied to the vagina or cervix. Whether the prostaglandins in amniotic fluid play any part in the mechanisms of the onset and progression of labour is unknown. Nevertheless, the concentrations of prostaglandins in amniotic fluid are quite an accurate index of important changes during labour, since abnormally low levels of prostaglandins are found in the liquor of women with clinically delayed labour that are destined to require oxytocin augmentation[9,16].

The possibility exists that in labour there is a shift in arachidonic acid metabolism away from the lipoxygenase pathways to the cyclo-oxygenase pathway. Although there may indeed be a relative shift in these pathways as suggested recently[17] (see later section on 'Sources of eicosanoids') it is not absolute. This obtains since it has been demonstrated that amniotic fluid concentrations of leukotriene B_4 (LTB_4), 15-hydroxyeicosatetraenoic acid (15-HETE) and 12-hydroxyeicosatetraenoic acid (12-HETE) are raised to varying extents during labour in women (R. Romero and M.D. Mitchell, unpublished observations). Hence, in labour, there is an increase in the rate of formation of lipoxygenase pathway products as well as cyclo-oxygenase pathway products of arachidonic acid metabolism. This is true even allowing for the possibility that 15-HETE in amniotic fluid may originate in a tissue where it is a product of the cyclo-oxygenase pathway[18].

EICOSANOIDS IN THE MATERNAL CIRCULATION

It is difficult to obtain reliable measurements of primary prostaglandins in peripheral plasma since not only do platelets have the ability to synthesize prostaglandins but also because concentrations of prostaglandins in the peripheral circulation are extremely low due to highly active metabolism by the lungs. These problems can be overcome, to some extent, in experimental animals by the use of chronically implanted vascular catheters in the venous drainage of an organ of interest e.g. the uterus. In sheep, for instance, there is considerable evidence that prostaglandin concentrations in utero-ovarian venous effluent are raised significantly during the 24 hours before delivery[19,20]. Similar data are now available for many other experimental animals. There is considerable evidence that these prostaglandins are the cause of the onset of labour.

The use of chronic catheterization techniques is obviously excluded in studies of human pregnancy and therefore two approaches have been adopted for the evaluation of eicosanoid production when only the peripheral circulation is available for sampling. The first approach adopted was the improvement of assay techniques such that peripheral plasma concentrations of PGE and PGF could be measured accurately and be consistent with levels that have been reported by the use of gas chromatography–mass spectrometry techniques[21,22]. Data obtained using such methods indicate that peripheral plasma concentrations of PGE_2 and $PGF_{2\alpha}$ do not change significantly during labour in women[22]. This finding is consistent with the known high capacity of the lungs to metabolize prostaglandins. Indeed, there is no conclusive proof for any human disease in which circulating levels of primary prostaglandins are elevated.

The second method adopted was the measurement of circulating metabolites of prostaglandins. This approach was suggested[21] because platelets cannot metabolize prostaglandins and circulating levels of metabolites are 10- to 30-fold greater than those of the primary prostaglandins. Hence, generation of prostaglandins during sampling and assay sensitivity were no longer major problems. The major circulating metabolite of $PGF_{2\alpha}$ is 13,14-dihydro-15-keto prostaglandin $F_{2\alpha}$ (PGFM). The plasma concentrations of PGFM change little during gestation with the possibility of a small rise during the final month of pregnancy; a significant increase in PGFM concentrations does however occur during labour[22,23] (Figure 5.2). It appears, therefore, that during labour there is an increasing rate of production of $PGF_{2\alpha}$, presumably by tissues within the uterus. This PGF is subsequently metabolized efficiently by the lungs such that only the levels of a metabolite can be detected in increased amounts in the peripheral circulation.

Since concentrations of both PGE_2 and $PGF_{2\alpha}$ are raised in amniotic fluid during labour and circulating levels of PGFM increase concomitantly it might

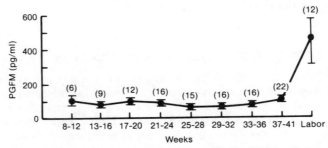

Figure 5.2 Peripheral plasma concentrations (mean $\pm$ SEM, no. of samples in parentheses) of 13,14-dihydro-15-keto-$PGF_{2\alpha}$ (PGFM) in 16 women throughout pregnancy and in labour (from 4, with permission)

be expected that levels of the comparable major circulating metabolite of PGE$_2$ would be raised also in the peripheral circulation. Unfortunately, 13,14-dihydro-15-keto-PGE$_2$ is unstable in aqueous media[24], and this caused many problems in developing radioimmunoassays for its measurement. The problem was overcome when two groups independently established that metabolites of PGE in the peripheral circulation could be converted to the same final product which is 11-deoxy-13,14-dihydro-15-keto-11,16-cyclo-prostaglandin E$_2$ (PGEM-II)[25,26]. Surprisingly, however, the circulating concentrations of this metabolite are not elevated to any great extent during labour[27]. These findings raised the possibility that the PGE being secreted towards the maternal circulation is metabolized to some other compound. Indeed, recently it has been found that PGE$_2$ can be converted to PGF$_{2\alpha}$ by enzymes in the decidua vera[28]. This finding is of importance because PGE$_2$ is approximately ten-fold more potent than PGF$_{2\alpha}$ in its actions on uterine contractility and cervical softening and effacement. Thus, this conversion is a protective mechanism. We have recently found that prostaglandin D$_2$ (PGD$_2$) can also be converted to prostaglandin F$_{2\alpha}$ by intrauterine human tissues of women at term of pregnancy (unpublished observations).

Measurements of PGD$_2$ in plasma are difficult due to its ability to bind to plasma proteins in a covalent manner. Such measurements would be of some considerable interest, however, since PGD$_2$ is not a good substrate for 15-hydroxyprostaglandin dehydrogenase[29,30] and thus, may be a circulating hormone. Recently, however, it has been demonstrated that circulating levels of PGD$_2$ are similar to those of PGE$_2$ and PGF$_{2\alpha}$[31]. In sheep, PGD$_2$ is a dilator of the uterine vasculature whilst being a mild constrictor of the peripheral vasculature[32]. Hence, this prostaglandin may have therapeutic potential in pathological conditions such as pregnancy-induced hypertension.

Obtaining an index of TxA$_2$ production by measurements of the degradation product TxB$_2$ in the peripheral circulation is also difficult. TxA$_2$ is produced in large amounts by platelets in response to many stimuli. TxA$_2$ also combines with plasma proteins in a covalent manner and, thus, it is difficult to draw meaningful conclusions from measurements of TxB$_2$ in the peripheral circulation. Measurements have been made, however, and to date they are suggestive of little change in TxB$_2$ concentrations in peripheral plasma throughout gestation or even in labour[33,34]. The question of TxA$_2$ production in pregnancy is not trivial since TxA$_2$ can contract the uterus and by way of its vasoconstrictive and proaggregatory activities can play a major role in uteroplacental pathology.

There is also considerable controversy concerning the measurement of 6-keto-PGF$_{1\alpha}$ (the degradation product of prostacyclin). Initially measurements using radioimmunoassay techniques and gas chromatography–mass spectrometry provided similar results with peripheral plasma concentrations of approximately 120 to 150 pg/ml. Subsequently, it has been reported that the circulating concentrations of 6-keto-PGF$_{1\alpha}$ are much closer to those of PGE$_2$ and PGF$_{2\alpha}$, i.e. 2–5 pg/ml. Once again, early studies provided evidence which suggested that little change occurred in the peripheral plasma concentrations of 6-keto-PGF$_{1\alpha}$ throughout pregnancy and indeed during labour[35]. Recent evidence from studies using a highly sensitive technique of mass spectrometry with negative ion chemical ionization detection suggests, however, that there is indeed a significant increase in the plasma concentrations of 6-keto-PGF$_{1\alpha}$ in late pregnancy with the possibility of a further elevation in labour[36].

In sheep, there is evidence that both utero-ovarian venous and cervical venous plasma concentrations of 6-keto-PGF$_{1\alpha}$ increase during the 24 to 48 hours before delivery[37,38]. Intrauterine production of prostacyclin is of some importance since in sheep it has been shown that prostacyclin is highly potent in its ability to inhibit uterine contractions[39]. In women, however, only mild inhibitory effects on uterine contractions have been found and most frequently no effect can be demonstrated[40-42]. There is however evidence from studies of other experimental animals showing that prostacyclin can potentiate the effects of contractile agents such as oxytocin[43]. Presently no data are available concerning the plasma concentrations of lipoxygenase products of arachidonic acid metabolism.

EICOSANOIDS IN THE FETAL CIRCULATION

There is considerable evidence that prostaglandins play many roles within the fetus. In particular it is well established that PGE$_2$ is the major factor in maintaining the patency of the ductus arteriosus during intrauterine life[44]. The ductus arteriosus is patent throughout intrauterine life, and the lungs receive a relatively small proportion of cardiac output. Thus, this is a situation when circulating prostaglandin concentrations are likely to be extremely high and there is the possibility that prostaglandins may act as circulating hormones in the fetus. Concentrations of PGE$_2$ and PGF$_{2\alpha}$ have been measured in the circulation of fetal sheep during late pregnancy and labour[45]. Although a slight increase in PGF$_{2\alpha}$ concentrations was shown, there was also a highly significant increase in PGE$_2$ concentrations during labour that was most interesting. Increased PGE$_2$ production with labour is of significance because PGE$_2$ is known to inhibit fetal breathing movements[46] and such movements occur with a decreased frequency during labour[47,48]. In fact, it has been suggested that the absence of fetal breathing movements in women in preterm labour is a predictor of 'true' preterm labour and that delivery will then eventuate[48,49]. The concentrations of 6-keto-PGF$_{1\alpha}$ in ovine fetal plasma are also increased significantly during labour[37]. The physiological significance of this increase in prostacyclin biosynthesis is unknown.

It has been shown that circulating concentrations of prostaglandins in the human fetus are extremely high during the first half of pregnancy[50]. The blood samples for this study were obtained by the technique of fetoscopy. At term of pregnancy umbilical plasma concentrations of prostaglandins have been measured[51,52] (Figure 5.3). PGE$_2$, PGF$_{2\alpha}$ and PGFM concentrations in umbilical plasma were all found to be raised above those found in the maternal circulation. Moreover, a significant arterio-venous difference across the umbilical circulation was demonstrated for PGE$_2$, venous levels being raised. Thus, it was suggested that the placenta is a major source of the PGE circulating in the fetus. The arterio-venous difference across the umbilical circulation for PGE$_2$ was found whether labour had occurred or not. It should

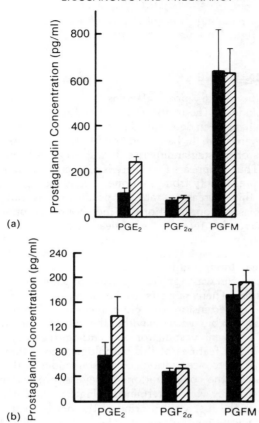

(a)

(b)

Figure 5.3 The concentrations of prostaglandins (mean $\pm$ SEM) in umbilical arterial (filled bars) and venous (hatched bars) plasma taken **a.** (upper panel) immediately after delivery of the fetus before clamping of the cord from twelve women after spontaneous labour and delivery, and **b.** (lower panel) from ten women immediately after delivery by elective Caesarean section (from 51,52, with permission)

be noted that this evidence is consistent with findings that circulating PGE_2 concentrations decrease rapidly in the neonatal period. Hence, the placenta may contribute (by way of PGE_2) to the patency *in utero* of the ductus arteriosus and physical separation of the newborn from the placenta in itself will contribute to the postnatal closure of this vessel. Obviously, the increased blood flow through the lungs and the concomitant increase in clearance of prostaglandins in the postnatal period play a major role in this mechanism.

The concentrations of 6-keto-$PGF_{1\alpha}$ and TxB_2 in umbilical plasma have also been determined[53]. Neither of these prostanoids have a significant arterio-venous difference across the umbilical circulation. Umbilical plasma concentrations of these prostanoids exceed or are similar to circulating concentrations in the mother, but the mode of delivery does not influence measured levels.

Measurements of circulating concentrations of arachidonate lipoxygenase metabolites in the fetus have yet to be reported.

EICOSANOIDS IN URINE

Measurements of the primary prostaglandins E_2 and $F_{2\alpha}$ in urine reflect only production by the kidney. The major urinary metabolites of PGE_2 and $PGF_{2\alpha}$ in men and women have been determined and methods for their measurement have also been established. It has been found that the concentrations of urinary metabolites of prostaglandins rise during pregnancy and particularly during labour[54,55]. Thus it appears that there is an increasing rate of secretion of prostaglandins, presumably from a uterine source, throughout pregnancy. The reason why this increasing rate of production is not reflected in measurements of plasma concentrations of metabolites of prostaglandins is uncertain. There have also recently been measurements of a major urinary metabolite of prostacyclin[56]. The production rate of this prostacyclin metabolite was again found to be increased with gestation although the effect of labour was not determined. Interestingly, the rate of production of this urinary metabolite of prostacyclin was significantly lower in patients with pregnancy-induced hypertension. There appears to be a consensus of opinion that pregnancy-induced hypertension (or pre-eclampsia) is associated with a deficiency in prostacyclin biosynthesis within the feto-placental unit[57]. A local deficiency in such a potent vasodilator and anti-aggregatory agent would account for many of the features of this pathological condition.

Little is known of the concentrations of prostaglandin in the urine of the fetus. In a recent study the concentrations of several prostaglandins in fetal urine at term of pregnancy were determined[58] (Figure 5.4). Fetal urine in this case was obtained as the first voided urine of the newborn which was thus formed *in utero*. Significant concentrations of PGE_2, $PGF_{2\alpha}$, PGFM and 6-keto-$PGF_{1\alpha}$ were found. Thus, it seems that prostaglandins in fetal urine do contribute to the prostaglandins that are found in amniotic fluid. Increased

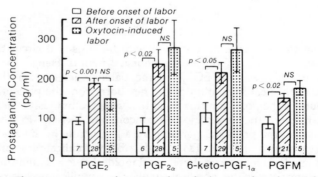

Figure 5.4 The concentrations of prostanoids in fetal urine of newborn infants delivered before or after the spontaneous onset of labour or after oxytocin-induced labour (from 58, with permission)

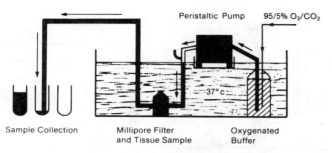

Figure 5.5 A diagrammatic representation of the method of tissue superfusion

concentrations of these prostaglandins with labour was found, although the increase observed was too small to account for a substantial fraction of the increased levels of prostaglandins in amniotic fluid during labour.

SOURCES OF EICOSANOIDS

In this section we will deal specifically with the sources of eicosanoids in the uterus. This seems a logical approach since circulating concentrations of eicosanoids are extremely low and hence, eicosanoids locally produced are the most likely to have significant effects within the uterus. The measurement of rates of production of eicosanoids by tissues has also been difficult. This is the case because trauma (e.g. in obtaining the tissue) is a major stimulus to the production of prostaglandins and, therefore, abnormally high rates of prostaglandin formation may be observed for some time after removal of tissue. Moreover it should be noted that prostaglandins are not stored in tissues, but are synthesized and secreted immediately. Hence, there is little to recommend the measurement of prostaglandins or other eicosanoids in tissues. Rather we must use methods for the measurement of prostaglandin production under dynamic conditions. Several methods have been used successfully to obtain such measurements. These methods include the use of cells separated from tissues and maintained either in monolayer culture or in suspension; alternatively whole tissue fragments have been maintained in organ culture. The most widely used technique is the incubation of an homogenate of a tissue or a subcellular fraction thereof, with precursor (radiolabeled or otherwise). Another popular method has been that of tissue superfusion. This technique permits the prostaglandins produced by the trauma of excision to be washed away and basal production rates of prostaglandins may then be established. A system for the method of tissue superfusion[59] is shown diagrammatically in Figure 5.5.

Using such a method the rates of production of a variety of prostanoids by intrauterine tissues obtained either before or after labour have been established[33,60,61] (Figure 5.6). Surprisingly, it has been found that the amnion, the inner fetal membrane, is a major site of the production of prostaglandins and specifically of PGE_2. Moreover, the rate of production of PGE_2 by amnion

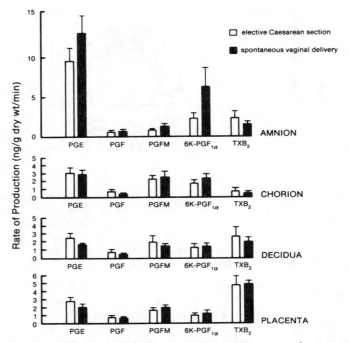

Figure 5.6 Rates of production of prostanoids by intrauterine tissues from women at term of pregnancy (after 33, 60, 61)

is increasing during labour. These findings have been confirmed and extended by several groups, e.g. refs 62–65. One of these groups found evidence additionally for increased production of prostaglandins also by chorion laeve[63] and decidua vera[65] with labour.

It has been established that in sheep there are increased rates of production of prostaglandins by not only fetal membranes but also maternal cotyledon and myometrium[1,19,59,66–69]. Evidence has been presented recently that the myometrium of women at term of pregnancy has increased activities of prostaglandin endoperoxide synthase and prostacyclin synthase[70]. Furthermore, it has been demonstrated that the production of prostacyclin in myometrium is not confined to vascular cells, but is also found in smooth muscle cells[71]. As mentioned earlier, although prostacyclin inhibits uterine activity in sheep evidence for its inhibitory activity in women is at present equivocal.

A key factor in the normal progression of labour and parturition is the softening and effacement of the uterine cervix. Cervical tissue can produce prostaglandins at high rates. In both human and ovine pregnancy there is evidence that the uterine cervix produces increased quantities of prostaglandins during the period of cervical softening, effacement and dilatation[72–77] (Figure 5.7). PGE_2 is used clinically for cervical ripening prior to the induction of

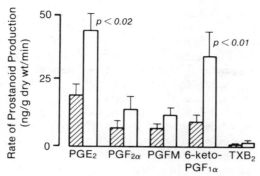

Figure 5.7 Mean prostanoid production rates by ovine cervical tissue during late pregnancy (hatched bars) and at delivery (open bars). Results are mean ± SEM, n = 7 to 10 observations (from 73 with permission)

labour and abortion[78]. This is a highly effective and successful treatment. Thus, the concept has been put forward that cervical ripening is a function of prostaglandins formed and acting locally[38]. The exact mechanisms by which prostaglandins and particularly PGE$_2$ influence cervical ripening are unknown. However, it has been shown that prostaglandins can enhance collagenolytic activity in the cervix and also have significant effects on the proteoglycan composition of the cervix, e.g. refs 38,78–81.

Another potential source of intrauterine prostaglandins is umbilical tissue. Prostaglandins may play a critical role in the regulation of the tone of the umbilical vessels since these vessels are not innervated and are required to close immediately at birth. It has been shown[82] that umbilical tissue has the capacity to produce a wide range of prostaglandins. The two major products within umbilical tissue are prostacyclin and PGE$_2$ (Figure 5.8) which have

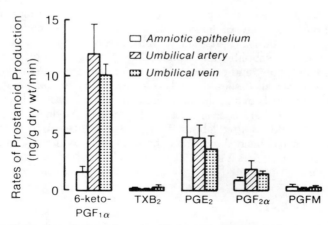

Figure 5.8 Rates of production of prostanoids (mean ± SEM, ng/g dry wt/min, n = 7) by umbilical tissues (from 82, with permission)

99

opposing actions on umbilical tone. Previously, it had been thought that TxB_2 was the major prostanoid formed by the umbilical tissue[83]. This was not the case, however, and it was later found there was a methodological discrepancy that accounted for this apparent high rate of production of TxB_2. This discrepancy resulted from the finding that addition of arachidonic acid, as substrate, to an incubation could alter the ratio of products formed; in this case favouring the formation of TxB_2 over that of 6-keto-$PGF_{1\alpha}$. It is now considered likely that the intramural production of prostacyclin and PGE_2 determines the tone of the umbilical vessels. The ratio of production of these two prostanoids would thus favour prostacyclin and maintenance of the patency of the umbilical vessels during intrauterine life. A change in that ratio at birth favouring PGE_2 (which is a constrictor of the umbilical vessels) would account for the rapid closure of the umbilical vessels.

There is evidence from studies using experimental animals that intrauterine tissues can metabolize arachidonic acid by way of lipoxygenase catalyzed pathways[84-86]. The production of these metabolites is of considerable significance since they are highly active biologically. For instance leukotriene B_4 is a calcium ionophore and its biosynthesis within the uterus could thus influence the activities of the phospholipases in uterine tissues that catalyze the hydrolysis of arachidonic acid from glycerophospholipids since these enzymes are calcium regulated. Moreover, other metabolites of arachidonic acid by way of lipoxygenase pathways, i.e. hydroperoxyeicosatetraenoic acids have many other biological activities including the inhibition of prostacyclin biosynthesis; other properties include chemotactic and chemokinetic abilities and, thus, these metabolites might recruit macrophages (which secrete PGE_2) into the intrauterine environment (for references see ref. 87).

Intrauterine tissues from women at term of pregnancy have been shown to have the enzymes necessary for the conversion of arachidonic acid into lipoxygenase pathway products[88-90]. The methodology used in these studies, however (thin layer chromatography), does not permit an effective separation of the lipoxygenase products of arachidonic acid metabolism. We have, therefore, recently undertaken a study in which we are evaluating arachidonic acid metabolism by way of lipoxygenase pathways in intrauterine tissues from women at term of pregnancy both before and after labour. The arachidonic acid metabolites are separated by the use of high-performance liquid chromatography and representative results are presented in Figure 5.9. It can be seen that all tissues studied have the ability to form one or more lipoxygenase products of arachidonic acid metabolism. It has not been possible to discern whether there is an increase in the rate of production in any one of these compounds during labour. It is of some interest to note that in another study it has been shown that the ratio of lipoxygenase products to cyclo-oxygenase products is shifted towards cyclo-oxygenase products during labour[17]. The data presented here are consistent with such a hypothesis.

FINAL COMMENTS

There is no question of the importance of eicosanoids formed within the uterus in the regulation of uteroplacental haemodynamics and the mechanisms

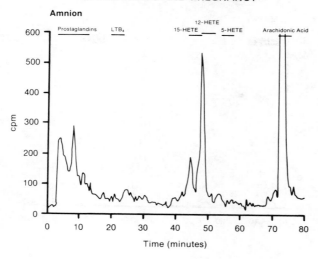

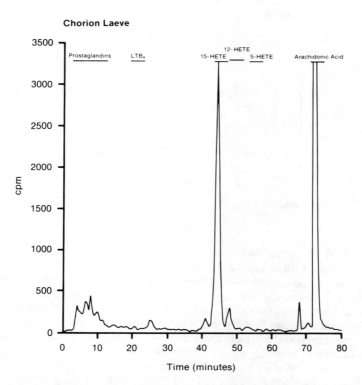

Figure 5.9 The formation of radiolabelled products upon incubation of intrauterine tissues from women delivered at term with [1-^{14}C]arachidonic acid. Separation was conducted by HPLC and fractions were collected at 30-second intervals

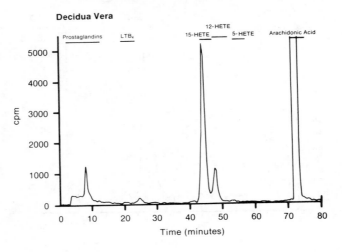

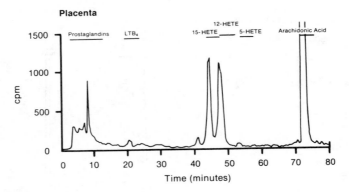

Figure 5.9   (continued)

that result in the onset of labour and delivery of the fetus. Neither is there any question that the results of studies designed to elucidate these mechanisms are not always consistent. Nevertheless, with time, a consensus is obtained on the major issues, e.g. the rate of production of prostaglandins by at least one intrauterine tissue (amnion) is raised during labour. The solution to the disparity of results can lie only in the improvement of techniques and caution in the interpretation of data. Data on the production of arachidonic acid metabolites by way of lipoxygenase enzymes are restricted presently. Nevertheless, there is every reason to believe that these substances will play a key role in the normal mechanisms of labour and may play greater roles in pathological states. It is increasingly likely that the mechanism of the onset of labour (and of preterm labour) will escape us until we understand more fully the mechanisms that regulate eicosanoid formation. Such information may also prove valuable, if not critical, in determining the causes of diseases of pregnancy such as pregnancy-induced hypertension.

ACKNOWLEDGEMENTS

I am grateful for the help and support of my colleagues who have participated in studies which have been described in this chapter. I thank Mrs. Joanne Hall for the typing of this manuscript. My own studies were supported in part by NIH HD 20747 and NIH HD 20779.

REFERENCES

1. Thorburn, G.D., Challis, J.R.G. and Robinson, J.S. (1977). Endocrine control of parturition. In Wynn, R.M. (ed.) *Biology of the Uterus*, pp. 653–732. (New York: Plenum Press)
2. Keirse, M.J.N.C. (1979). Endogenous prostaglandins in human parturition. In Keirse, M.J.N.C., Anderson, A.B.M. and Bennbroek Gravenhorst, J. (eds.) *Human Parturition*, pp. 101–142. (The Hague: Martinus Nijhoff)
3. Challis, J.R.G. and Patrick, J.E. (1980). The production of prostaglandins and thromboxanes in the feto-placental unit and their effects on the developing fetus. *Semin. Perinatol.*, **4**, 23–33
4. Mitchell, M.D. (1981). Prostaglandins during pregnancy and the perinatal period. *J. Reprod. Fertil.*, **62**, 305–315
5. Mitchell, M.D. (1984). The mechanism(s) of human parturition. *J. Dev. Physiol.*, **6**, 107–118
6. Karim, S.M.M. (1966). The identification of prostaglandins in human amniotic fluid. *J. Obstet. Gynaecol. Br. Commonw.*, **73**, 903–908
7. Karim, S.M.M. and Devlin, J. (1967). Prostaglandin content of amniotic fluid during pregnancy and labour. *J. Obstet. Gynaecol. Br. Commonw.*, **74**, 230–234
8. Turnbull, A.C., Anderson, A.B.M., Flint, A.P.F., Jeremy, J.Y., Keirse, M.J.N.C. and Mitchell, M.D. (1977). Human parturition. In Knight, J. and O'Connor, M. (eds.) *The Fetus and Birth*, pp. 427–452. (Amsterdam: Elsevier)
9. Keirse, M.J.N.C., Mitchell, M.D. and Turnbull, A.C. (1977). Changes in prostaglandin F and 13,14-dihydro-15-keto-prostaglandin F concentrations in amniotic fluid at the onset of and during labour. *Br. J. Obstet. Gynaecol.*, **8**, 743–746
10. Mitchell, M.D., Keirse, M.J.N.C., Brunt, J.D., Anderson, A.B.M. and Turnbull, A.C. (1979). Concentrations of the prostacyclin metabolite 6-keto-prostaglandin $F_{1\alpha}$ in amniotic fluid during late pregnancy and labour. *Br. J. Obstet. Gynaecol.*, **86**, 350–353
11. Mitchell, M.D., Keirse, M.J.N.C., Anderson, A.B.M. and Turnbull, A.C. (1978). Thromboxane B_2 in amniotic fluid before and during labour. *Br. J. Obstet. Gynaecol.*, **85**, 442–445
12. Challis, J.R.G. (1985). Factors responsible for parturition. In Beard, R.W. and Sharp, F. (eds.) *Preterm Labour and its Consequences*, pp. 61–69. (London: Royal College of Obstetricians and Gynaecologists)
13. TambyRaja, R.L., Salmon, J.A., Karim, S.M.M. and Ratnam, S.S. (1977). F Prostaglandin levels in amniotic fluid in premature labour. *Prostaglandins*, **13**, 339–348
14. Olund, A., Kindahl, H., Oliw, E., Lindgren, J.A. and Larson, B. (1980). Prostaglandins and thromboxanes in amniotic fluid during rivanol-induced abortion and labour. *Prostaglandins*, **19**, 791–803
15. MacKenzie, I.Z. and Mitchell, M.D. (1981). Serial determinations of prostaglandin E levels in amniotic fluid following the vaginal administration of a prostaglandin E_2 gel. *Prostagl. Med.*, **7**, 43–47
16. Reddi, K., Kambaran, S.R., Norman, R.J., Joubert, S.M. and Philpott, R.H. (1984). Abnormal concentrations of prostaglandins in amniotic fluid during delayed labour in multigravid patients. *Br. J. Obstet. Gynaecol.*, **91**, 781–787
17. Myatt, L., Rose, M.P. and Elder, M.G. (1985). Lipoxygenase products of arachidonic acid in human fetal membranes. Presented at the *32nd Annual Meeting of the Society for Gynecologic Investigation*, March 20-23, Phoenix
18. Bailey, J.M., Bryant, R.W., Whiting, J. and Salata, K. (1983). Characterization of 11-HETE and 15-HETE, together with prostacyclin as major products of the cyclooxygenase pathway in cultured rat aorta smooth muscle cells. *J. Lipid Res.*, **24**, 1419–1428

19. Liggins, G.C. and Grieves, S.A. (1971). Possible role for prostaglandin $F_{2\alpha}$ in parturition in sheep. *Nature*, **232**, 629–631
20. Thorburn, G.D., Nicol, D.H., Bassett, J.M., Shutt, D.A. and Cox, R.I. (1972). Parturition in the goat and sheep: Changes in corticosteroids, progesterone, oestrogens and prostaglandin F. *J. Reprod. Fertil. Suppl.*, **16**, 61–84
21. Samuelsson, B. (1973). Biosynthesis and metabolism of prostaglandins. In *Les Prostaglandines*, pp. 21–41 (Paris: INSERM)
22. Mitchell, M.D., Flint, A.P.F., Bibby, J., Brunt, J., Arnold, J.M., Anderson, A.B.M. and Turnbull, A.C. (1978). Plasma concentrations of prostaglandins during late human pregnancy: influence of normal and pre-term labour. *J. Clin. Endocrinol. Metabol.*, **46**, 947–951
23. Green, K., Bygdeman, M., Toppozada, M. and Wiqvist, N. (1974). The role of prostaglandin $F_{2\alpha}$ in human parturition. *Am. J. Obstet. Gynecol.*, **120**, 25–31
24. Mitchell, M.D., Sors, H. and Flint, A.P.F. (1977). Instability of 13,14-dihydro-15-keto-prostaglandin E_2. *Lancet*, **2**, 588
25. Fitzpatrick, F.A., Aguirre, R., Pike, J.E. and Lincoln, F.H. (1980). The stability of 13,14-dihydro-15-keto-PGE$_2$. *Prostaglandins*, **19**, 917–931
26. Granstrom, E., Hamberg, M., Hansson, G. and Kindahl, H. (1980). Chemical instability of 15-keto-13,14-dihydro-PGE$_2$: the reason for low assay reliability. *Prostaglandins*, **19**, 933–957
27. Mitchell, M.D., Ebenhack, K., Kraemer, D.L., Cox, K., Cutrer, S. and Strickland, D.M. (1982). A sensitive radioimmunoassay for 11-deoxy-13,14-dihydro-15-keto-11,16-cyclo-prostaglandin E_2: application as an index of prostaglandin E_2 biosynthesis during human pregnancy and parturition. *Prostagl. Leukotr. Med.*, **9**, 549–557
28. Schlegel, W., Kruger, S. and Korte, K. (1984). Purification of prostaglandin E_2-9-oxo-reductase from human decidua vera. *FEBS Lett.*, **171**, 141–144
29. Sun, F.F., Armour, S.B., Bockstanz, V.R. and McGuire, J.C. (1976). Studies on 15-hydroxy-prostaglandin dehydrogenase from monkey lung. In Samuelsson, B. and Paoletti, R. (eds.) *Advances in Prostaglandin and Thromboxane Research*, Vol. 1, pp. 163–169. (New York: Raven Press)
30. Ruckrich, M.F., Schlegel, W. and Jung, A. (1976). Prostaglandin endoperoxide analogues and prostaglandin D_2 as substrates of human placental 15-hydroxy prostaglandin dehydrogenase. *FEBS Lett.*, **68**, 59–62
31. Barrow, S.E., Heavey, D.J., Ennis, M., Chappell, C.G., Blair, I.A. and Dollery, C.T. (1984). Measurement of prostaglandin D_2 and identification of metabolites in human plasma during intravenous infusion. *Prostaglandins*, **28**, 743–754
32. Clarke, K.E., Austin, J.E. and Seeds, A.E. (1982). Effect of bisenoic prostaglandins and arachidonic acid on the uterine vasculature of pregnant sheep. *Am. J. Obstet. Gynecol.*, **142**, 261–268
33. Mitchell, M.D., Bibby, J.G., Hicks, B.R., Redman, C.W.G., Anderson, A.B.M. and Turnbull, A.C. (1978). Thromboxane B_2 and human parturition: concentrations in the plasma and production in vitro. *J. Endocrinol.*, **78**, 435–441
34. Ylikorkala, O. and Viinikka, L. (1980). Thromboxane A_2 in pregnancy and puerperium. *Br. Med. J.*, **281**, 1601–1602
35. Mitchell, M.D. (1981). Prostacyclin during human pregnancy and parturition. In Lewis, P.J. and O'Grady, J. (eds.) *Clinical Pharmacology of Prostacyclin*, pp. 121–129. (New York: Raven Press)
36. Barrow, S.E., Blair, I.A., Waddell, K.A., Shepherd, G.L., Lewis, P.J. and Dollery, C.T. (1983). Prostacyclin in late pregnancy: analysis of 6-oxo-prostaglandin $F_{1\alpha}$ in maternal plasma. In Lewis, P.J., Moncada, S. and O'Grady, J. (eds.) *Prostacyclin in Pregnancy*, pp. 79–85. (New York: Raven Press)
37. Mitchell, M.D., Anderson, A.B.M., Brunt, J.D., Clover, L., Ellwood, D.A., Robinson, J.S. and Turnbull, A.C. (1979). Concentrations of 6-oxo-prostaglandin F in the maternal and foetal plasma of sheep during spontaneous and induced parturition. *J. Endocrinol.*, **83**, 141–148
38. Ellwood, D.A., Anderson, A.B.M., Mitchell, M., Murphy, G. and Turnbull, A.C. (1981). Prostanoids, collagenase and cervical softening in the sheep. In Ellwood, D.A. and Anderson, A.B.M. (eds.) *The Cervix in Pregnancy and Labour: Clinical and Biochemical Investigations*, pp. 57–73. (Edinburgh: Churchill Livingstone)
39. Lye, S.J. and Challis, J.R.G. (1982). Inhibition by PGI$_2$ of myometrial activity *in vivo* in non-pregnant ovariectomized sheep. *J. Reprod. Fertil.*, **66**, 311–315

40. Omini, L., Folco, G.C., Pasargiklian, R., Fano, M. and Berti, F. (1979). Prostacyclin (PGI$_2$) in pregnant human uterus. *Prostaglandins*, **17**, 113–120

41. Makarainen, L. and Ylikorkala, O. (1982). Lack of effect of circulating prostacyclin on contractility of the non-pregnant human uterus. *Br. J. Obstet. Gynaecol.*, **89**, 402–407

42. Wilhelmsson, L., Wikland, M. and Wiqvist, N. (1981). PGH$_2$, TxA$_2$ and PGH$_2$ have potent and differentiated actions on human uterine contractility. *Prostaglandins*, **21**, 277–286

43. Williams, K.I., El Tahir, K.E.H. and Marcinkiewicz, E. (1979). Dual actions of prostacyclin (PGI$_2$) on the rat pregnant uterus. *Prostaglandins*, **17**, 667–672

44. Coceani, F., Olley, P.M. and Bodach, E. (1976). Prostaglandins: a possible regulator of muscle tone in the ductus arteriosus. In Samuelsson, B. and Paoletti, R. (eds.) *Adv. Prostagl. Thrombox. Res.*, **1**, pp. 417–424. (New York: Raven Press)

45. Challis, J.R.G., Dilley, S.R., Robinson, J.S. and Thorburn, G.D. (1976). Prostaglandins in the circulation of the fetal lamb. *Prostaglandins*, **11**, 1041–1052

46. Kitterman, J.A., Liggins, G.C., Fewell, J.E. and Tooley, W.H. (1983). Inhibition of breathing movements in fetal sheep by prostaglandins. *J. Appl. Physiol. Resp. Env. Exer. Physiol.*, **54**, 687–692

47. Richardson, B., Natale, R. and Patrick, J. (1979). Human fetal breathing activity during electively induced labour at term. *Am. J. Obstet. Gynecol.*, **133**, 247–255

48. Boylan, P., O'Donovan, P. and Owens, O.J. (1985). Fetal breathing movements and the diagnosis of labour: a prospective analysis of 100 cases. *Obstet. Gynecol.*, **66**, 517–520

49. Castle, B.M. and Turnbull, A.C. (1983). The presence or absence of fetal breathing movements predicts the outcome of pre-term labour. *Lancet*, **2**, 471–473

50. MacKenzie, I.Z., MacLean, D.A. and Mitchell, M.D. (1980). Prostaglandins in the human fetal circulation in mid-trimester and term pregnancy. *Prostaglandins*, **20**, 649–654

51. Mitchell, M.D., Brunt, J., Bibby, J., Flint, A.P.F., Anderson A.B.M. and Turnbull, A.C. (1978). Prostaglandins in human umbilical circulation at birth. *Br. J. Obstet. Gynaecol.*, **85**, 114–118

52. Bibby, J.G., Brunt, J.D., Hodgson, H., Mitchell, M.D., Anderson, A.B.M. and Turnbull, A.C. (1979). Prostaglandins in umbilical plasma at elective caesarean section. *Br. J. Obstet. Gynaecol.*, **86**, 282–284

53. Mitchell, M.D., Sellers, S.M., Menchini, M., Aynsley-Green, A. and Turnbull, A.C. (1981). 6-keto-prostaglandin F$_{1\alpha}$ and thromboxane B$_2$ in human umbilical and neonatal circulations. *IRCS J. Med. Sci.*, **9**, 222–223

54. Hamberg, M. (1974). Quantitative studies on prostaglandin synthesis in man III. Excretion of the major urinary metabolites of prostaglandins F$_{1\alpha}$ and F$_{2\alpha}$ during pregnancy. *Life Sci.*, **14**, 247–252

55. Satoh, K., Takehiko, Y., Fukuoka, H., Kinoshita, K., Kaneko, Y., Tsuchiya, M. and Sakamoto, S. (1979). Prostaglandin F$_{2\alpha}$ metabolite levels in plasma, amniotic fluid, and urine during pregnancy and labour. *Am. J. Obstet. Gynecol.*, **133**, 886–890

56. Goodman, R.P., Killam, A.P., Brash, A.R. and Branch, R.A. (1982). Prostacyclin production during pregnancy: comparison of production during normal pregnancy and pregnancy complicated by hypertension. *Am. J. Obstet. Gynecol.*, **142**, 817–822

57. Makila, U.M., Viinikka, L. and Ylikorkala, O. (1984). Evidence that prostacyclin deficiency is a specific feature in preeclampsia. *Am. J. Obstet. Gynecol.*, **148**, 772–774

58. Casey, M.L., Cutrer, S. and Mitchell, M.D. (1983). Origin of prostanoids in human amniotic fluid: the fetal kidney as a source of amniotic fluid prostanoids. *Am. J. Obstet. Gynecol.*, **147**, 547–551

59. Mitchell, M.D. and Flint, A.P.F. (1978). Prostaglandin production by intrauterine tissues from periparturient sheep: use of a superfusion technique. *J. Endocrinol.*, **76**, 111–121

60. Mitchell, M.D., Bibby, J., Hicks, B.R. and Turnbull, A.C. (1978). Specific production of prostaglandin E by human amnion in vitro. *Prostaglandins*, **15**, 377–382

61. Mitchell, M.D., Bibby, J.G., Hicks, B.R. and Turnbull, A.C. (1978). Possible role for prostacyclin in human parturition. *Prostaglandins*, **16**, 931–937

62. Okazaki, T., Casey, M.L., Okita, J.R., MacDonald, P.C. and Johnston, J.M. (1981). Initiation of human parturition XII. Biosynthesis and metabolism of prostaglandins in human fetal membranes and uterine decidua. *Am. J. Obstet. Gynecol.*, **139**, 373–381

63. Olson, D., Skinner, K. and Challis, J.R.G. (1983). Prostaglandin output in relation to parturition by cells dispersed from human intrauterine tissues. *J. Clin. Endocrinol. Metab.*, **57**, 694–699

64. Kinoshita, K., Satoh, K. and Sakamoto, S. (1984). Human amniotic membrane and prostaglandin biosynthesis. *Bio. Res. Pregn. Perinatol.*, **5**, 61–67
65. Skinner, K.A. and Challis, J.R.G. (1985). Changes in the synthesis and metabolism of prostaglandins by human fetal membranes and decidua at labor. *Am. J. Obstet. Gynecol.*, **151**, 519–523
66. Evans, C.A., Kennedy, T.G., Patrick, J.E. and Challis, J.R.G. (1981). Uterine prostaglandin concentrations in sheep during late pregnancy and adrenocorticotropin-induced labour. *Endocrinology*, **109**, 1533–1538
67. Evans, C.A., Kennedy, T.G. and Challis, J.R.G. (1982). Gestational changes in prostanoid concentrations in intrauterine tissues and fetal fluids from pregnant sheep and the relation to prostanoid output in vitro. *Biol. Reprod.*, **27**, 1–11
68. Olson, D.M., Lye, S.J., Skinner, K. and Challis, J.R.G. (1984). Early changes in concentrations in ovine maternal and fetal plasma, amniotic fluid and from dispersed cells of intrauterine tissues before the onset of ACTH-induced pre-term labour. *J. Reprod. Fertil.*, **71**, 45–55
69. Olson, D.M., Lye, S.J., Skinner, K. and Challis, J.R.G. (1985). Prostanoid concentrations in maternal/fetal plasma and amniotic fluid and intrauterine tissue prostanoid output in relation to myometrial contractility during the onset of adrenocorticotropin-induced preterm labor in sheep. *Endocrinology*, **116**, 389–397
70. Moonen, P., Klok, G. and Keirse, M.J.N.C. (1984). Increase in concentrations of prostaglandin endoperoxide synthase and prostacyclin synthase in human myometrium in late pregnancy. *Prostaglandins*, **28**, 309–321
71. Keirse, M.J.N.C., Moonen, P. and Klok, G. (1984). Prostaglandin synthase in pregnant human myometrium is not confined to the utero-placental vasculature. *IRCS Med. Sci.*, **12**, 824–825
72. Ellwood, D.A., Mitchell, M.D., Anderson, A.B.M. and Turnbull, A.C. (1980). *In vitro* production of prostanoids by the human cervix during pregnancy: preliminary observations. *Br. J. Obstet. Gynaecol.*, **87**, 210–214
73. Ellwood, D.A., Mitchell, M.D., Anderson, A.B.M. and Turnbull, A.C. (1980). Specific changes in the *in vitro* production of prostanoids by the ovine cervix at parturition. *Prostaglandins*, **19**, 479–488
74. Hillier, K. and Wallis, R.M. (1981). Prostaglandins, steroids and the human cervix. In Ellwood, D.A. and Anderson, A.B.M. (eds.) *The Cervix in Pregnancy and Labour: Clinical and Biochemical Investigations*, pp. 144–162. (Edinburgh: Churchill Livingstone)
75. Tanaka, M., Morita, I., Hirakawa, S. and Murota, S. (1981). Increased prostacyclin synthesising activity in human ripening uterine cervix. *Prostaglandins*, **21**, 83–86
76. Mitsuhashi, N. and Kato, J. (1984). Bioconversion of arachidonic acid by human uterine cervical tissue and endocervix in late pregnancy. *Endocrinol. Jpn.*, **31**, 533–538
77. Christensen, N.J., Belfrage, P., Bygdeman, M., Floberg, J., Mitsuhashi, N. and Green, K. (1985). Bioconversion of arachidonic acid in human pregnant uterine cervix. *Acta Obstet. Gynecol. Scand.*, **64**, 259–265
78. Mackenzie, I.Z. (1981). Clinical studies on cervical ripening. In Ellwood, D.A. and Anderson, A.B.M. (eds.) *The Cervix in Pregnancy and Labour: Clinical and Biochemical Investigations*, pp. 163–186. (Edinburgh: Churchill Livingstone)
79. Hillier, K. and Wallis, R.M. (1982). Collagen solubility and tensile properties of the rat uterine cervix in late pregnancy: effects of arachidonic acid and prostaglandin $F_{2\alpha}$. *J. Endocrinol.*, **95**, 341–347
80. Norstrom, A., Wilhelmsson, L. and Hamberger, L. (1983). Experimental studies on the influence of prostaglandins on the connective tissue of the human cervix uteri. *Acta Obstet. Gynecol. Scand. Suppl.*, **113**, 167–170
81. Uldbjerg, N., Ekman, G., Malmstrom, A., Ulmsten, U. and Wingerup, L. (1983). Biochemical changes in human cervical connective tissue after local applications of prostaglandin E_2. *Gynecol. Obstet. Invest.*, **15**, 291–299
82. Mitchell, M.D., Jamieson, D.R.S., Sellers, S.M. and Turnbull, A.C. (1980). 6-keto-PGF$_{1\alpha}$: Concentrations in human umbilical plasma and production by umbilical vessels. In Samuelsson, B., Ramwell, P.W. and Paoletti, R. (eds.) *Advances in Prostaglandin and Thromboxane Research, Vol. 7*, pp. 891–895. (New York: Raven Press)
83. Tuvemo, T., Strandberg, K., Hamberg, M. and Samuelsson, B. (1976). Maintenance of the tone of human umbilical artery by prostaglandin and thromboxane formation. In

Samuelsson, B. and Paoletti, R. (eds.) *Adv. Prostaglandins Thromboxane Research, Vol. 1*, pp. 425–428. (New York: Raven Press)

84. Elliot, W.J., McLaughlin, L.L., Bloch, M.H. and Needleman, P. (1984). Arachidonic acid metabolism by rabbit fetal membranes of various gestational ages. *Prostaglandins*, **27**, 27–36

85. Bloch, M.H., McLaughlin, L.L., Crowley, J., Needleman, P. and Morrison, A.R. (1985). Arachidonic acid metabolic pathway of the rabbit placenta. *Prostaglandins*, **29**, 203–216

86. Pakrasi, P.L., Becka, R. and Dey, S.K. (1985). Cyclooxygenase and lipoxygenase pathways in the preimplantation rabbit uterus and blastocyst. *Prostaglandins*, **29**, 481–495

87. Mitchell, M.D., Strickland, D.M., Brennecke, S.P. and Saeed, S.A. (1983). New aspects of arachidonic acid metabolism and human parturition. In MacDonald, P.C. and Porter, J.C. (eds.) *Inhibition of Parturition: Prevention of Prematurity*, pp. 145–153. Report of the Fourth Ross Conference on Obstetric Research. (Columbus: Ross Laboratories)

88. Saeed, S.A. and Mitchell, M.D. (1982). Formation of arachidonate lipoxygenase metabolites by human fetal membranes, uterine decidua vera and placenta. *Prostagl. Leukotr. Med.*, **8**, 635–640

89. Saeed, S.A. and Mitchell, M.D. (1982). New aspects of arachidonic acid metabolism in human uterine cervix. *Eur. J. Pharmacol.*, **81**, 515–516

90. Saeed, S.A. and Mitchell, M.D. (1983). Lipoxygenase activity in human uterine and intrauterine tissues: new prospects for control of prostacyclin production in pre-eclampsia. *Clin. Exp. Hypert., Part B*, **82**, 103–111

6
Regulation of eicosanoid biosynthesis during pregnancy and parturition

M. D. Mitchell

INTRODUCTION

In the previous chapter we reviewed the information available on the production of eicosanoids during pregnancy and parturition and how this is reflected in changes in eicosanoid concentrations in biological fluids. In order to understand more fully the roles that eicosanoids play during gestation and in the onset of labour we must first have a greater understanding of the regulation of eicosanoid biosynthesis at these times. Other reviews are available concerning the basic mechanisms that control eicosanoid biosynthesis[1-4] and the reader is encouraged to consult them. In this chapter, I will attempt to delineate those regulatory mechanisms that are considered most significant in, or specific to, pregnancy and parturition.

REGULATION OF ARACHIDONIC ACID MOBILIZATION

The release of arachidonic acid from glycerophospholipids is considered to be the rate-limiting step in eicosanoid formation (Figure 6.1). Arachidonic acid, as with other polyunsaturated fatty acids will typically be esterified at the sn-2 position of a glycerophospholipid (Figure 6.2). Thus, the most direct mechanism for the release of arachidonic acid would be through the action of phospholipase A_2. Another mechanism for the release of arachidonic acid that may be even more important is through the action initially of phospholipase C followed by the actions of diacylglycerol lipase and monoacylglycerol lipase. Before discussing the mechanisms that may regulate the activities of these enzymes we will review briefly the information concerning arachidonic acid in uterine tissues.

Arachidonic acid (the precursor of prostaglandins of the 2-series) is present in uterine tissues in vastly greater amounts than dihomo-γ-linolenic acid (the precursor of prostaglandins of the 1-series)[5]. Hence, the emphasis on

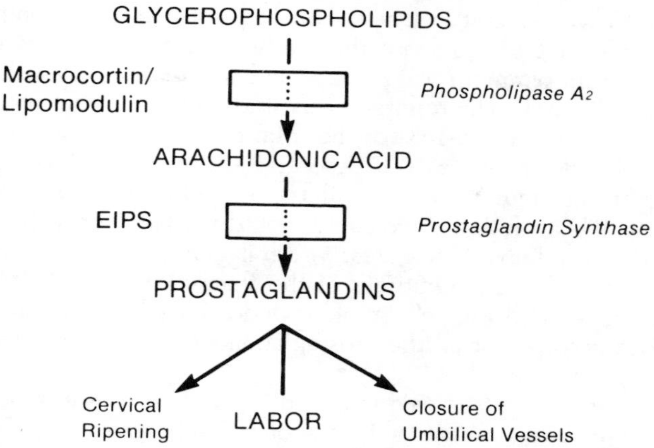

GLYCEROPHOSPHOLIPIDS

Macrocortin/
Lipomodulin   *Phospholipase A₂*

ARACHIDONIC ACID

EIPS   *Prostaglandin Synthase*

PROSTAGLANDINS

Cervical   **LABOR**   Closure of
Ripening   Umbilical Vessels

Figure 6.1. A simplified representation of some aspects of arachidonic acid metabolism. EIPS: endogenous inhibitor of prostaglandin synthase

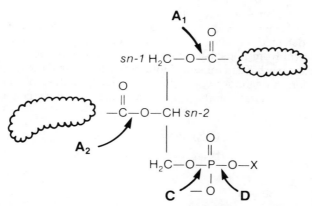

Figure 6.2. The structure of a generalized glycerophospholipid. The various alcohols that may be found in phosphomonoester linkage are depicted as X. The sites of hydrolysis catalyzed by the various phospholipases are indicated by the letters A_1, A_2, C and D. A saturated fatty acid is typically esterified at the *sn*-1 position and a polyunsaturated fatty acid commonly esterified at the *sn*-2 position. The fatty acids are represented by ⟨⟩ (from ref. 12 with permission)

arachidonic acid as a substrate for eicosanoid biosynthesis. The relative abundance of arachidonic acid in uterine tissues is higher than in many other tissues; it accounts for 7–20% of the non-esterified fatty acids. Concentrations of non-esterified arachidonic acid in amniotic fluid increase several-fold during labour[6,7]. This increase exceeds those of other fatty acids and indicates a degree of specificity in the mobilization of arachidonic acid.

It has been shown that there is a significantly lower arachidonic acid content in fetal membranes (amnion and chorion) from women in labour compared with women not in labour[8]. Subsequently, a more comprehensive study was conducted to compare the arachidonic acid contents of amnion (and chorion) from women not in labour and women in early labour (cervix less than 4 cm dilated)[9]. The results of this study indicated that before labour, arachidonic acid constitutes 14% of the total fatty acids in amnion and after labour this value decreases to 10%. Separation of the total glycerophospholipids of amnion into individual classes has revealed a significant change with early labour in the arachidonic acid content of (diacyl) phosphatidylethanolamine and phosphatidylinositol (Figure 6.3). Similar changes have been observed in chorion, although the magnitudes of the changes are less in this tissue. It has been calculated that this release of arachidonic acid from fetal membranes is sufficient to account for all the prostaglandins formed during the onset of labour.

How is the release of arachidonic acid from these glycerophospholipids controlled? Regulation of the activities of phospholipases A_2 and C is an obvious method. In amnion there is a phospholipase A_2 that is calcium-dependent and has a substrate preference for phosphatidylethanolamine that contains arachidonic acid[10]. This is consistent with the release of arachidonic acid from phosphatidylethanolamine in amnion during labour. There is also a phosphatidylinositol-specific phospholipase C in amnion that is calcium dependent[11]. Moreover, diacylglycerol and monoacylglycerol lipase activities have been detected in amnion[12]. This is consistent with the release of arachidonic acid from phosphatidylinositol during early labour.

The simplest mechanism for arachidonic acid release (and thence prostaglandin generation) in labour would be increased activities of the enzymes described above. Assay of the specific activities of these enzymes, under

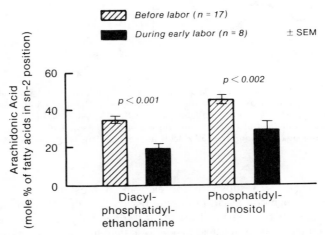

Figure 6.3 Arachidonic acid content of (diacyl) phosphatidylethanolamine and phosphatidylinositol of amnion. The arachidonic acid contents of (diacyl) phosphatidylethanolamine and phosphatidylinositol are expressed as mole percentages of total acids in the *sn*-2 position of each lipid. Early labour is defined as a cervical dilatation of 4 cm or less (from ref. 12, with permission)

optimal conditions, at term before and after labour, however, has not revealed a significant change in the specific activities of the enzymes in uterine tissues[13].

The optimal conditions used in the assay of phospholipase activities included concentrations of Ca^{2+} that were far greater than those found in the cytosol of amnion cells under normal conditions. Thus, it is possible that, *in vivo*, changes in the activities of phospholipases could occur that account for the mobilization of arachidonic acid. Such changes could result from the action of a regulatory factor that either raises the cytosolic concentration of Ca^{2+} in amnion cells or increases the sensitivity of the phospholipases to Ca^{2+}. It has been suggested that both basal and stimulated prostaglandin production by amnion cells are extremely dependent upon extracellular calcium[14,15]. In these studies not only a calcium channel blocker but also trifluoperazine (a calmodulin antagonist) had significant inhibitory effects on prostaglandin biosynthesis.

Several substances have been identified in amniotic fluid that could influence intracellular Ca^{2+} concentrations in amnion. For instance, mean concentrations of 1,25-dihydroxyvitamin D_3 in amniotic fluid are increased during late gestation and this hormone is known to affect Ca^{2+} fluxes[16]. Another intriguing substance that has the properties of a calcium ionophore[17] and is found in amnion cell culture media and in amniotic fluid[18] is leukotriene B_4 (LTB$_4$). Intriguingly LTB$_4$ may actually be synthesized in amnion[18,19] and, hence, may have an autocrine action. Perhaps the most likely candidate for the role of Ca^{2+} regulator in amnion at term is platelet activating factor (PAF; 1-O-alkyl-2-acetyl-sn-glycero-3-phosphocholine). PAF is known to cause a rapid increase in the cytosolic concentration of Ca^{2+} in platelets; this results in activation of phospholipases, release of arachidonic acid and generation of prostaglandins[20]. It has also been suggested that PAF may induce the biosynthesis of lipoxygenase products of arachidonic acid metabolism which may act as mediators of its actions[21,22]. PAF has been identified in the amniotic fluid of women in labour at term, but is not found in the liquor of women at term but not in labour[23]. Moreover, the concentration of PAF in amnion tissue from women in labour at term is 2 to 3-fold greater than that of women at term but not in labour[24]. Finally, PAF acts on fresh amnion tissue to increase the rate of prostaglandin biosynthesis substantially[24]. Hence, presently, PAF best fulfils the requirements for a regulator of cytosolic Ca^{2+} concentrations in amnion at term that may result in the cascade of events of parturition.

It should be noted that Ca^{2+} may also have effects on arachidonic acid metabolism that are independent of actions on phospholipase activities. For instance it may act through the actions of the phospholipid requiring, Ca^{2+}-dependent protein kinase known[25] as protein kinase C. Protein kinase C has been implicated in the control of thromboxane A_2 biosynthesis in platelets by way of an action on arachidonic acid mobilization[26]. Furthermore, amnion tissue has been shown to have protein kinase C activity[27]. The possibility that protein kinase C may play a part in the release of arachidonic acid for eicosanoid biosynthesis at term was strengthened by our recent finding that phorbol esters (which activate protein kinase C) stimulate PGE$_2$ production in human amnion cells (unpublished observations).

There is an ever increasing number of hormones that may have actions to increase the mobilization of arachidonic acid, possibly via activation of the phosphatidylinositol cycle. This effect can be of varying importance in the known actions of this group of hormones. Examples of these hormones include oxytocin[28], bradykinin[29], vasopressin[30], angiotensin II[31], catecholamines[32] and possibly even PGE_2[33]. Conversely, it has suggested that relaxin[34] and glucocorticosteroids[35-38] have inhibitory actions on phospholipase activities. In the case of glucocorticosteroids this inhibitory action is mediated by way of induction of the biosynthesis of an antiphospholipase protein now known as lipomodulin. This protein has recently been sequenced[39] and thus the potential for its production by uterine tissues can now be evaluated (see Figure 6.1).

Substances have been reported to be present within the uterus that have actions on phospholipase activities; these substances have yet to be fully characterized. Amniotic fluid contains a substance that can stimulate fibroblast phospholipase A_2 activity[40]. Moreover, this action can be enhanced by the presence of soluble constituents of meconium. Information on the characteristics of these substances remains limited, but they have obvious potential for a role in the regulation of arachidonic acid mobilization by amnion as well as possible roles in pathologies such as meconium aspiration syndromes. Recently, two substances have been found in amniotic fluid that inhibit phospholipase activities of endometrial cells[41]. These substances have apparent molecular weights of 150-165 000 and 70-80 000 daltons. Whether these substances are synthesized in amnion is uncertain, but conditioned media from amnion cells can inhibit endometrial cell prostaglandin biosynthesis[42]. If these inhibitory substances were to be present in reduced concentrations at the time of the onset of labour this could constitute the equivalent of the release of a brake on arachidonic acid mobilization and result subsequently in the onset of labour.

INHIBITION OF EICOSANOID BIOSYNTHESIS

The concept has been advanced that there is tonic inhibition of prostaglandin biosynthesis during pregnancy and that the onset of labour is associated with, and may require, withdrawal of such inhibition[43]. The hypothesis was based on the observation that extra-amniotic administration of arachidonic acid would not induce labour in rhesus monkeys and that the arachidonic acid was not converted substantially into prostaglandins. Consistent with such an hypothesis it has been found that decidua of early pregnancy has a dramatically reduced prostaglandin content compared with endometrium[44]. The discovery of an endogenous inhibitor of prostaglandin synthase (EIPS) in plasma of several animal species[45] led to speculation that it may play a role in the suppression of prostaglandin biosynthesis during pregnancy (see Figure 6.1). EIPS is a heat-labile protein of mol.wt. = 70-100 000 daltons; it's activity is increased significantly by glucocorticosteroid treatment.

There is no change in plasma EIPS activity in early human pregnancy or during gestation until term (Figure 6.4)[46]. At term there is a small but significant reduction in plasma EIPS activity that does not persist in labour[47].

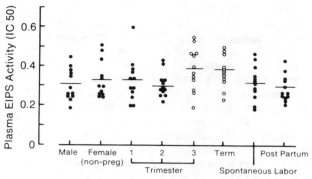

Figure 6.4 Human plasma EIPS activity in relation to pregnancy parturition and the puerperium. NB IC50 is inversely related to inhibitory potency (from ref. 47, with permission)

It has been suggested that this slight decline in plasma EIPS activity may play a permissive, rather than a direct role in the onset of labour. The return of plasma EIPS activity to normal levels during labour may represent a feedback regulation possibly by prostaglandins. Interestingly, EIPS activity is low in the fetal circulation[48], consonant with the high circulating levels of prostaglandins in the fetus. The large maternal-fetal gradient for EIPS also suggests that EIPS does not cross the placenta.

It seems likely that the amnion plays a key role in the mechanism of the onset of labour by way of its secretion of prostaglandins[49]. Amnion, however, is avascular and factors that are important in the regulation of prostaglandin biosynthesis in this tissue are probably located in amniotic fluid, rather than plasma. Hence, EIPS activity has been determined in amniotic fluid. EIPS activity is present in human amniotic fluid and its concentration declines

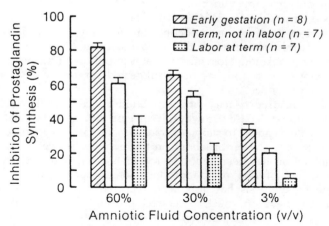

Figure 6.5 Inhibition of prostaglandin synthesis by human amniotic fluid in relation to gestation and labour. (from ref. 50, with permission)

slightly from early gestation until term (Figure 6.5)[50]. This change probably reflects the increased volume of the amniotic sac. In labour, however, there is a significant reduction in EIPS activity in amniotic fluid. This change may be of importance in the onset of labour since it reflects withdrawal of an inhibitory influence on prostaglandin biosynthesis. Recently, EIPS-like activity has been suggested to be present in amnion at term before the onset of labour[51]. This activity was reported to be completely absent in amnion obtained after labour. Whether amnion is a source of EIPS is still uncertain since the methods used do not distinguish between synthesis of EIPS and binding or association. Nevertheless, amnion has been shown to secrete a factor(s) that can inhibit endometrial prostaglandin biosynthesis[42]. The level at which this inhibition occurs (Figure 6.1) and the relationship of this factor(s) to EIPS are unknown.

Ovine allantoic fluid contains a substance(s) that inhibits prostaglandin synthase of endometrial cotyledonary tissue[52]. The activity of this inhibitory substance is high in the second half of pregnancy (100–130 days gestation) but is undetectable near term (140 days gestation). Another substance with inhibitory properties has been isolated from bovine maternal caruncle (placental) tissue[53,54]. The inhibitory action was determined using prostaglandin production by bovine luteal cells. This inhibitory activity was high throughout most of pregnancy (120–250 days gestation) but was undetectable at term (260–280 days gestation). These findings are consistent with the hypothesis that the onset of labour is preceded by, or associated with, the withdrawal of inhibitory influences on prostaglandin biosynthesis.

A slightly different factor has been found in rat plasma. This factor not only inhibits prostaglandin biosynthesis, but also enhances prostaglandin catabolic activity. The substance has been designated as reciprocal coupling factor[55,56]. There is no convincing evidence at present that this substance has a role in pregnancy or parturition. An uncharacterized activity has been found as a soluble product of the decidua, which can induce dose-related inhibition of amnion cell prostaglandin biosynthesis (Romero, R. and Mitchell, M.D. unpublished observations). Whether this factor acts locally on chorion or myometrium or even has an autocrine function is uncertain. It is possible, however, that this substance can diffuse to amnion and have an action at this key site for prostaglandin biosynthesis that is important in the onset of labour. Such transport and action has been suggested for prolactin[57] and will be discussed in a later section.

There is a relative paucity of information concerning the inhibition of arachidonate lipoxygenase pathways. It appears that a substance(s) in plasma and amniotic fluid can act to suppress arachidonate-15-lipoxygenase activity[58]. The influence of gestation or labour on this activity has yet to be reported. Product inhibition has been reported for 15-lipoxygenase activity[59] and an inhibitory effect of one of the products of 15-lipoxygenase activity on leukotriene biosynthesis has also been reported[60]. Also, in cervical tissue prostaglandins have an effect to redirect prostaglandin biosynthesis away from the cyclo-oxygenase pathway[61]. Whether this action results in increased lipoxygenase product formation is uncertain.

Placental and umbilical tissue production of prostaglandins (particularly prostacyclin) is significantly reduced in women with pregnancy-induced hypertension[62,63]. It has been hypothesized that this reflects aberrant arachidonic acid metabolism resulting in over-production of hydroperoxy and hydroxyeicosatetraenoic acids (HPETEs and HETEs)[64]. These products are known to inhibit prostacyclin formation[65,66] and recently 15-HETE was shown to inhibit cyclo-oxygenase activity[67]. Thus, more substrate would be available to the lipoxygenase enzymes with the potential for formation of greater amounts of HPETEs and HETEs and, thence, further inhibition of prostacyclin formation.

STIMULATION OF EICOSANOID BIOSYNTHESIS

There is a considerable body of evidence that is suggestive of a critical role for increased amnion prostaglandin production in the mechanism of the onset of human labour[49]. The avascular nature of amnion has led to an examination of amniotic fluid for substances that might exert such a stimulatory action. This in turn has focussed attention on fetal urine since, at term, amniotic fluid is composed principally of the products of fetal urination. It has been found that human fetal urine (and amniotic fluid) contains a substance(s) that stimulates prostaglandin endoperoxide synthase[68]. The activity of this substance is greater in urine of fetuses of women that have laboured than in urine of fetuses of women that have not laboured (Figure 6.6). Hence, this substance may represent a potential trigger for the onset of labour.

The prostaglandin endoperoxide synthase stimulatory factor has a mol.wt. < 500 and acts in a manner different from other known cofactors for prostaglandin endoperoxide synthase[69]. If whole amniotic fluid is tested on prostaglandin endoperoxide synthase an inhibitory action (of EIPS) prevails (see previous section). Separation of EIPS from this stimulatory substance in amniotic fluid has revealed that both inhibitory and stimulatory activities change significantly with labour; inhibitory activity declines and stimulatory activity increases[70]. This result confirmed previous findings with regard to a decline in EIPS activity in amniotic fluid during labour[50].

Actions of EIPS or this stimulant of prostaglandin endoperoxide synthase on PGE production by amnion tissue or cells have yet to be described.

Cytosolic fractions prepared from uterine tissues have been shown to contain substances that increase the activity of prostaglandin synthase[71]. The substances exhibited various degrees of specificity with respect to the tissues acted upon and the prostaglandin whose synthesis was stimulated. Similar observations on cytosols from other tissues had been made earlier[72,73]. An unusual factor has been described to be present in the cytosolic fraction of human placenta[74]. This factor is heat stable, inhibits thromboxane A_2 synthesis and directs prostaglandin H_2 (endoperoxide) placental microsome metabolism towards prostaglandin E_2. Such a factor could play a significant role in uteroplacental haemodynamics. Substances derived from cytosols that act on different parts of prostaglandin synthetase quite likely are not secreted but have regulatory actions within the tissue of origin.

It is important to establish whether substances that may alter arachidonic

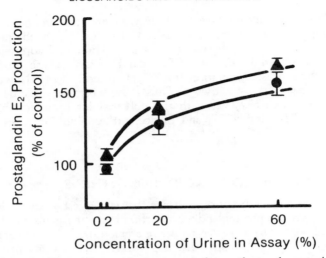

Figure 6.6 The effect of human fetal urine on the synthesis of prostaglandin E_2 by prostaglandin synthase from bovine seminal vesicles. Values shown are means ($\pm$ SEM) for urine samples from ($\blacktriangle$) newborns delivered at term after spontaneous labour ($n = 10$) and ($\bullet$) newborns delivered at Caesarean sections scheduled at term before the onset of labour (from ref. 68, with permission)

acid metabolism can act on intact cells and thus can travel to and act on a secondary tissue. Since amnion is a key tissue in the mechanism of the onset of labour and it is avascular, studies have been directed towards the effects of amniotic fluid and fetal urine (see previous section) on amnion cell prostaglandin biosynthesis. Excitingly, it has been found that human fetal urine contains a substance that increases the rate of production of prostaglandin E_2 in amnion by 5 to 50-fold (Figure 6.7)[75]. This substance is apparently secreted by the fetal kidney and probably adult kidney also; it has a mol.wt. of 18 000 and has properties consistent with those of a growth factor[76]. Importantly, this prostaglandin stimulatory substance acts by way of the epidermal growth factor (EGF) receptor and can induce anchorage-independent growth in NRK cells. Thus, this substance is probably an alpha transforming growth factor. Further discussion of the effects of EGF itself on prostaglandin biosynthesis in amnion will be described in the next section. The activity of the prostaglandin synthesis stimulatory substance in amniotic fluid does not change substantially from early gestation until term[77]. Nevertheless, the activity of this substance is markedly enhanced in the presence of a calcium ionophore. It is likely that this substance accounts for the stimulatory action of amniotic fluid on not only cells, but also fresh amnion tissue that is minced and superfused (Figure 6.8)[78] and possibly myometrial and decidual tissue slices[79]. Since the prostaglandin synthesis stimulatory substance is formed in the fetus and communicates with amnion where it enhances prostaglandin E_2 production, it is a strong candidate for a vital role in the mechanism that controls the onset of labour. Moreover, this factor may provide a link between fetal growth and development and the mechanism of parturition.

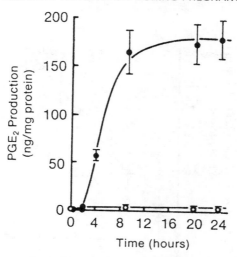

Figure 6.7   Time course of stimulation by human fetal urine of prostaglandin E₂ production in amnion cells. Medium was collected at various times after treatment with water (○) or human fetal urine (●) (from ref. 75, with permission)

A substance that is less well characterized has been found in the plasma of normal and pregnant women; it stimulates prostacyclin biosynthesis[80,81]. Normal activity of this substance has been reported in women with pregnancy-induced hypertension, a disease characterized by lack of prostacyclin generation by blood vessels. Moreover, greatly reduced activities of this substance are found near term, a time when prostacyclin synthesis is increased. No explanations have been forthcoming to explain these apparent contradictions. Two reports of inhibitors of prostacyclin biosynthesis will be mentioned here for completeness. One is associated with the IgG fraction of plasma containing the lupus anticoagulant of a woman with a history of recurrent arterial thrombosis[82]. The patient had lost two pregnancies due to intrauterine death at 23 and 24 weeks gestation. Another prostacyclin inhibitory factor has been described in the plasma of a patient with thrombotic thrombocytopenic purpura[83]. This factor, however, is of low molecular weight. Further information will be required in order to evaluate the possible roles of such factors in pregnancy but the potential to regulate the production of such a powerful vasodilator is clearly of significance.

There is little information concerning endogenous stimulants of arachidonate lipoxygenase activities. Nevertheless, it has been shown that human plasma and amniotic fluid contain substances that can stimulate arachidonate-15-lipoxygenase activity[58]. Moreover, it is possible that factors that inhibit prostaglandin biosynthesis at the level of cyclo-oxygenase activity will enhance lipoxygenase product formation by providing more available substrate for lipoxygenase enzymes.

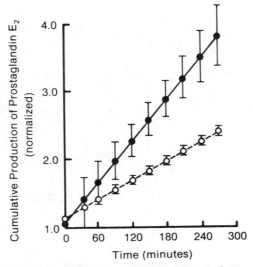

Figure 6.8 Effects of amniotic fluid (AF) on prostaglandin E_2 production by human amnion. Regression lines represent cumulative normalized production of prostaglandin E_2 vs. time after baseline. At time $t = 0$ Medium + AF (30 % v/v) was superfused into test samples. Error bars indicate 95 % confidence limits. Correlation coefficients and regression slopes are:

(●) Medium plus AF $r = 0.67$, df $= 68$, $p < 0.001$
                                  slope $= 1.02 \times 10^{-2}$

(○) Medium alone $r = 0.93$, df $= 68$, $p < 0.001$
                                  slope $= 4.65 \times 10^{-3}$

(from ref. 78, with permission)

EFFECTS OF HORMONES AND OTHER SUBSTANCES

A number of hormones were described earlier that have actions that result in decreased eicosanoid biosynthesis. Glucocorticosteroids are, perhaps, the best known and have the most well characterized mechanism (see earlier section)[35-38]. Relaxin also has been reported to have inhibitory actions on prostaglandin biosynthesis[34] although part of its actions to inhibit uterine activity may result from a stimulatory effect on prostacyclin biosynthesis in myometrium[84]. Prolactin has been suggested to have a key inhibitory influence on prostaglandin biosynthesis in amnion[57]. The source of the prolactin has been suggested to be decidua and it has been shown that disruption of the contact between fetal membranes and decidua will markedly alter amnion prostaglandin production. The latter effect was attributed to the impairment of prolactin transport from decidua to amnion[57,85]. It should be noted that prolactin concentrations in amniotic fluid decline in labour[86] and thus, this forms another potential withdrawal of inhibitors associated with parturition.

Melatonin is an indoleamine that has some structural similarity to indomethacin and was shown recently to inhibit platelet thromboxane biosynthesis[87]. Moreover, it has been demonstrated that melatonin treatment of uterine horns *in vitro* will diminish uterine prostaglandin production[88]. This inhibitory action within the hypothalamo-pituitary axis would be of significance in reproduction because of the effects of prostaglandins on pituitary hormone secretion[89]. One of the hormones that was first established to have an inhibitory effect on prostaglandin biosynthesis within the uterus was progesterone[90] although part of its actions may result from its stimulatory effect on prostaglandin catabolism[91]; the inhibitory action has been suggested to be the result of stabilization of lysosomal membranes with a concomitant decrease in available phospholipase A_2 activity[92]. Progesterone has a slightly more complicated set of actions than simply inhibition of prostaglandin biosynthesis. It has been shown that treatment with progesterone followed by its withdrawal and subsequent oestrogen treatment results in maximal production of prostaglandins[93]. Progesterone, under these conditions, has a priming action with respect to prostaglandin biosynthesis possibly by inducing an accumulation of substrate[94]. Oestrogen alone, however, has stimulatory actions on prostaglandin biosynthesis that can be blocked by concomitant administration of progesterone[95,96]. These actions of progesterone and oestrogen can be discerned both *in vivo* and *in vitro*.

Catecholoestrogens are not only stimulatory of prostaglandin biosynthesis, but also can redirect the pathways in favour of prostaglandin $F_{2\alpha}$ at the expense of prostacyclin[97,98]. Prostaglandins themselves can redirect the eicosanoid pathways in cervical tissue in favour of non cyclo-oxygenase products[61]. Also, prostaglandins can act to promote the mobilization of arachidonic acid and thus provide substrate for even higher rates of prostaglandin biosynthesis[33]. In tissues other than those of the uterus both leukotriene C_4 and D_4 can enhance prostaglandin and thromboxane production[99]. Oxytocin can also act to enhance prostaglandin production both *in vivo* and *in vitro*[28,100]. This action provides two myometrial contractile substances at the same site. Hence, this is a mechanism that may result in the acceleration of labour and may have particular significance for the second and third stages of labour.

Catecholamines have been demonstrated to have actions as cofactors for prostaglandin synthase[2]. Additionally, however, β-adrenergic agents have been demonstrated to mobilize arachidonic acid and thence increase prostaglandin production in amnion[15,101]. Receptors for β-adrenergic agents are present on amnion[102] and catecholamine concentrations in amniotic fluid increase in the third trimester of pregnancy[103,104]. It is uncertain what effects these agents have on myometrial prostaglandin production since in general they are potent inhibitors of uterine contractions.

Two substances that have been shown to be present in amniotic fluid can have highly significant stimulatory actions on prostaglandin biosynthesis. One of these substances is uric acid which likely acts as a hydroxyl radical scavenger and by this action may prolong cyclo-oxygenase activity[105]. The other substance is EGF which was shown to stimulate prostaglandin biosynthesis in a kidney cell line[106], but more recently has been demonstrated to induce massive secretion of prostaglandin E_2 by amnion cells[107]. The latter action is concentration-dependent and has maximal effects in the concentration range found in human amniotic fluid i.e. $1-9$ ng/ml[108]. EGF has other actions

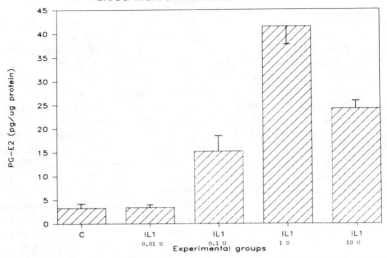

Figure 6.9 The effect of interleukin 1 on prostaglandin E_2 production by amnion cells

that promote lung maturation[109] and increase adrenal steroidogenesis[110]. Hence, this substance has the potential to play an important role in fetal development and parturition.

Infections in pregnancy can lead to labour and delivery of the fetus. The mechanism is unknown. One hypothesis was provided by a study that demonstrated that bacteria have phospholipase activity[111]. Hence, the bacterial infection could provide an enzyme that would act in most tissues to generate substrate for prostaglandin biosynthesis and the prostaglandin formed subsequently would induce labour. Recently, it has been shown that bacterial products will indeed act on amnion tissue to increase greatly prostaglandin E_2 production[112].

Recently, it has been suggested that a host product secreted in response to the bacterial infection could increase prostaglandin production[113]. It was shown that endotoxin added to human amnion cells causes an increase in prostaglandin E_2 production. An even more striking increase in prostaglandin E_2 production can be elicited by conditioned media from monocytes treated with endotoxin. This is a general method for interleukin 1 production. Interleukin 1, in purified form, will induce a concentration-related increase in prostaglandin E_2 production by amnion cells (Figure 6.9)[113]. Hence, it has been suggested that interleukin 1 may mediate the induction of labour associated with intra-amniotic infections.

What other mechanisms can alter eicosanoid biosynthetic pathways? The result of what is presumably such a mechanism is presented in Figure 6.10[114]. In labour there is a preferential drive through the pathways of prostaglandin formation that favours the uterotonic prostaglandins (E_2 and $F_{2\alpha}$) over the myometrial relaxant prostacyclin. A similar mechanism has been suggested to be active during labour in sheep[115]. The factors that cause this effect are unknown although it is known that oestrogens can modify the type of

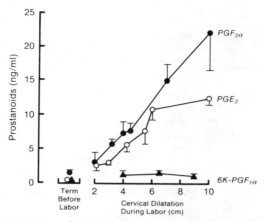

Figure 6.10 Concentrations of prostaglandin E_2 (PGE$_2$), prostaglandin $F_{2\alpha}$(PGF$_{2\alpha}$) and 6-keto-prostaglandin $F_{1\alpha}$ (6K-PGF$_{1\alpha}$) in amniotic fluid of women during late pregnancy and labour at term (after ref. 114, with permission)

prostaglandins formed. Oestrogens also can stimulate not only cyclo-oxygenase activity directly but also lipoxygenase enzyme activities as demonstrated in uterine tissues[116]. Another intriguing possible level of regulation is in the relative utilization of arachidonic acid by the cyclo-oxygenase and lipoxygenase pathways. It has been suggested that labour is associated with a preferential drive of substrate through the cyclo-oxygenase pathway[117].

The production ratio of prostaglandins E_2 and $F_{2\alpha}$ can be influenced by several factors of which NaCl is an example that is of importance for renal function[118]. It has been demonstrated that at least one intrauterine tissue (endometrium/decidua) has prostaglandin-E_2-9-keto-reductase activity[119]. Hence, PGE$_2$ can be converted to PGF$_{2\alpha}$. This action is an attenuation mechanism since PGE$_2$ is ten times more potent than PGF$_{2\alpha}$ in its actions to induce uterine contractions and cervical ripening[120].

FINAL COMMENTS

The regulation of eicosanoid biosynthesis has implications for numerous biological functions. Certainly these regulatory mechanisms play a critical part in the maintenance of pregnancy, cardiovascular adaptations of pregnancy, the onset and progression of labour and many other physiological and pathophysiological events associated with pregnancy. The complexity and variety of points of control in the eicosanoid biosynthetic pathways would seemingly reflect a requirement for precise regulation that may vary between individual eicosanoids and tissues. Our ability to detect certain pathological events and to improve treatment regimes may well be linked closely to an improvement in our understanding of the regulation of eicosanoid biosynthesis during pregnancy and parturition.

ACKNOWLEDGEMENTS

I am grateful for the help and support of my colleagues who have participated in studies which have been described in this chapter. I thank Mrs. Joanne Hall for the typing of this manuscript. My own studies were supported in part by NIH HD 20747 and NIH HD 20779.

REFERENCES

1. Gibson, K.H. (1977). Prostaglandins, thromboxanes, PGX: biosynthetic products from arachidonic acid. *Chem. Soc. Rev.*, **6**, 489–510
2. Samuelsson, B., Goldyne, M., Granstrom, E., Hamberg, M., Hammarstrom, S. and Malmsten, C. (1978). Prostaglandins and thromboxanes. *Annu. Rev. Biochem.*, **47**, 997–1029
3. Lands, W.E.M. (1979). The biosynthesis and metabolism of prostaglandins. *Annu. Rev. Physiol.*, **41**, 633–652
4. Hammarstrom, S. (1983). Leukotrienes, *Annu. Rev. Biochem.*, **52**, 355–377
5. Keirse, M.J.N.C. (1979). Endogenous prostaglandins in human parturition. In Keirse, M.J.N.C., Anderson, A.B.M. and Bennebroek Gravenhorst, J. (eds.) *Human Parturition*, pp. 101–142. (The Hague: Martinus Nijhoff)
6. MacDonald, P.C., Schultz, F.M., Deunhoelter, J.H., Gant, N.F., Jimenez, J.M., Pritchard, J.A., Porter, J.C. and Johnston, J.M. (1974). Initiation of human parturition. I. Mechanism of action of arachidonic acid. *Obstet. Gynecol.*, **44**, 629–636
7. Keirse, M.J.N.C., Hicks, B.R., Mitchell, M.D. and Turnbull, A.C. (1977). Increase of the prostaglandin precursor, arachidonic acid, in amniotic fluid during spontaneous labour. *Br. J. Obstet. Gynaecol.*, **84**, 937–940
8. Schwarz, B.E., Schultz, F.M., MacDonald, P.C. and Johnston, J.M. (1975). Initiation of human parturition: III. Fetal membrane content of prostaglandin E_2 and $F_{2\alpha}$ precursor. *Obstet. Gynecol.*, **46**, 564–568
9. Okita, J.R., MacDonald, P.C. and Johnston, J.M. (1982). Mobilization of arachidonic acid from specific glycerophospholipids of human fetal membranes during early labour. *J. Biol. Chem.*, **257**, 14029–14034
10. Okazaki, T., Okita, J.R., MacDonald, P.C. and Johnston, J.M. (1978). Initiation of human parturition: X. Substrate specificity of phospholipase A_2 in human fetal membranes. *Am. J. Obstet. Gynecol.*, **130**, 432–438
11. DiRenzo, G.C., Johnston, J.M., Okazaki, T., Okita, J.R., MacDonald, P.C. and Bleasdale, J.E. (1981). Phosphatidylinositol-specific phospholipase C in fetal membranes and uterine decidua. *J. Clin. Invest.*, **67**, 847–856
12. Bleasdale, J.E. and Johnston, J.M. (1985). Prostaglandins and human parturition: regulation of arachidonic acid metabolism. In Scarpelli, E.M. and Cosmi, E.V. (eds.) *Reviews in Perinatal Medicine* Vol. 5, pp. 151–191. (New York: Alan R. Liss Inc.)
13. Okazaki, T. Sagawa, N., Bleasdale, J.E., Okita, J.R., MacDonald, P.C. and Johnston, J.M. (1981). Initiation of human parturition: XIII. Phospholipase C, phospholipase A_2, and diacylglycerol lipase activities in fetal membranes and decidua vera tissues from early and late gestation. *Biol. Reprod.*, **25**, 103–109
14. Olson, D.M., Opavsky, M.A. and Challis, J.R.G. (1983). Prostaglandin synthesis by human amnion is dependent upon extracellular calcium. *Can. J. Physiol. Pharmacol*, **61**, 1089–1092
15. Warrick, C., Skinner, K., Mitchell, B.F. and Challis, J.R.G. (1985). Relation between cyclic adenosine monophosphate and prostaglandin output by dispersed cells from human amnion and decidua. *Am. J. Obstet. Gynecol.*, **153**, 66–71
16. Lazebnik, R., Eisenberg, Z., Lazebnik, N., Spirer, Z. and Weisman, Y. (1983). Vitamin D metabolites in amniotic fluid. *J. Clin. Endocrinol. Metab.*, **56**, 632–634
17. Serhan, C.N., Fridovich, J., Goetzl, E.J., Dunham, P.B. and Weissmann, G. (1982). Leukotriene B_4 and phosphatidic acid are calcium ionophores: studies employing arsenazo III in liposomes. *J. Biol. Chem.*, **257**, 4746–4752
18. Mitchell, M.D. (1986). Regulation of eicosanoid biosynthesis in amnion by epidermal

growth factor. Presented at the *Annual Meeting of the Endocrine Society*, June 25–27, Anaheim

19. Mitchell, M.D., Grzyboski, C.F. and Hunter, J.A. (1986). Arachidonic acid (AA) metabolism by lipoxygenase pathways in intrauterine tissues of pregnant women. Presented at the *33rd Annual Meeting of the Society for Gynecologic Investigation*, March 19–22, Toronto

20. Roukin, R., Tense, M., Mencia-Huerta, J.M., Arnoux, B., Ninio, E. and Beneveniste, J. (1983). A chemically defined monokine: Macrophage-derived platelet-activating factor (PAF-Acether). *Lymphokines*, **8**, 240–276

21. Lee, T.-C., Malone, B. and Snyder, F. (1983). Stimulation of calcium uptake by 1-alkyl-2-acetyl-*sn*-glycero-3-phosphocholine (platelet activating factor) in rabbit platelets: possible involvement of the lipoxygenase pathway. *Arch. Biochem. Biophys.*, **223**, 33–39

22. Bonnet, J., Thibaudeau, D. and Bessin, P. (1983). Dependency of the PAF-acether induced bronchospasm on the lipoxygenase pathway in the guinea pig. *Prostaglandins*, **26**, 457–466

23. Billah, M.M. and Johnston, J.M. (1983). Identification of phospholipid platelet-activating factor (1-0-alkyl-2-acetyl-*sn*-glycero-3-phosphocholine) in human amniotic fluid and urine. *Biochem. Biophys. Res. Commun.*, **113**, 51–58

24. Billah, M.M., DiRenzo, G.C., Ban, C., Truong, C.T., Hoffman, D.R., Anceschi, M.M., Bleasdale, J.E. and Johnston, J.M. (1985). Platelet-activating factor metabolism in human amnion and the responses of this tissue to extracellular platelet-activating factor. *Prostaglandins*, **30**, 841–850

25. Nishizuka, Y. (1984). The role of protein kinase C in cell surface signal transduction and tumor promotion. *Nature*, **308**, 693–698

26. Takai, Y., Kishimoto, A., Kawahara, Y., Minakuchi, R., Sano, K., Kikkawa, U., Mori, T., Yu, B., Kaibuchi, K. and Nishizuka, Y. (1981). Calcium and phosphatidylinositol turnover as signalling for trans-membrane control of protein phosphorylation. *Adv. Cyclic. Nucleot. Res.*, **14**, 301–313

27. Okazaki, T., Ban, C. and Johnston, J.M. (1984). The identification and characterization of protein kinase C activity in fetal membranes. *Arch. Biochem. Biophys.*, **229**, 27–32

28. Williams, K.I. and El Tahir, K.E.H. (1980). Effects of uterine stimulant drugs on prostacyclin production by the pregnant rat myometrium I. oxytocin, bradykinin and $PGF_{2\alpha}$. *Prostaglandins*, **19**, 31–38

29. Bareis, D.L., Manganiello, V.C., Hirata, F., Vaughan, M. and Axelrod, J. (1983). Bradykinin stimulates phospholipid methylation, calcium influx, prostaglandin formation and cAMP accumulation in human fibroblasts. *Proc. Natl. Acad. Sci USA*, **80**, 2514–2518

30. Zusman, R.M., Keiser, H.R. and Handler, J.S. (1977). Vasopressin-stimulated prostaglandin E biosynthesis in the toad urinary bladder. *J. Clin. Invest.*, **60**, 1339–1347

31. Danon, A., Chang, L., Sweetman, B., Nies, A. and Oates, J. (1975). Synthesis of prostaglandins by the rat renal papilla in vitro; mechanism of stimulation by angiotensin II. *Biochim. Biophys. Acta*, **388**, 71–83

32. Campos, G.A., Liggins, G.C. and Seamark, R.F. (1980). Differential production of PGF and 6-keto-$PGF_{1\alpha}$ by the rat endometrium in response to oxytocin, catecholamines and calcium ionophore. *Prostaglandins*, **20**, 297–310

33. Hodges, V.A., Treadwell, C.T. and Vahouny, G.V. (1978). Prostaglandin E_2 - induced hydrolysis of cholesterol esters in rat adrenocortical cells. *J. Steroid. Biochem.*, **9**, 1111–1118

34. Williams, K.I. and El Tahir, K.E.H. (1982). Relaxin inhibits prostacyclin release by the rat pregnant myometrium. *Prostaglandins*, **24**, 129–136

35. Flower, R.J. and Blackwell, G.J. (1979). Anti-inflammatory steroids induce biosynthesis of a phospholipase A_2 inhibitor which prevents prostaglandin generation. *Nature*, **278**, 456–459

36. Blackwell, G.J., Carnuccio, R., DiRosa, M., Flower, R.J., Parente, L. and Persico, P. (1980). Macrocortin: a polypeptide causing the antiphospholipase effect of glucocorticoids. *Nature*, **287**, 147–149

37. Hirata, F., Schiffmann, E., Venkatasubramanian, K., Salomon, D. and Axelrod, J. (1980). A phospholipase inhibitory protein in rabbit neutrophils induced by glucocorticoids. *Proc. Natl. Acad. Sci. USA*, **77**, 2533–2536

38. Hirata, F. (1981). The regulation of lipomodulin, a phospholipase inhibitory protein, in rabbit neutrophils by phosphorylation. *J. Biol. Chem.*, **256**, 7730–7733

39. Wallner, B.P., Mattaliano, R.J., Hession, B., Cate, R.L., Tizard, R., Sinclair, L.K., Foeller, C., Pingchang, E., Browning, J.L., Ramachandran, K.L. and Pepinsky, R.B. (1986). Cloning and expression of human lipocortin, a phospholipase A_2 inhibitor with potential anti-inflammatory activity. *Nature*, **320**, 77—81

40. Roscher, A.A. and Rosegger, H. (1983). Effect of meconium and amniotic fluid on activation of phospholipase A_2 in cultured human fibroblasts. *IRCS Med. Sci.*, **11**, 494—495

41. Wilson, T., Liggins, G.C., Aimer, G.P. and Skinner, S.J.M. (1985). Partial purification and characterization of two compounds from amniotic fluid which inhibit phospholipase activity in human endometrial cells. *Biochem. Biophys. Res. Commun.*, **131**, 22—29

42. Manzai, M. and Liggins, G.C. (1984). Inhibitory effects of dispersed amnion cells on production rates of prostaglandin E and F by endometrial cells. *Prostaglandins*, **28**, 297—307

43. Robinson, J.S., Chapman, R.L.K., Challis, J.R.G., Mitchell, M.D. and Thorburn, G.D. (1978). Extra-amniotic arachidonic acid administration and the suppression of uterine prostaglandin synthesis during pregnancy in the rhesus monkey. *J. Reprod. Fertil.*, **54**, 369—373

44. Maathuis, J.B. and Kelly, R.W. (1978). Concentrations of prostaglandins $F_{2\alpha}$ and E_2 in endometrium throughout the human menstrual cycle, after the administration of clomiphene or an oestrogen-progestogen pill and in early pregnancy. *J. Endocrinol.*, **77**, 361—371

45. Saeed, S.A., McDonald-Gibson, W.J., Cuthbert, J., Copas, J.L., Schneider, C., Gardiner, P.J., Butt, N.M. and Collier, H.O.J. (1977). Endogenous inhibitor of prostaglandin synthetase. *Nature*, **270**, 32—36

46. Brennecke, S.P., Lenton, E.A., Turnbull, A.C. and Mitchell, M.D. (1982). Inhibition of prostaglandin synthase by maternal plasma factors in early human pregnancy. *Br. J. Obstet. Gynaecol.*, **89**, 612—616

47. Brennecke, S.P., Bryce, R.L., Turnbull, A.C. and Mitchell, M.D. (1982). The prostaglandin synthase inhibitory ability of maternal plasma and the onset of labour. *Eur. J. Obstet. Gynec. Reprod. Biol.*, **14**, 81—88

48. Mitchell, M.D., Brennecke, S.P., Denning-Kendall, P.A., McDonald-Gibson, W.J., Saeed, S.A. and Collier, H.O.J. (1981). Comparisons between the abilities of various human and ovine plasmas to inhibit prostaglandin synthesis. *Prostagl. Med.*, **6**, 495—501

49. Mitchell, M.D. (1984). The mechanism(s) of human parturition. *J. Dev. Physiol.*, **6**, 107—118

50. Saeed, S.A., Strickland, D.M., Young, D.C., Dang, A. and Mitchell, M.D. (1982). Inhibition of prostaglandin synthesis by human amniotic fluid: Acute reduction in inhibitory activity of amniotic fluid obtained during labour. *J. Clin. Endocrinol. Metab.*, **55**, 801—803

51. Mortimer, G., Hunter, I.C., Stimson, W.H. and Govan, A.D.T. (1985). A role for amniotic epithelium in control of human parturition. *Lancet*, **1**, 1074—1075

52. Leach-Harper, C.M. and Thorburn, G.D. (1983). Inhibition of prostaglandin synthesis by ovine allantoic fluid: acute reduction in inhibitory activity during late gestation. *Can. J. Physiol. Pharmacol.*, **62**, 1152—1157

53. Shemesh, M., Hansel, W., Strauss, III, J., Rafaeli, A., Lavi, S. and Mileguir, R. (1983). Control of prostanoid synthesis in bovine trophoblast and placentome. *Anim. Reprod. Sci.*, **10**, 1—18

54. Shemesh, M., Hansel, W. and Strauss,III,J.F. (1984). Modulation of bovine placental prostaglandin synthesis by an endogenous inhibitor. *Endocrinology*, **115**, 1401—1405

55. Moore, P.K. and Hoult, J.R.S. (1980). Anti-inflammatory steroids reduce tissue PG synthetase activity and enhance PG breakdown. *Nature*, **288**, 269—270

56. Moore, P.K. and Hoult, J.R.S. (1980). Pathophysiological states modify levels in rat plasma of factors which inhibit synthesis and enhance breakdown of PG. *Nature*, **288**, 271—279

57. Tyson, J.E., McCoshen, J.A. and Dubin, N.H. (1985). Inhibition of fetal membrane prostaglandin production by prolactin: relative importance in the initiation of labour. *Am. J. Obstet. Gynecol.*, **151**, 1032—1038

58. Mitchell, M.D. and Corbin, J. (1985). Arachidonate lipoxygenase activity modulating factors in human plasma and amniotic fluid. *Prostagl. Leukotr. Med.*, **17**, 359—364

59. Funk, M.O., Kim, S.H.S. and Alteneder, A.W. (1981). Factors affecting the initial rate of lipoxygenase catalysis. *Biochem. Biophys. Res. Commun.*, **98**, 922—929

60. Vanderhoek, J.Y., Bryant, R.W. and Bailey, J.M. (1980). Inhibition of leukotriene biosynthesis by the leukocyte product 15-hydroxy-5,8,11,13-eicosatetraenoic acid. *J. Biol. Chem.*, **255**, 10 064–10 066

61. Christenson, N.J. and Bygdeman, M. (1985). The effect of prostaglandins on the bioconversion of arachidonic acid in cervical tissue in early human pregnancy. *Prostaglandins*, **29**, 291–302

62. Goodman, R.P., Killiam, A.P., Brash, A.R. and Branch, R.A. (1982). Prostacyclin production during pregnancy: comparison of production during normal pregnancy and pregnancy complicated by hypertension. *Am. J. Obstet. Gynecol.*, **142**, 817–822

63. Makila, U.M., Viinikka, L. and Ylikorkala, O. (1984). Evidence that prostacyclin deficiency is a specific feature in preeclampsia. *Am. J. Obstet. Gynecol.*, **148**, 772–774

64. Saeed, S.A. and Mitchell, M.D. (1983). Lipoxygenase activity in human uterine and intrauterine tissues: new prospects for control of prostacyclin production in pre-eclampsia. *Clin. Exp. Hyperten., Part B.*, **82**, 103–111

65. Moncada, S., Gryglewski, R., Bunting, S. and Vane, J.R. (1976). A lipid peroxide inhibits the enzyme in blood vessel microsomes that generates from prostaglandin endoperoxides the substance (prostaglandin X) which prevents platelet aggregation. *Prostaglandins*, **12**, 715–737

66. Turk, J., Wyche, A. and Needleman, P. (1980). Inactivation of prostacyclin synthetase by platelet lipoxygenase products. *Biochem. Biophys. Res. Commun.*, **95**, 1628–1634

67. Yamarja Setty, B.N. and Stuart, M.J. (1986). 15-hydroxy-5,8,11,13-eicosatetraenoic acid inhibits human vascular cyclooxygenase: Potential role in diabetic vascular disease. *J. Clin. Invest.*, **77**, 202–211

68. Strickland, D.M., Saeed, S.A., Casey, M.L. and Mitchell, M.D. (1983). Stimulation of prostaglandin biosynthesis by urine of the human fetus may serve as a trigger for parturition. *Science*, **220**, 521–522

69. Mitchell, M.D., Craig, D.A., Saeed, S.A. and Strickland, D.M. (1985). Endogenous stimulant of prostaglandin endoperoxide synthase activity in human amniotic fluid. *Biochem. Biophys. Acta.*, **833**, 379–385

70. Cohen, D.K., Craig, D.A., Strickland, D.M., McCubbin, J.H. and Mitchell, M.D. (1985). Prostaglandin biosynthesis stimulatory and inhibitory substances in human amniotic fluid during pregnancy and labour. *Prostaglandins*, **30**, 13–20

71. Saeed, S.A. and Mitchell, M.D. (1982). Stimulants of prostaglandin biosynthesis in human fetal membranes, uterine decidua vera and placenta. *Prostaglandins*, **24**, 475–484

72. Samuelsson, B. (1973). Biosynthesis and metabolism of prostaglandins. *Prog. Biochem. Pharmacol.*, **13**, 59–70

73. Samuelsson, B. (1973). Biosynthesis and metabolism of prostaglandins. In *Les Prostaglandines*, pp. 21–41. (Paris: INSERM)

74. Dembele-Duchesne, M.J., Thaler-Dao, H., Chavis, C. and Crastes-de-Paulet, A. (1981). Some new prospects in the mechanism of control of arachidonate metabolism in human placenta and amnion. *Prostaglandins*, **22**, 979–1002

75. Casey, M.L., MacDonald, P.C. and Mitchell, M.D. (1983). Stimulation of prostaglandin E$_2$ production in amnion cells in culture by a substance(s) in human fetal and adult urine. *Biochem. Biophys. Res. Commun.*, **114**, 1056–1063

76. Berchuck, A., Casey, M.L., Mitchell, M.D. and MacDonald, P.C. (1985). The PGE synthesis stimulatory substance (PSSS) in fetal urine is a transforming growth factor. Presented at the *32nd Annual Meeting of the Society for Gynecologic Investigation*, March 20–23, Phoenix

77. Mitchell, M.D., MacDonald, P.C. and Casey, M.L. (1984). Stimulation of prostaglandin E$_2$ synthesis in human amnion cells maintained in monolayer culture by a substance(s) in amniotic fluid. *Prostagl. Leukotr. Med.*, **15**, 399–407

78. Strickland, D.M. and Mitchell, M.D. (1986). Stimulation of PGE production in superfused human amnion by human amniotic fluid. *Gynecol. Obstet. Invest.*, (In press)

79. Rehnstrom, J., Ishikawa, M., Fuchs, F. and Fuchs, A.-R. (1983). Stimulation of myometrial and decidual prostaglandin production by amniotic fluid from term, but not mid trimester pregnancies. *Prostaglandins*, **26**, 973–981

80. Remuzzi, G., Zoja, C., Marchesi, D., Schieppati, A., Mecca, G., Mirsiani, R., Donati, M.B. and DeGaetano, G. (1981). Plasmatic regulation of vascular prostacyclin in pregnancy. *Br. Med. J.*, **282**, 512–514

81. Dadak, C., Hoche, C. and Sinzinger, H. (1984). Prostacyclin synthesis stimulating plasma factor in pregnancy and puerperium. *Obstet. Gynecol.,* **64,** 72–76

82. Carreras, L.O., Machin, S.J., Deman, R., Defreyn, G., Vermylen, J., Spitz, B. and Van Assche, A. (1981). Arterial thrombosis, intrauterine death and 'lupus' anticoagulant: detection of immunoglobulin interfering with prostacyclin formation. *Lancet,* **1,** 244–246

83. Machin, S.J., Very, B.A., Parry, H. and Marrow, W.J.W. (1982). A plasma factor inhibiting prostacyclin-like activity in thrombotic-thrombocytopenic purpura. *Acta Haematol.,* **67,** 8–12

84. Richardson, M., Mitchell, M.D., MacDonald, P.C. and Casey, M.L. (1984). Effect of relaxin on prostacyclin production by human myometrial cells in monolayer culture. Presented at the *31st Annual Meeting of the Society for Gynecologic Investigation,* March 21–24, San Francisco

85. McCoshen, J.A., Tagger, O.Y., Wodzicki, A. and Tyson, J.E. (1982). Choriodecidual adhesion promotes decidual prolactin transport by human fetal membrane. *Am. J. Physiol.,* **243,** R552–R557

86. Rigg, L.A. and Yen, S.S.C. (1977). Multiphasic prolactin secretion during parturition in human subjects. *Am. J. Obstet. Gynecol.,* **128,** 215–218

87. Leach, C.M. and Thorburn, G.D. (1980). A comparison of the inhibitory effects of melatonin and indomethacin on platelet aggregation and thromboxane release. *Prostaglandins,* **20,** 51–56

88. Gimeno, M.F., Landia, A., Sterin-Speziale, N., Cardinal, D.P. and Gimeno, A.L. (1980). Melatonin blocks in vitro generation of prostaglandin by the uterus and hypothalamus. *Eur. J. Pharmacol.,* **62,** 309–317

89. Behrman, H.R. (1979). Prostaglandins in hypothalamo-pituitary and ovarian function. *Annu. Rev. Physiol.,* **41,** 685–700

90. Blatchley, F.R. and Poyser, N.L. (1974). The effect of oestrogen and progesterone on the release of prostaglandins from the uterus of the ovariectomised guinea-pig. *J. Reprod. Fertil.,* **40,** 205–209

91. Bedwani, J.R. and Marley, P.B. (1975). Enhanced inactivation of prostaglandin E_2 by the rabbit lung during pregnancy or progesterone treatment. *Br. J.Pharmacol.,* **53,** 547–554

92. Szego, C.M. (1974). The lysosome as a mediator of hormone action. *Rec. Prog. Horm. Res.,* **30,** 171–233

93. Louis, T.M., Parry, D.M., Robinson, J.S., Thorburn, G.D. and Challis, J.R.G. (1977). Effects of exogenous progesterone and oestradiol on prostaglandin F and 13,14-dihydro-15-oxo-prostaglandin $F_{2\alpha}$ concentrations in uteri and plasma of ovariectomized ewes. *J. Endocrinol.,* **73,** 427–439

94. Brinsfield, T.H. and Hawk, H.W. (1973). Control by progesterone of the concentration of lipid droplets in epithelial cells of the sheep endometrium. *J. Anim. Sci.,* **36,** 919–922

95. Pakrasi, P.L., Cheng, H.C. and Dey, S.K. (1983). Prostaglandins in the uterus: Modulation by steroid hormones. *Prostaglandins,* **26,** 991–1009

96. Abel, M. and Baird, D.T. (1980). The effect of 17β-estradiol and progesterone on prostaglandin production by human endometrium maintained in organ culture. *Endocrinology,* **106,** 1599–1606

97. Kelly, R.W. and Abel, M.H. (1980). Catechol oestrogens stimulate and direct prostaglandin synthesis. *Prostaglandins,* **20,** 613–626

98. Needleman, S.W. and Parks, W.M. (1982). Catechol oestrogens and thrombosis: differential effect of 2-hydroxyestradiol and estradiol on prostacyclin release. *Prostaglandins,* **26,** 317–320

99. Omini, C., Folco, G.C., Vigano, T., Rossoni, G. and Berti, F. (1981). Leukotriene-C_4 induces generation of PGI_2 and TxA_2 in guinea-pig in vivo. *Pharmacol. Res. Comm.,* **13,** 633–640

100. Mitchell, M.D., Flint, A.P.F. and Turnbull, A.C. (1975). Stimulation by oxytocin of prostaglandin F levels in uterine venous effluent in pregnant and puerperal sheep. *Prostaglandins,* **9,** 47–56

101. Di Renzo, G.C., Anceschi, M.M. and Bleasdale, J.E. (1984). Beta-adrenergic stimulation of prostaglandin production by human amnion tissue. *Prostaglandins,* **27,** 37–49

102. Di Renzo, G.C., Venincasa, M.D. and Bleasdale, J.E. (1984). The identification and characterization of β-adrenergic receptors in human amnion tissue. *Am. J. Obstet. Gynecol.,* **148,** 398–405

103. Phillippe, M. and Ryan, K.J. (1981). Catecholamines in human amniotic fluid. *Am. J. Obstet. Gynecol.*, **139**, 204–208
104. Divers, W.A., Wilks, M.M., Babaknia, A. and Yen, S.S.C. (1981). An increase in catecholamines and metabolites in the amniotic fluid compartment from middle to late gestation. *Am. J. Obstet. Gynecol.*, **139**, 483–486
105. Deby, C. and Deby-Dupont, G. (1981). Mechanism of intervention of uric acid metabolism in PG biosynthesis. *Agents Actions*, **11**, 651–652
106. Levine, L. and Hassid, A. (1977). Epidermal growth factor stimulates prostaglandin biosynthesis by canine kidney (MDCK) cells. *Biochem. Biophys. Res. Commun.*, **76**, 1181–1187
107. Mitchell, M.D. and Casey, M.L. (1984). Role of growth factors in PGE formation in human amnion cells in monolayer culture. Presented at the *31st Annual Meeting of the Society for Gynecologic Investigation*, March 21–24, San Francisco
108. Ladda, R.L., Bullock, L.P., Giannopoulos, T. and McCormick, L. (1979). Radioreceptor assay for epidermal growth factor. *Anal. Biochem.*, **93**, 286–294
109. Sundell, H.W., Gray, M.E., Serenius, F.S., Escobedo, M.B. and Stahlman, M.T. (1980). Effects of epidermal growth factor on lung maturation in fetal lambs. *Am. J. Pathol.*, **100**, 707–726
110. Singh-Asa, P. and Waters, M.J. (1983). Stimulation of cortisol biosynthesis by epidermal growth factor. *Mol. Cell. Endocrinol.*, **30**, 189–199
111. Bejar, R., Curbelo, V., Danes, C. and Gluck, L. (1981). Premature labour. II. Bacterial sources of phospholipase. *Obstet. Gynecol.*, **57**, 479–482
112. Lamont, R.F., Rose, M. and Elder, M.J. (1985). Effect of bacterial products on prostaglandin E production by amnion cells. *Lancet*, **2**, 1331–1333
113. Romero, R., Durum, S., Dinarello, C., Hobbins, J.C. and Mitchell, M.D. (1986). Cellular and biochemical mechanisms for the onset of labor in intraamniotic infections. Presented at the *6th Annual Meeting of the Society of Perinatal Obstetricians*, January 30–31, San Antonio
114. Mitchell, M.D. (1981). Prostaglandins during pregnancy and the perinatal period. *J. Reprod. Fertil.*, **62**, 305–315
115. Challis, J.R.G. (1985). Factors responsible for parturition. In Beard, R.W. and Sharp, F. (eds.) *Preterm Labour and its Consequences*, pp. 61–69. (London: Royal College of Obstetricians and Gynaecologists)
116. Guivernau, M., Terragno, A. and Terragno, N.A. (1981). Estrogens induce lipoxygenase pathway activation in two target organs, uterus and gingival tissue. Presented at an *International Conference on Leukotrienes and other Lipoxygenase Products*, May, Florence
117. Myatt, L., Rose, M.P. and Elder, M.G. (1985). Lipoxygenase products of arachidonic acid in human fetal membranes. Presented at the *32nd Annual Meeting of the Society for Gynecologic Investigation*, March 20–23, Phoenix
118. Weber, P.C., Larson, C. and Scherer, B. (1977). Prostaglandin E_2-9-ketoreductase as a mediator of salt intake-related prostaglandin–renin interaction. *Nature*, **266**, 65–66
119. Schlegel, W., Kruger, S. and Korte, K. (1986). Purification of prostaglandin E_2-9-oxo-reductase from human decidua vera. *FEBS Lett.*, **171**, 141–144
120. Thiery, M. (1979). Induction of labor with prostaglandins. In Keirse, M.J.N.C., Anderson, A.B.M. and Bennebroek-Gravenhorst, J. (eds.) *Human Parturition*, pp. 155–164. (The Hague: Martinus Nijhoff)

7
Eicosanoids and pregnancy-related hypertension

S. W. Walsh

INTRODUCTION

Pregnancy-related hypertension, or pre-eclampsia, is considered one of the most significant health problems in human pregnancy[1-5]. It complicates approximately 5% of pregnancies, and is a leading cause of fetal growth retardation, indicated premature delivery and maternal death. It is primarily characterized by proteinuria and increased vasoconstriction leading to maternal hypertension and reduced uteroplacental blood flow. Platelet aggregation, thrombocytopenia, anasarca and hyperreflexia, occasionally manifested as convulsions (eclampsia), may be associated with the disease process. Because pre-eclampsia only occurs during pregnancy or in the presence of placental tissue (i.e. hydatidiform mole)[5] it is logical that the causative factors of pre-eclampsia originate in the placenta. Few investigators, however, have concentrated their efforts on placental production of chemical messengers that could cause the clinical disorders of pre-eclampsia.

CARDIOVASCULAR AND HORMONAL CHANGES IN PREGNANCY-RELATED HYPERTENSION

A number of cardiovascular changes normally occur during human pregnancy[6]. Heart rate increases by 10–15 %, cardiac output by 30–50%, and blood volume by up to 48%. Blood pressure changes are small in normotensive women, but generally there is a slight decrease of 2–3 mmHg in systolic and 5–10 mmHg in diastolic pressures. Normal blood pressures during the third trimester average 95/50 mmHg in a lateral position and 106/65 mmHg in a supine position. Women with essential hypertension may actually show a significant decrease in blood pressure during the first two trimesters. These facts indicate that normal pregnancy is associated with an increase in the production of a vasodilatory agent.

Pregnancy-related hypertension is characterized by the development of hypertension (maternal systemic arterial blood pressure $\geq 140/90$ mmHg) and proteinuria (urinary protein > 0.3 g/d) during pregnancy or in the early puerperium in women who were normotensive before the pregnancy[1-5]. Blood pressure usually returns to normotensive levels within 10 days following parturition. The aetiology of pregnancy-related hypertension is not known but it is likely due, in part, to a decreased production of a vasodilator.

The plasma concentrations of a number of hormones have been determined in pregnancy-related hypertension, but the changes or lack of changes do not provide any easy explanations to account for the clinical symptoms of this disorder. One might expect an increase in hypertensive hormones but this does not occur. The renin–angiotensin system is paradoxically suppressed. Renin activity, aldosterone levels and angiotensinase activity are usually lower than during normal pregnancy[2,7]. There are no differences in the plasma concentrations of renin substrate, progesterone, cortisol, corticosterone or antidiuretic hormone (ADH) between normal and pre-eclamptic pregnancies. Urinary levels of epinephrine and norepinephrine are increased in pre-eclamptic patients[2] but plasma catecholamine levels are not[7].

Angiotensin II levels in the plasma are increased over the non-pregnant state in both normal and pre-eclamptic pregnancies[2], but the vascular responsiveness to angiotensin II is greatly increased in pre-eclampsia so this hormone may have a role in the vasoconstriction of pregnancy-related hypertension. The classic work of Gant and associates[8] demonstrated that the dose of angiotensin II required to elicit a pressor response of 20 mmHg in diastolic blood pressure was significantly less than normal as early as the 23–26 weeks of pregnancy in women destined to develop hypertension. This study is significant for at least two reasons. One, it demonstrated the increased vascular responsiveness of pre-eclamptic women, and two, it showed that this increased responsiveness was present as early as the second trimester, long before any clinical symptoms were manifest.

The mechanism for the increased responsiveness is not known, but it has been suggested that defective prostaglandin production or a loss of response to prostaglandins contributes to the development of pregnancy-related hypertension[2,9,10]. Everett and colleagues[9] showed that the dose of angiotensin II necessary to cause a 20 mmHg rise in diastolic blood pressure in pregnant women was significantly reduced in women treated with prostaglandin synthetase inhibitors. In other words, by inhibiting prostaglandin synthesis the investigators mimicked the increased vascular responsiveness of pre-eclampsia.

PROSTAGLANDINS E AND F

Because of the vascular effects of prostaglandins E and F, the initial eicosanoid studies focused on these prostanoids as causative agents in pregnancy-related hypertension. Prostaglandin E_2 (PGE_2) is a vasodilator and prostaglandin $F_{2\alpha}$ ($PGF_{2\alpha}$) is a vasoconstrictor, so a decrease in PGE_2 and/or an increase in $PGF_{2\alpha}$ production during pregnancy would contribute to the development of hypertension. Unfortunately, the data published on them for pre-eclampsia are inconsistent and conflicting. Demers and Gabbe[11] measured placental tissue levels and found PGE_2 levels were reduced while PGF levels were elevated in pre-eclampsia as compared to normal pregnancy. Robinson and co-workers[12] also measured placental tissue levels and reported that both PGE and PGF were decreased in women with pre-eclampsia. Hillier and Smith[13] on the other hand, found no difference between normal and pre-eclamptic placentas with respect to the levels of these prostanoids. Pedersen et al.[7] measured urinary concentrations of PGE and PGF. They reported that the concentrations of both were higher during normal pregnancy when compared to the nonpregnant state, but that in pre-eclamptic pregnancy the urinary concentrations of PGE but not PGF were reduced. To add even more confusion, Valenzuela et al.[14] found the plasma levels of both PGE and PGF were increased in patients with pregnancy related hypertension. The inconsistencies in the information for prostaglandins E and F make it difficult to formulate a consistent hypothesis with respect to them as causal agents in pre-eclampsia.

PROSTACYCLIN

Prostacyclin is a potent vasodilator, an inhibitor of platelet aggregation[15-17], and an inhibitor of uterine contractility[18-20], so its combined effects would seem to favour increased uteroplacental blood flow. A deficiency in its production during pregnancy would contribute to the clinical manifestations of pre-eclampsia. The role of prostacyclin in pregnancy has been extensively reviewed[21]. During normal pregnancy the production of prostacyclin is increased because maternal plasma concentrations of its stable metabolite, 6-keto-prostaglandin $F_{1\alpha}$ (6-keto-$PGF_{1\alpha}$), as well as its urinary metabolites, are higher during late pregnancy than during early pregnancy or the non-pregnant state[22-24]. Various tissues of human pregnancy are known to produce prostacyclin, such as the placenta[25-33]; umbilical, placental and uterine vessels[29,34-37]; ductus arteriosus[35]; amnion, chorion and decidua[26,29,32]; and myometrium[18,38].

A considerable amount of data indicates that prostacyclin production is decreased in pre-eclampsia. The first evidence came in 1980 from studies on vascular tissues by Remuzzi et al.[39], Bussolino et al.[40] and Downing et al.[41]. Remuzzi and colleagues[39] reported that prostacyclin production was decreased in umbilical arteries and placental veins obtained from five patients with severe pre-eclampsia. Bussolino et al.[40] examined vascular prostacyclin production in vessels obtained from normal and pre-eclamptic pregnancies. They found that prostacyclin production was decreased in placental veins, subcutaneous vessels and uterine vessels in severely pre-eclamptic patients. Downing et al.[41] examined the enzymatic kinetics of prostacyclin synthase in umbilical arteries. They found that the enzyme activity was the same in normal and hypertensive cords but the hypertensive cords contained less enzyme. Additional studies confirmed the decreased vascular production of prostacyclin in hypertensive pregnancies[42-44]. Prostacyclin production is, therefore, decreased in umbilical arteries, placental veins, uterine vessels and subcutaneous vessels obtained from pre-eclamptic women as compared to normally pregnant women.

Other studies also confirm decreased prostacyclin production in pre-eclampsia. For example, urinary metabolite concentrations are depressed[23] as are amniotic fluid concentrations of prostacyclin's stable metabolite, 6-keto-$PGF_{1\alpha}$[45] and amniotic fluid concentrations of prostacyclin-like activity[46]. Plasma levels of prostacyclin in pre-eclampsia have been reported to be decreased[47,48], unchanged[49] or increased compared to normal pregnancy[50]. However, there is considerable controversy as to the plasma concentrations of prostacyclin and whether it is a circulating hormone[51-58].

Prostacyclin was first identified in the human placenta by Myatt and Elder[25] and subsequently confirmed by others[26-33]. Placental prostacyclin is present early in gestation and increases sharply between weeks 6-12 of pregnancy[28]. We were the first to report in 1983 that placental production of prostacyclin is significantly decreased in pre-eclampsia (Figure 7.1)[59,32,33]. Placental prostacyclin production is also decreased in pregnancies complicated by fetal growth retardation[43,60,61]. The significance of placentally produced prostacyclin should not be underestimated. Although prostacyclin production rates by umbilical vessels, for example, are several fold higher than by whole placental tissues when expressed on a per mg basis, this does not diminish the potential role of placentally produced prostacyclin to locally inhibit platelet aggregation and maintain placental vascular vasodilatation. Comparison of production rates on a per mg whole tissue basis between a purely vascular tissue and the placenta is misleading because the placenta is composed of several different tissues, including trophoblast, stroma and vascular tissue. Prostacyclin is likely produced primarily by the endothelial cells of the placental vessels, but the trophoblast also produces prostacyclin[28,60,61]. Although the production rate is small when expressed per mg of wet tissue per hour, the large placental mass makes it a formidable endocrine organ during pregnancy. A placental production rate of 6.7 to 7.2 pg mg h is equivalent to approximately 94 to 97 μ g per placenta per day[32,33]. This is certainly a high enough production rate to produce physiological effects, and to affect fetal and/or maternal circulating levels provided the placenta or lungs do not first bind or metabolize the prostacyclin.

An alternative hypothesis to placentally produced prostacyclin being a circulating hormone is that the placenta produces chemical messengers that do circulate and stimulate prostacyclin production locally in various tissues of the body. A deficiency in the placental production of these messengers in pre-eclampsia would, therefore, cause decreased prostacyclin production in extra-placental tissues, as well as in the placenta. With less prostacyclin being produced in pre-eclampsia, the vasoconstrictor effects of angiotensin II, thromboxane and catecholamines would not be efficiently opposed leading to hypertension. The renin-angiotensin system is paradoxically suppressed in pre-eclampsia but angiotensin II levels are still elevated over the non-pregnant state[2,7]. Prostacyclin stimulates this system[62,63] so defective prostacyclin production might also explain why angiotensin II levels are lower in pre-eclampsia than in normal pregnancy.

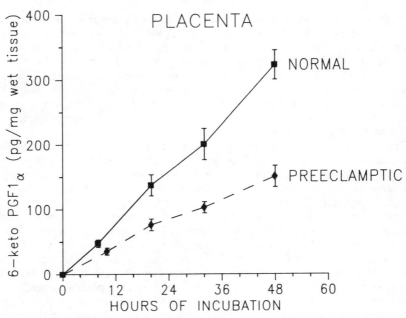

Figure 7.1 Production rates of prostacyclin by normal and pre-eclamptic term placental tissues, as estimated by the concentrations of its stable metabolite, 6-keto prostaglandin $F_{1\alpha}$, in the incubation media. Pre-eclamptic vs. normal production rate = 3.0 ± 0.3 vs 6.7 ± 0.5 pg/mg wet tissue/h, $p < 0.001$, or 44 μg/day vs. 97 μg/day. Data represent mean $\pm$ SE ($n = 10$ vs. 11). From Walsh, S.W., *Am. J. Obstet. Gynecol.*, **152**, 335–340, 1985

THROMBOXANE

The production of thromboxane is increased during normal pregnancy because maternal plasma levels of its stable metabolite, thromboxane B_2 (TxB$_2$), are higher during late pregnancy than during mid pregnancy or the non-pregnant state[64,65]. Thromboxane opposes the actions of prostacyclin. Thromboxane is a potent vasoconstrictor, a stimulator of platelet aggregation[15–17] and a stimulator of uterine contractility[19]. Its combined actions would presumably lead to a decrease in uteroplacental blood flow. It occurred to us that the deficiency in prostacyclin production by pre-eclamptic placentas could be coupled to enhanced production of thromboxane similar to the imbalances in these eicosanoids that have been suggested for other pathological states[15,66]. Since the placenta was known to produce thromboxane[64], we investigated the simultaneous production rates of prostacyclin and thromboxane in normal and pre-eclamptic placentas. In the spring of 1984 we presented the first evidence that a production imbalance exists in the pre-eclamptic placenta for these eicosanoids[67]. The pre-eclamptic placenta produced over three times as much thromboxane as the normal placenta, but less than one half as much prostacyclin (Figures 7.1 and 7.2). Perhaps even more interesting were the production rate ratios of thromboxane to prostacyclin (Figure 7.3). The normal placenta produced approximately equivalent amounts of thromboxane and prostacyclin so their biological actions on vascular tone, platelet aggregation and uterine contractility would be balanced. The pre-eclamptic placenta, however, produced over seven times as much thromboxane as prostacyclin so the balance of biological actions would be tipped heavily in favour of thromboxane (Figure 7.4)[33]. This imbalance in itself can account for the major clinical symptoms of pre-eclampsia.

The thromboxane study validated the prostacyclin data. Decreased prostacyclin production by the pre-eclamptic placenta could hardly be due to non-specific factors or an overall reduction in metabolic capability of the placenta when thromboxane production was simultaneously increased. To assure we were measuring prostacyclin and thromboxane production rather than tissue release, and to assure that the production rates were not limited by precursor availability, placental tissues were also incubated with indomethacin or arachidonic acid, respectively (Figure 7.5)[32,33]. Indomethacin inhibited prostacyclin and thromboxane production in both normal and pre-eclamptic tissues. Addition of arachidonic acid did not significantly affect prostacyclin or thromboxane production in either normal or pre-eclamptic placentas. These data indicate that the placenta actively produces prostacyclin and thromboxane,

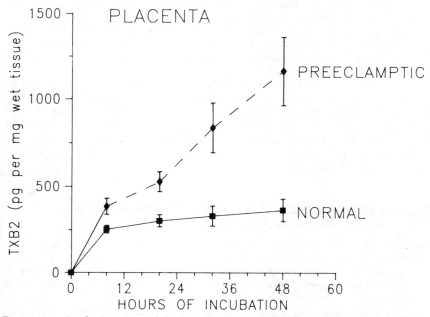

Figure 7.2 Production rates of thromboxane by normal and pre-eclamptic term placental tissues, as estimated by the concentrations of its stable metabolite, thromboxane B_2 (TxB_2), in the incubation media. Pre-eclamptic vs. normal production rate = 22.9 $\pm$ 4.7 vs 6.3 $\pm$ 1.5 pg/mg wet tissue/h, $p < 0.01$, or 335 μg/day vs. 92 μg/day. Data represent mean $\pm$ SE ($n = 10$ vs. 11). From Walsh, S.W., *Am. J. Obstet. Gynecol.*, **152**, 335–340, 1985

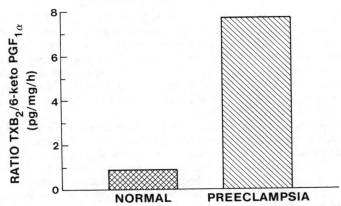

Figure 7.3 Ratios of placental production rates of thromboxane to prostacyclin (TxB$_2$/6)keto PGF$_{1\alpha}$) in normal and pre-eclamptic pregnancies. From Walsh, S.W., *Am. J. Obstet. Gynecol.,* **152**, 335–340, 1985

and that their production rates are not affected by an increased availability of arachidonic acid. Therefore in pre-eclampsia, one cannot explain decreased placental prostacyclin production by deficient arachidonic acid availability, nor can one explain increased thromboxane production by enhanced arachidonic acid availability. Placental prostacyclin and thromboxane production rates are most likely controlled by the amounts or activities of the enzymes necessary for their biosynthesis.

Few research groups have concentrated on simultaneous measurements of prostacyclin and thromboxane in pre-eclampsia. Amniotic fluid levels, umbilical, uterine venous and peripheral plasma levels, and placental release have been determined[30,45,68–70]. In each case the data show an imbalance in the ratio of thromboxane to prostacyclin that favours thromboxane. The thromboxane pathway of platelets is also enhanced in pre-eclamptic women with small-for-gestational age infants[71].

EFFECTS OF PROSTACYCLIN AND THROMBOXANE ON FETOPLACENTAL BLOOD FLOW

Based on the known biological actions of prostacyclin and thromboxane, it is probable that the production imbalance of increased thromboxane/decreased prostacyclin by the pre-eclamptic placenta results in placental vasoconstriction and reduced fetoplacental blood flow. The only information pertaining to the primate placenta, however, is from *in vitro* studies. In experiments using the perfused human placenta, a thromboxane mimic caused vasoconstriction and prostacyclin attenuated the vasoconstrictor effects of angiotensin II when infused into the fetal side of the placenta[72]. In studies using isolated human placental arteries, prostacyclin vasodilated the vessels[73].

The primate placenta is relatively impermeable to transplacental passage

NORMAL PREGNANCY

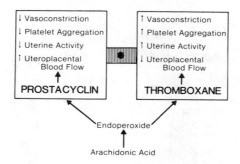

PREECLAMPSIA

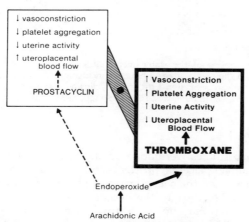

Figure 7.4 Comparison of the balance in the biological actions of prostacyclin and thromboxane in normal pregnancy with the imbalance of increased thromboxane/decreased prostacyclin in pre-eclamptic pregnancy. The heavy type and box for thromboxane suggest an exacerbation of its actions in pre-eclampsia, whereas the lighter type and box for prostacyclin suggest a diminution of its actions. From Walsh, S.W., *Am. J. Obstet. Gynecol.*, **152**, 335–340, 1985

of the eicosanoids. In the study above by Glance and colleagues[72] no placental vascular effects were observed when the cyclo-oxygenase compounds were infused from the maternal side of the placenta indicating that neither prostaglandins nor thromboxane cross from the maternal to the fetal side. This was confirmed by the same investigators in studies using radioactive prostaglandins E_2 and $F_{2\alpha}$[74]. The fact that prostacyclin does not cross the human placenta explains why maternal infusion of prostacyclin does not change fetal or placental blood flow in pre-eclampsia[75], and is ineffective as a treatment for pre-eclampsia[47,76,77]. Maternal prostacyclin infusion treats the mother but not the fetus or placenta.

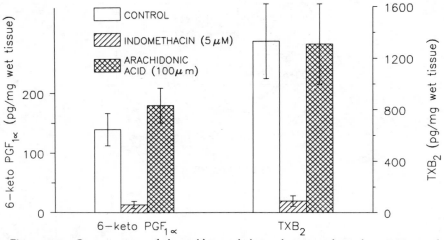

Figure 7.5 Concentrations of the stable metabolites of prostacyclin (6-keto $PGF_{1\alpha}$) and thromboxane (TxB_2) in the media after 48 hours of incubation of term pre-eclamptic placental tissues. Data represent mean $\pm$ SE, $n = 5$ for prostacyclin and $n = 6$ for thromboxane. Modified from Walsh, S.W., *Am. J. Obstet. Gynecol.*, **152**, 335–340, 1985 and Walsh *et al.*, *Am. J. Obstet. Gynecol.*, **151**, 110–115, 1985

The only *in vivo* studies were done on sheep, but contrary to the *in vitro* findings for the human placenta, prostacyclin in conjunction with angiotensin II further vasoconstricted the sheep maternal placenta[78], and had no effect by itself when infused directly into the uterine artery[79]. The maternal placenta of the sheep, however, may not be a good model for the primate placenta because of physiological and/or anatomical differences. The sheep has an epitheliochorial, cotyledonary type of placenta with a distinct maternal placenta. The primate has an haemochorial, discoidal type of placenta with no distinct maternal placenta[80,81]. Teleologically one might consider the maternal cotyledonary placenta of the sheep to be homologous to the decidua of the primate, and the sheep fetal cotyledonary placenta to be homologous to the primate discoidal placenta. If one accepts this reasoning, then in sheep, the fetal rather than the maternal placenta might be the better model for the primate placenta. In one study, a large bolus injection of prostacyclin (180 μg/kg) to the ovine fetus lowered its blood pressure by 30 %, decreased vascular resistance of the fetal membranes but did not significantly change placental vascular resistance[82], perhaps because the fetal placenta was already maximally dilated. Rankin *et al.*[82] found that prostacyclin attenuated the vasoconstrictor effects of norepinephrine in the sheep maternal placenta, but they did not do the same experiment for the fetal placenta. Fetal sheep infusions of thromboxane or leukotrienes have not as yet been done to test their vasoactive effects on the fetal placenta.

The increased vascular congestion and platelet aggregation of human pre-eclamptic placentas[1,2,83,84] might also be explained by the local placental imbalance of increased thromboxane, decreased prostacyclin. Because the human placenta produces these eicosanoids, one would expect their concentrations in the placental vasculature to be considerably higher than in the maternal peripheral circulation leading to an intensification of their effects in the placental blood vessels. In pre-eclampsia, the effects of thromboxane to increase vasoconstriction and platelet aggregation would predominate causing a decrease in placental blood flow (Figure 7.4). *In vivo*, it is probable that the increased platelet aggregation leads to thromboxane concentrations locally in the pre-eclamptic placental vasculature that are higher than those produced by the placenta *in vitro* because platelets produce thromboxane during the aggregation process. Aggregated platelets adhering to placental vascular walls cannot account for the placental thromboxane production *in vitro* because the platelets would have released their thromboxane during the aggregation process. As discussed later, the trophoblast appears to be a rich source of thromboxane in the human placenta.

We have considered placentally produced prostacyclin and thromboxane to be primarily important in the local regulation of uteroplacental blood flow[32,33]. However, systemic effects in the mother and fetus of these placentally produced eicosanoids cannot be ruled out. They are apparently secreted into the maternal and fetal circulations because their concentrations are considerably higher in the uterine and umbilical veins than in the maternal peripheral circulation[69]. In patients with pre-eclampsia an imbalance of increased thromboxane/decreased prostacyclin exists in the vessels draining the placenta, an imbalance that persists in the maternal peripheral circulation[69]. The thromboxane/prostacyclin imbalance of pre-eclampsia could reduce the blood flow from the placenta to the fetus because thromboxane constricts and prostacyclin dilates the umbilical artery[85,86]. Additionally, the distribution of blood flow within the fetus could be altered because the increased ratio of thromboxane to prostacyclin could cause vasoconstriction of the ductus arteriosus and pulmonary vasculature[87–89].

LIPOXYGENASE COMPOUNDS

Prostacyclin and thromboxane are products of the cyclo-oxygenase pathway of arachidonic acid metabolism. Arachidonic acid (or eicosatetraenoic acid) can also be metabolized by the lipoxygenase enzymes leading to the biologically active hydroperoxyeicosatetraenoic acids (HPETEs), hydroxyeicosatetraenoic acids (HETEs) and leukotrienes (LTs) (Figure 7.6). There are at least four lipoxygenase enzymes (5-, 11-, 12- and 15-lipoxygenase). The 5-lipoxygenase is the primary pathway to the leukotrienes. Arachidonic acid is first converted to the HPETEs and then to either HETEs or leukotrienes[90,91]. There is, thus, competition between the cyclo-oxygenase and lipoxygenase pathways for arachidonic acid, and the possibility that imbalances exist in the production of lipoxygenase, as well as cyclo-oxygenase, products in pre-eclampsia.

HUMAN PLACENTA

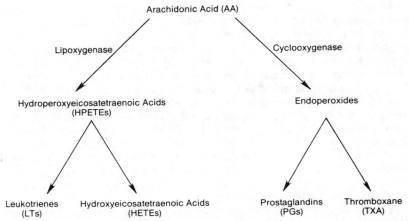

Figure 7.6 Metabolism of arachidonic acid by the cyclo-oxygenase and lipoxygenase pathways. There are at least four lipoxygenase enzymes (5-, 11-, 12- and 15-lipoxygenase). The 5-lipoxygenase is the primary pathway to formation of the leukotrienes

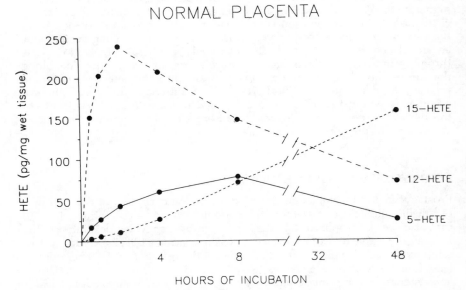

Figure 7.7 Patterns of 5-, 12- and 15-HETE concentrations in the media during 48 hours of incubation of normal human term placental tissues

5-HETE, 12-HETE and LTB$_4$ have been identified by HPLC in the human placenta with the amount of 12-HETE greater than either 5-HETE or LTB$_4$[92,93]. Since placental production rates of lipoxygenase compounds had not previously been determined, we measured the production for three of the HETEs (5-, 12- and 15-HETE) in order to estimate the activities of the 5-, 12- and 15-lipoxygenase enzymes[94]. The normal term placenta produced 5-HETE for the first eight hours of incubation and 12-HETE for the first two hours (Figure 7.7). Production then either stopped or the rate of metabolism exceeded the rate of production for each because their concentrations in the incubation media declined. The production of 15-HETE was different from 5- and 12-HETE, but similar to prostacyclin and thromboxane in that concentrations in the incubation media increased progressively during the entire 48 hours of incubation.

To see if the placental production rates of the HETEs were influenced by precursor availability, arachidonic acid was added to the incubation media. Addition of arachidonate greatly increased 5-, 12- and 15-HETE production[95] but did not prevent the decline in 5- and 12-HETE concentrations by 48 hours of incubation. The results for 5-HETE are shown in Figure 7.8. The human placenta, therefore, contains an abundance of the lipoxygenase enzymes and HETE production can be greatly stimulated by increased availability of precursor. This is in sharp contrast to placental prostacyclin and thromboxane production for which addition of arachidonate does not affect the production rates (Figure 7.5)[32,33]. Therefore, the production rates of prostacyclin and

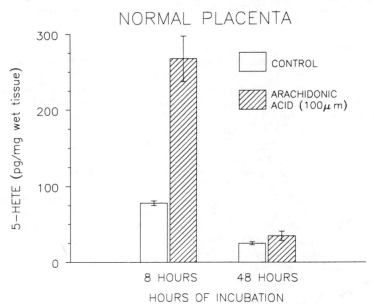

Figure 7.8 Concentrations of 5-HETE in the media after 8 and 48 hours of incubation of human placental tissues with or without arachidonic acid (100 μmol/l). Data represent mean $\pm$ SE, $n = 3$ or 5, respectively

thromboxane in the placenta appear to be enzyme limited, whereas the production rates for the HETEs appear to be precursor limited.

The pattern of 5- and 12-HETE production is interesting in that it was inversely related to the production pattern of 15-HETE, prostacyclin and thromboxane. When concentrations of the latter three compounds were low, concentrations of 5- and 12-HETE were high. But as 15-HETE and cyclo-oxygenase production concentrations increased, 5- and 12-HETE concentrations decreased. The reason for this might, in part, have been the gradually rising levels of 15-HETE in the incubation media. 15-HETE is a potent inhibitor of 5-HETE, 12-HETE and LTB$_4$ production by rabbit polymorphonuclear neutrophils and of 12-HETE, but not thromboxane, production by human platelets[96]. Inhibitory effects of cyclo-oxygenase metabolites on the lipoxygenase enzymes are discussed later.

The physiological functions of the HETEs in the placenta are not known but the HETEs, as well as the HPETEs and leukotrienes, do exert biological actions in other tissues, some of which may be important to placental function and pregnancy. It is known that both 5-HETE and LTB$_4$ stimulate leukocytic chemotaxis and chemokinesis, increase aggregation of leukocytes, stimulate the uptake of calcium and D-glucose by neutrophils and eosinophils, increase bronchial constriction and mucus secretion, increase vasodilatation and enhance vascular permeability[97]. Cardiovascular effects of the leukotrienes are discussed in the next section.

The human placenta, therefore, metabolizes arachidonic acid by both the cyclo-oxygenase and lipoxygenase pathways leading to biologically active compounds that could exert effects locally in the placenta and uterus, and perhaps systemically in the mother and fetus as well. The activities of the two pathways, however, are quite dissimilar. Prostacyclin and thromboxane are produced continually during a 48-hour *in vitro* incubation period. In contrast, 5-HETE and 12-HETE are rapidly produced initially by the placenta with peak concentrations in the incubation media reached at 8 hours and 2 hours, respectively. But then production slows or ceases and the placenta metabolizes the 5- and 12-HETE present since their concentrations gradually decline by 48 hours. This pattern is specific for 5- and 12-HETE because the concentrations of 15-HETE increase gradually over the entire 48-hour incubation period similar to prostacyclin and thromboxane.

The pre-eclamptic placenta produced less 5-HETE and less 12-HETE than the normal placenta at term, but its production of 15-HETE was approximately the same (Figure 7.9). The pre-eclamptic placenta not only produced less 5-HETE but its capacity to produce it was of a shorter duration than the normal placenta. The concentrations of 5-HETE in the incubation media of pre-eclamptic placentas increased for only 2 hours as compared to 8 hours for normal placentas. Production by the pre-eclamptic placenta then dramatically slowed or ceased as concentrations of 5-HETE in the incubation media plateaued to eight hours and then declined. Increased metabolism of 5- and 12-HETE by the pre-eclamptic placenta cannot explain the lower concentrations in the incubation media, because the pre-eclamptic placenta metabolized 5- and 12-HETE at a slower rate than the normal placenta (Figure 7.10). The term pre-eclamptic placenta is, thus, deficient in the 5- and 12-lipoxygenase

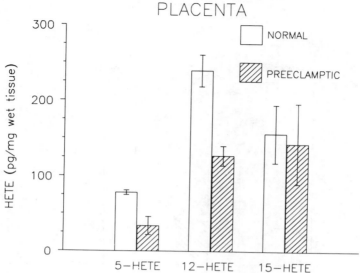

Figure 7.9 Peak concentrations of the HETEs in the incubation media of normal versus pre-eclamptic placentas. 5-HETE concentrations increased until eight hours of incubation and then declined. 12-HETE concentrations increased until two hours and then declined. 15-HETE concentrations continued to increase throughout the entire 48-hour incubation period. Data represent mean ± SE, $n = 4$ for 5-HETE; $n = 10$ vs. 6 for 12-HETE; $n = 5$ vs. 3 for 15-HETE

enzymes.

Deficiency of 5-lipoxygenase may be particularly important because it is the primary enzymatic pathway to the potent, biologically active leukotrienes[90,91]. With respect to pre-eclampsia, deficient placental leukotriene production may contribute to hypertension by depriving the pre-eclamptic patient of placental messengers that normally lower maternal systemic arterial pressure during pregnancy. Both LTC_4 and LTD_4 lower systemic arterial blood pressure in several species[98] including man[99], and injection of LTB_4, LTC_4 or LTD_4 into the lower vena cava to mimic the systemic route of placentally produced hormones lowers both systolic and diastolic blood pressures in pregnant rhesus monkeys (Figure 7.11)[100]. The mechanism of action is not known but it is likely that the leukotrienes stimulate prostacyclin production by endothelial cells either in the lungs or locally in the systemic vasculature, thereby lowering systemic arterial blood pressure. LTC_4 promotes prostacyclin synthesis by human endothelial cells[101], and both LTC_4 and LTD_4 increase prostacyclin release by bovine aortic endothelial cells[102].

Although it might be argued that leukotrienes are local mediators of physiological responses and do not function as circulating hormones, this may not be entirely true during pregnancy because of supplemental production by the placenta. Even small amounts entering the systemic circulation from the placenta could affect maternal cardiovascular status because blood pressure was lowered in pregnant rhesus monkeys with a rather low dose of leukotriene

PLACENTA

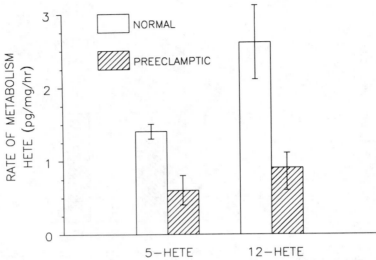

Figure 7.10 Rate of metabolism of 5-HETE and 12-HETE by normal versus pre-eclamptic placentas. Data represent mean ± SE, $n = 4$ for 5-HETE; $n = 10$ vs. 6 for 12-HETE

(0.5 μg/kg), and the effects were manifest with the first passage of leukotriene through the maternal arterial system (i.e. first effects after 20 to 30 seconds) (Figure 7.11)[100]. Apparently, the vascular receptors have a high affinity for leukotrienes and are rapidly responsive to circulating levels. The role of leukotrienes in normal and pre-eclamptic pregnancies, however, is speculative and must be viewed with caution until placental leukotriene production rates and circulating concentrations are determined.

CARDIOVASCULAR EFFECTS OF LEUKOTRIENES

The leukotrienes exert biological actions in various tissues of the body as reviewed by several authors[90,91,98,103–105]. They produce contraction of a number of smooth muscle tissues including the small airways of the lung, the ileum, the stomach, the gallbladder and the uterus. In the cardiovascular system leukotrienes often produce opposite effects in different vascular beds and in different species[98,106]. LTC_4 and LTD_4 produce vasoconstriction and cause plasma leakage in guinea-pig skin and the hamster cheek pouch, but they are potent vasodilators in human skin. Leukotrienes are potent vasoconstrictors in the coronary circulation of guinea-pigs, rats, rabbits, cats, dogs, pigs and sheep. LTC_4 and LTD_4 are the most active. LTB_4 does not appear to affect the coronary circulation in any species. Coronary vasoconstriction reduces the contractile force of the heart leading to a decrease in cardiac output. In some instances leukotrienes might directly affect inotropic

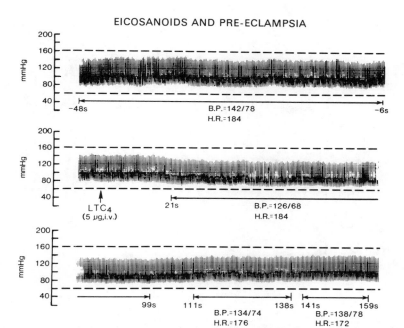

Figure 7.11 Effect of injection of LTC$_4$ (5 μg) into the lower vena cava to mimic the systemic route of placentally produced hormones on maternal systemic arterial blood pressure in the pregnant rhesus monkey. Similar blood pressure lowering effects were observed for LTD$_4$ and LTB$_4$

and chronotropic properties of the heart causing tachycardia and arrythmias[104].

Systemically, LTC$_4$ and LTD$_4$ lower arterial blood pressure in most species[98,106], including man[99]. In male monkeys, LTC$_4$ causes transient pulmonary and systemic hypertension, followed by a prolonged hypotensive period associated with decreased cardiac output[107]. In pregnant and pospartum rhesus monkeys, intravenous infusion of LTB$_4$, LTC$_4$ or LTD$_4$ lowers both systolic and diastolic blood pressures as discussed in the previous section (Figure 7.11)[100], indicating both decreased cardiac output and systemic vasodilatation.

Little is known about the effects of leukotrienes on the fetal or placental vasculatures. In newborn lambs and piglets, LTD$_4$ increases pulmonary and systemic vascular resistance[108,109], whereas blockage of the leukotriene receptors with FPL 57231 decreases pulmonary and systemic arterial pressures in late gestational sheep fetuses[110]. Human newborns with pulmonary hypertension and persistent fetal circulation have LTC$_4$ and LTD$_4$ present in their tracheal lavage, while normal newborns do not[111]. Leukotriene inhibition with the receptor blocker, FPL 57231, increases pulmonary blood flow and decreases pulmonary vascular resistance in fetal lambs[110], and it prevents and reverses hypoxic pulmonary vasoconstriction in newborn lambs[112]. In the rabbit, FPL 55712 dilates the maternal placenta[113].

The mechanisms of action of leukotrienes on the vasculature are poorly understood, but as cited in the review articles referenced above cyclo-oxygenase compounds are often involved as intermediate messengers,

NORMAL PLACENTA

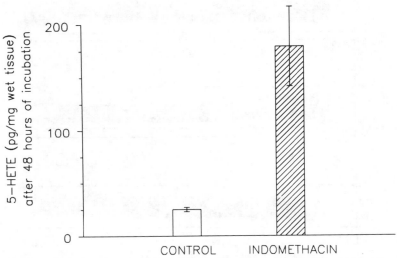

Figure 7.12 5-HETE concentrations in the media after 48 hours of incubation of normal placental tissues either with or without indomethacin. Data represent mean $\pm$ SE, $n = 4$

especially prostacyclin and thromboxane. Indomethacin blocks or attenuates the actions of leukotrienes in various tissues. Human vascular tissues produce thromboxane as well as prostacyclin, although the amount of thromboxane is relatively small compared to prostacyclin[114]. Leukotrienes have been shown to stimulate both prostacyclin[101,102] and thromboxane[115] by vascular tissue, so leukotrienes may vasodilate some vascular beds by stimulating prostacyclin synthesis and vasoconstrict other vascular beds by stimulating thromboxane synthesis. Differential effects may depend on the endogenous amount of leukotriene released or the dose of exogenous leukotriene administered.

REGULATION OF PLACENTAL LIPOXYGENASE COMPOUNDS BY CYCLO-OXYGENASE COMPOUNDS

It is quite possible that one or more of the cyclo-oxygenase metabolites endogenously inhibit the lipoxygenase enzymes in the human placenta. This is suggested by the inverse relationship in the placental incubation concentrations of prostacyclin and thromboxane versus 5- and 12-HETE (Figures 7.1, 7.2, 7.7) and by the fact that the addition of indomethacin to inhibit the cyclo-oxygenase pathway results in greatly increased HETE concentrations in the incubation media[95]. Data for 5-HETE are shown in Figure 7.12. The increased HETE concentrations cannot be explained simply by a shunting of arachidonic acid from the cyclo-oxygenase to the lipoxygenase pathway. Addition of arachidonate increases placental production of the

HETEs, but as long as prostaglandins and thromboxane are present the concentrations of 5- and 12-HETE in the incubation media decline by 48 hours[95] (Figure 7.8). This suggests that cyclo-oxygenase metabolites not only inhibit the lipoxygenase enzymes but also stimulate the metabolism of 5- and 12-HETE.

In other tissues and species there is evidence that the cyclo-oxygenase compounds inhibit lipoxygenase enzymes. For example, in sensitized guinea-pig lungs indomethacin potentiates leukotriene release, as does selective inhibition of thromboxane with imidazole or of prostacyclin with 15-HPETE[116]. Addition of thromboxane B_2 or prostacyclin, on the other hand, inhibits leukotriene release. In these studies PGF and PGE did not have inhibitory effects. In rat peritoneal cells indomethacin increases and prostacyclin, but not thromboxane, inhibits the release of leukotrienes induced by IgG_a[117]. Because the β-receptor agonist, isoprenaline, also inhibits leukotriene release, Burka and Garland[117] suggest the mechanism of prostacyclin inhibition is by increasing c-AMP because c-AMP inhibits the production and release of lipoxygenase compounds[104]. In human polymorphonuclear leukocytes, ibuprofen stimulates 15-HETE but inhibits 5-HETE formation[118].

Indomethacin might affect the placental lipoxygenase pathways by mechanisms other than inhibition of the cyclo-oxygenase enzyme. Indomethacin also inhibits phosphodiesterase[119] which would increase c-AMP levels. Since c-AMP inhibits the lipoxygenase pathway, this mechanism would not explain increased HETE production in the human placenta after indomethacin. Another possible mechanism is that indomethacin might inhibit the placental metabolism of the HETEs thereby leading to increased concentrations. Indomethacin inhibits 15-hydroxyprostaglandin dehydrogenase[120]. This might explain an increase in 15-HETE concentrations, but not increases in 5- and 12-HETE because they do not have an hydroxyl group associated with carbon 15.

REGULATION OF PLACENTAL PROSTACYCLIN AND THROMBOXANE: CAUSES FOR THE IMBALANCE IN PRE-ECLAMPSIA

Steroids

Because the placenta produces both steroids and eicosanoids, it is possible that the local production of oestrogen and progesterone exert autocrine and/or paracrine effects on eicosanoid production. Steroids are known to affect prostaglandin production in reproductive tissues[121] but little is known about their effects in the placenta.

We first determined the production rates of oestradiol and progesterone by whole placental tissues to see if any abnormalities existed in the pre-eclamptic placenta[122]. Tissues were incubated both without and with precursor. Oestradiol production rates were similar in both normal and pre-eclamptic placentas, regardless of whether dehydroepiandrosterone sulphate (DHEAS) (100 μmol/l) was added as a precursor or not. Addition of an aromatase inhibitor along with DHEAS suppressed oestradiol production. Progesterone production was significantly higher in pre-eclamptic placentas than in normal placentas without addition of precursor (Figure 7.13). Incubation with addition of pregnenolone as substrate (100 μmol/l) greatly increased progesterone production and eliminated the difference between normal and pre-eclamptic placentas. Addition of pregnenolone sulphate, however, restored the difference.

The data indicate that progesterone concentrations are significantly higher in the pre-eclamptic placenta than in the normal placenta. One possible explanation is that the pre-eclamptic placenta contains more pregnenolone sulphatase so it converts pregnenolone sulphate more efficiently into progesterone. Another possibility is that the pre-eclamptic placenta contains larger stores of cholesterol than normal. This is suggested by the experiment in which progesterone concentrations were measured without addition of precursor. Perhaps the pre-eclamptic placenta has more LDL receptors than normal so its endogenous stores of cholesterol are increased[123]. Still another possibility is that metabolism of progesterone is decreased in the pre-eclamptic placenta leading to increased concentrations in the incubation media. This might contribute to placental vasoconstriction because one of progesterone's metabolites, 5α-dihydroprogesterone, but not progesterone, antagonizes the vasoconstrictor effects of angiotensin II in women with mild pre-eclampsia[124].

To see if increased progesterone concentrations in the pre-eclamptic placenta might be involved in the imbalance of prostacyclin and thromboxane, we added progesterone alone or with oestradiol to the incubation media and measured eicosanoid production rates[122]. Since maternal circulating levels and urinary metabolites of progesterone are not different between normal and

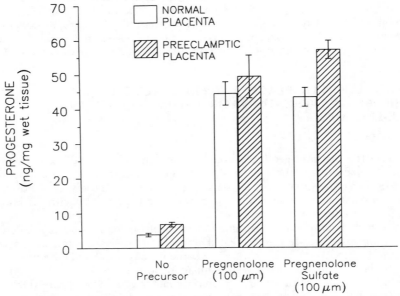

Figure 7.13 Concentrations of progesterone in the media after three hours incubation of placental tissues either with or without precursor added to the incubation media. Data represent mean $\pm$ SE, $n = 8$ for no precursor, $n = 5$ for precursor

pre-eclamptic patients[2,125] we considered that steroidal effects would be exerted locally within the placenta. Because the placenta produces both steroids and eicosanoids, it seemed reasonable that the steroid concentrations within the placenta would be quite high and fully saturate any receptors mediating their effects. For this reason, a relatively high dose of steroid (100 μmol/l) was used. Addition of progesterone significantly decreased prostacyclin production by both normal (Figure 7.14) and pre-eclamptic placentas. Addition of oestradiol alone had no statistically significant effect but combined with progesterone suppressed prostacyclin even more than progesterone alone. Neither steroid significantly affected thromboxane production indicating their effects are specific for prostacyclin. Myatt and associates reported that oestradiol stimulated and progesterone inhibited prostacyclin production by dispersed term placental cells in culture, whereas the combination of oestradiol plus progesterone inhibited prostacyclin[61,126]. This is similar to what we found in the whole tissue incubation studies except oestradiol alone did not increase prostacyclin.

Therefore, one potential explanation for decreased prostacyclin production in pre-eclampsia is that increased placental progesterone concentrations locally suppress its synthesis. The synergistic effect of oestradiol when combined with progesterone is, perhaps in part, due to its ability to increase receptors for progesterone.

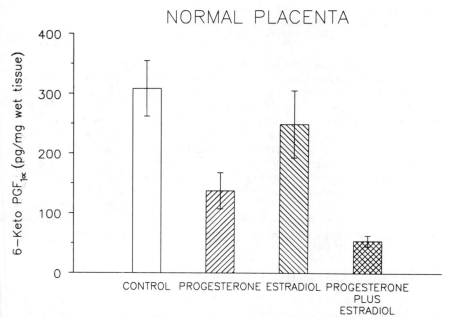

Figure 7.14 Effects of progesterone and oestradiol (100 μmol/l each) on placental production of prostacyclin as estimated by its stable metabolite 6-keto PGF$_{1\alpha}$. Data represent the concentrations in the incubation media after 48 hours of incubation (mean $\pm$ SE, $n = 5$)

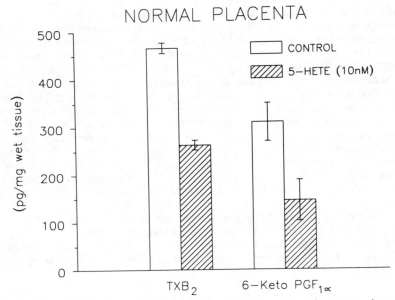

Figure 7.15 5-HETE inhibition of placental prostacyclin and thromboxane production as estimated by their stable metabolites, 6-keto PGF$_{1\alpha}$ and TxB$_2$, respectively. Tissues were incubated for 48 hours. Data represent mean $\pm$ SE, $n = 3$

There are several possible mechanisms for steroidal regulation of eicosanoids. (1) Steroids may influence the rate of metabolic inactivation. Oestrogen and progesterone increase the activity of prostaglandin dehydrogenase (PGDH) in uterine tissues of pseudopregnant rats[127]. Prostacyclin and thromboxane, however, are relatively poor substrates for this enzyme[128,129], and oestrogen and progesterone reportedly inhibit, not stimulate, PGDH in the human placenta[130]. (2) Steroids may regulate the synthesis or activity of inhibitory or stimulatory proteins. The human placenta contains a protein that inhibits prostaglandin synthesis[131] and both stimulatory and inhibitory proteins exist in amniotic fluid[132–135]. (3) Steroids may affect the release of arachidonic acid. Progesterone has been shown to inhibit the release of arachidonic acid from human endometrial and decidual cells[136]. (4) Steroids may directly affect the activity or synthesis of eicosanoid synthases.

Lipoxygenase compounds

Lipoxygenase compounds might also regulate placental prostacyclin and thromboxane production. 12-HPETE inhibits human platelet thromboxane synthase[137], and 15-HPETE inhibits vascular or endothelial cell prostacyclin synthase[15]. 5-HETE inhibits prostacyclin synthesis in the bovine corpus luteum[138], and it inhibits both thromboxane and prostacyclin production in the human placenta (Figure 7.15). Leukotriene receptor blockade increases thromboxane biosynthesis in rat peritoneal mononuclear cells[104]. LTC_4 or LTD_4, on the other hand, stimulate prostacyclin and thromboxane production in the guinea-pig lung[139] and in human and bovine aortic endothelial cells[101,102,115]. These observations demonstrate that lipoxygenase compounds can affect cyclo-oxygenase product production. It may, therefore, be pertinent that 5-HETE and 12-HETE production rates are higher in the normal placenta than in the pre-eclamptic placenta.

Imbalances of the placental lipoxygenase pathways in pre-eclampsia could contribute to the imbalance of increased thromboxane/decreased prostacyclin production if one considers the possibility that eicosanoids are compartmentalized within different tissues of the placenta (Figure 7.16). For example, 5-HETE and thromboxane may be produced primarily by the trophoblastic cells, but prostacyclin primarily by the endothelial cells. In the normal placenta 5-HETE could locally inhibit thromboxane production in the trophoblast without affecting prostacyclin production in the endothelium. In pre-eclampsia the deficit of 5-HETE would allow thromboxane production to increase unchecked. This could explain the progressive increase in thromboxane concentrations in the incubation media of pre-eclamptic placentas and the plateau in concentrations after eight hours of incubation in normal placentas (Figure 7.2)[33].

Compartmentalization of prostacyclin and thromboxane production within the placenta is a reasonable hypothesis supported by preliminary data obtained

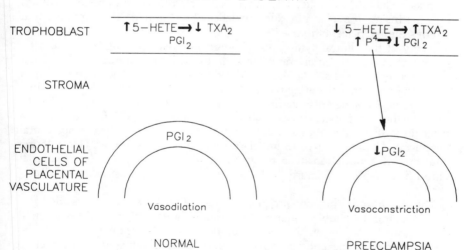

HUMAN PLACENTA

TROPHOBLAST	↑ 5−HETE → ↓ TXA₂ PGI₂	↓ 5−HETE → ↑ TXA₂ ↑ P⁴ → ↓ PGI₂

STROMA

ENDOTHELIAL CELLS OF PLACENTAL VASCULATURE

PGI₂

↓PGI₂

Vasodilation

Vasoconstriction

NORMAL

PREECLAMPSIA

Figure 7.16 Hypothetical model for compartmentalization of eicosanoids within the human placenta, and a possible mechanism for the imbalance of increased thromboxane and decreased prostacyclin production in pre-eclampsia. In the normal placenta 5-HETE suppresses thromboxane (TxA_2) production locally in the trophoblast without affecting prostacyclin (PGI_2) production in the endothelium. In pre-eclampsia decreased 5-HETE concentrations allow thromboxane production to increase unchecked, and increased progesterone (P_4) concentrations inhibit prostacyclin production

in collaboration with Dr D. Michael Nelson at Washington University School of Medicine in St. Louis. Dr Nelson has essentially pure human trophoblastic cell cultures[140] from which we have preliminary measurements of prostacyclin and thromboxane concentrations in the culture media. The trophoblastic cells produced both thromboxane and prostacyclin, but thromboxane concentrations were 10–16 times greater than those for prostacyclin. We have not yet cultured placental endothelial cells, but the placental vessels are known to produce prostacyclin[34,36,39] so if the placental endothelial cells are similar to every other vascular tissue studied they will be the major source of prostacyclin in the placenta.

Prostacyclin and thromboxane are compartmentalized in other areas of the body. In the lung, prostacyclin is produced by the pulmonary vessels (endothelial cells) and thromboxane by the parenchymal tissue (alveolar interstitial cells)[139]. In the general circulation, prostacyclin is produced by endothelial cells of blood vessels and thromboxane by platelets[15–17].

ORIGIN OF PREGNANCY-RELATED HYPERTENSION – DEFICIENT TROPHOBLASTIC PRODUCTION OF PROSTACYCLIN?

The aetiology of pregnancy-related hypertension is not known but at least two factors must be involved. One is the placenta because pre-eclampsia only occurs in the presence of the placenta, or in the presence of placental tissue such as hydatidiform mole[5]. The other factor is a reduction in maternal blood flow perfusing the placenta due to deficient erosion of the uterine spiral arteries during placentation.

Many of the clinical symptoms of pregnancy-related hypertension can be produced in experimental animal models by reducing uteroplacental blood flow. In pregnant rhesus monkeys, reducing the abdominal aorta to one third of its original diameter during the last month of gestation causes hypertension, proteinuria, focal necrosis in the liver, renal histological changes similar to those in human pre-eclampsia, and diffuse haemorrhagic infarctions in the placenta[141]. In late gestational sheep, gradual embolization of the uteroplacental vascular bed by injection of 15 μm diameter microspheres results in intrauterine fetal growth retardation[142]. In pregnant rabbits, reduction of uterine arterial blood flow increases maternal arterial blood pressure and produces proteinuria[143].

During normal human pregnancy the spiral arteries are eroded by the invading trophoblast during the establishment of the uteroplacental circulation[144–146]. The erosion is so complete that the entire portion of the spiral arteries in the endometrium (or decidua) is eliminated[80]. The uterine content of sympathetic neurotransmitters is also decreased producing a functional denervation[147,148]. Therefore, the uterine blood vessels have decreased vascular tone and are probably maximally dilated during normal pregnancy. In pre-eclampsia there is less erosion of the spiral arteries so they are thicker, their lumens are narrower with atherosclerotic lesions, and they have higher vascular tone than the vessels of normal pregnancy[83,144–146].

Blood flow through the uterus and into the intervillous space of the placenta is, thus, reduced[144,149]. The higher uterine content of the catecholamines (norepinephrine, dopamine) in pre-eclampsia[148] is probably due to the persistence of the spiral arteries since the uterine vasculature is richly supplied with adrenergic nerves[150]. This makes the uterine vasculature of the pre-eclamptic patient responsive to vasoconstrictive stimuli which further reduces uterine blood flow and perfusion of the placenta.

An hypothesis that would be difficult to test but is interesting to consider is that the initial defect in pre-eclampsia is deficient prostacyclin production by the invading trophoblast during establishment of the uteroplacental circulation. It has been suggested that the ability of invading tissue to colonize vascular tissue is related to its ability to produce prostacyclin and, hence, avoid being immobilized by platelet aggregates[151]. Prostacyclin is well known for its ability to prevent platelet aggregation, but one of the original discoveries by Sir John Vane and Dr Salvador Moncada was that prostacyclin can also disaggregate platelets that are already clumped together[15,152,153]. Prostacyclin's ability to inhibit cell-to-cell interactions appears to be widespread. For example, it prevents metastatic tumour colony formation by preventing the tumour cells from adhering to microvascular endothelium[154], and it inhibits white-cell adherence to vessel walls[152]. Perhaps trophoblastic secretion of prostacyclin is necessary for the trophoblast to invade the spiral arteries, to disaggregate the vascular cells and prevent reformation of the spiral arteries in the decidua.

In pre-eclampsia with deficient prostacyclin production, the invading trophoblast would not erode the spiral arteries efficiently leading to their persistence in the decidua causing reduced uteroplacental blood flow. This hypothesis implies a genetic defect in the coding for trophoblastic prostacyclin production. Recently, Chesley and Cooper[155] provided evidence that pre-eclampsia—eclampsia occurs at a frequency in sisters, daughters and granddaughters that closely accords with the frequency predicted by the hypothesis that a single recessive gene determines development of the disorder. Therefore, the genotype of a woman is involved in the aetiology of pre-eclampsia, so defective genetic coding for placental prostacyclin production could be present from the time of conception in women destined to develop pre-eclampsia.

TREATMENT OF PREGNANCY-RELATED HYPERTENSION BASED ON AN EICOSANOID IMBALANCE

The treatment of pregnancy-related hypertension based on aberrant eicosanoid production is a relatively new concept and still in its infancy. After the discovery in 1980 that prostacyclin production was reduced in pre-eclampsia, some investigators attempted to treat the disorder by administering prostacyclin to the mother. Because prostacyclin is unstable, a constant intravenous infusion was needed. At least seven severely hypertensive patients, reported in three different studies, have been treated with prostacyclin after failure of conventional medication[47,76,77]. In each case, maternal blood pressure decreased but none of the patients carried their pregnancies to term. Prostacyclin infusions lasted from five hours to 11 days depending on the patient. Maternal side effects included nausea, vomiting, facial flushing and headache. All patients were delivered prematurely by caesarean section. Fetal bradycardia was observed in two of the pregnancies and only four babies survived.

If prostacyclin deficiency is a characteristic of pre-eclampsia, then why is maternal infusion of prostacyclin ineffective as treatment? The answer may be that prostacyclin does not cross the placenta. In an experiment using the perfused human placenta, prostacyclin attenuated the vasoconstrictor effects of angiotensin II when infused into the fetal side of the placenta demonstrating its ability to vasodilate the placental vasculature[72]. When the same experiment was done from the maternal side, prostacyclin was without effect indicating that it did not cross from the maternal to the fetal side of the placenta. This explains why maternal infusion of prostacyclin does not change fetal or placental blood flow in pre-eclampsia[75]. Maternal prostacyclin infusion treats the mother but not the fetus or placenta.

Thromboxane synthase inhibitors have also been considered as potential treatments. Systemic administration of dazoxiben to four pre-eclamptic women not only decreased thromboxane concentrations in the mother's blood, but also increased prostacyclin levels[156], presumably by shunting endoperoxide from thromboxane synthesis in platelets to prostacyclin synthesis in endothelial cells[66,157]. Maternal blood pressure dropped after treatment, but only one patient continued to term. The other three pregnancies were terminated prematurely due to fetal distress or death. Only two of four babies survived.

Treatment of pre-eclampsia with thromboxane synthase inhibitors would seem to be better than treatment with prostacyclin alone because it not only decreases thromboxane but simultaneously increases prostacyclin in the mother's blood. To see if a similar shift would occur in the placenta, we incubated placental tissues with a thromboxane synthase inhibitor, U-63,557A (Upjohn) (Figure 7.17). Addition of U-63,557A inhibited thromboxane production in both normal and pre-eclamptic placentas. Placental prostacyclin production, however, was not affected. Therefore, prostacyclin production is regulated differently in the placenta than in the systemic circulation in that inhibition of thromboxane synthesis to increase endoperoxide availability does not result in an augmentation of placental prostacyclin production. These data support the conclusions drawn from the arachidonic acid studies (Figure 7.5) that placental prostacyclin and thromboxane production rates are limited by the amount or activity of the placental enzymes, not by the amount of precursor present.

The data also emphasize that the effective treatment of pre-eclampsia will have to address placental, as well as systemic, issues. Treatment with thromboxane synthase inhibitors might decrease thromboxane production both systemically and in the placenta, but increase prostacyclin production only systemically. Placental prostacyclin synthesis will have to be stimulated directly by increasing the amount or activity of enzyme.

One of the most promising potential treatments for pregnancy-related hypertension was recently reported by Beaufils and colleagues[158]. These investigators divided 102 patients at high risk for pre-eclampsia into two groups. The treatment group received 300 mg dipyridamole and 150 mg

PREECLAMPTIC PLACENTA

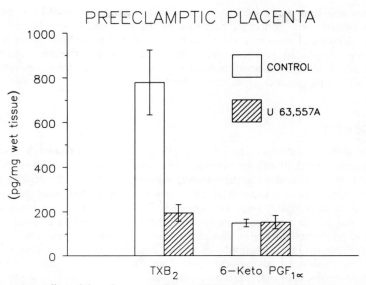

Figure 7.17 Effect of thromboxane synthase inhibitor (U63,557A, Upjohn) on pre-eclamptic placental production of thromboxane and prostacyclin as estimated by their stable metabolites, TxB_2 and 6-keto $PGF_{1\alpha}$, respectively. Tissues were incubated for 48 hours. Data represent mean $\pm$ SE, $n = 6$

aspirin daily from three months' gestation onward, whereas the control group received no treatment. Hypertension occurred in six patients in the control group and none in the treated group. Major complications such as fetal death or severe growth retardation occurred in nine patients in the control group and none in the treated group. No serious adverse effects were observed in the treatment group. The reason low dose aspirin in combination with dipyridamole may be effective in treating pregnancy-related hypertension is that dipyridamole enhances the effectiveness of prostacyclin by inhibiting phosphodiesterase to increase c-AMP[153,159], and low dose aspirin inhibits thromboxane synthesis in platelets without affecting prostacyclin production by vascular endothelial cells[15-17,160-162].

The problems with the study by Beaufils and colleagues[158] are that all but three patients were multiparous and the patients selected had previous complicated pregnancies or vascular risk factors such as known essential hypertension or familial hypertension. According to many authorities pre-eclampsia is defined as the development of hypertension with proteinuria, oedema, or both, induced by pregnancy[1-5]. Patients with pre-existing hypertension are, therefore, excluded. Pre-eclampsia is also considered primarily a disorder of primigravidas. It can be argued that hypertension in a multiparous patient is due to either pre-existing hypertension or is an indication that the patient is predisposed to developing essential hypertension later in life. The study by Beaufils and colleagues is encouraging, but must be confirmed in controlled studies with primigravid patients.

At the present time it is necessary to learn more about eicosanoid production in both normal and abnormal pregnancies, to understand the factors that regulate eicosanoid production, and to explore the changes that occur in the regulatory factors in pre-eclampsia. By understanding the regulation of eicosanoids, it should be possible to intervene therapeutically to specifically correct abnormal production in particular tissues.

POSTSCRIPT

Since the writing of this review, Dr H.C.S. Wallenburg and associates reported a prospective, controlled, double-blind trial using low-dose aspirin for the treatment of pre-eclampsia in primigravid patients at risk for pre-eclampsia[163]. Forty-six normotensive women at 28 weeks gestation who were judged to be at risk of developing hypertension later in their pregnancies because of an increased blood pressure response to intravenously infused angiotensin II were studied. Twenty-three of the patients received 60 mg aspirin daily until delivery. The other 23 patients received placebo. In the placebo group, seven women developed pre-eclampsia, four developed pregnancy-induced hypertension (defined as hypertension without proteinuria in this study), and one patient became eclamptic. In the low-dose aspirin group, only two women developed mild pre-eclampsia. There were no adverse effects of low-dose aspirin treatment in either the mothers or infants. The investigators attributed their success to the fact that low-dose aspirin inhibits thromboxane production without affecting prostacyclin production. Therefore, the imbalance of increased thromboxane/decreased prostacyclin was attenuated.

The study by Wallenburg et al. is indeed encouraging and should stimulate additional clinical trials. It remains to be determined if low-dose aspirin must be given chronically or if it will also be effective in treating pre-eclampsia acutely. In addition, mechanisms for stimulating endogenous prostacyclin production are needed.

ACKNOWLEDGEMENTS

This work was supported by Grant HD20973 from the National Institute of Child Health and Human Development, and by gifts from The Upjohn Company, Kalamazoo, Michigan and Merck Frosst Canada Inc., Pointe Claire-Dorval, Quebec.

REFERENCES

1. Chesley, L.C. (1978). *Hypertensive Disorders in Pregnancy.* (New York: Appleton–Century–Crofts)
2. Dennis, E.J., III, McFarland, K.F. and Hester, L.L., Jr. (1982). The pre-eclampsia-eclampsia syndrome. In Danforth, D.N. (ed.) *Obstetrics and Gynecology,* 4th Edn., pp. 455–474. (Philadelphia: Harper and Row)
3. MacGillivray, I. (1983). *Pre-eclampsia: the Hypertensive Disease of Pregnancy.* (Philadelphia: W.B. Saunders Co.)
4. Roberts, J.M. (1984). Pregnancy-related hypertension. In Creasy, R.K. and Resnik, R. (eds.)

Maternal—Fetal Medicine: Principles and Practice, pp. 703—752. (Philadelphia: W.B. Saunders Co.)

5. Pritchard, J.A., MacDonald, P.C. and Gant, N.F. (1985). *Williams Obstetrics*, 17th Edn. (Norwalk, CT: Appleton—Century—Crofts)

6. Quilligan, E.J. (1982). Maternal physiology. In Danforth, D.N. (ed.) *Obstetrics and Gynecology*, 4th Edn., pp. 326—341. (Philadelphia: Harper and Row)

7. Pedersen, E.B., Christensen, N.J., Christensen, P., Johannesen, P., Kornerup, H.J., Kristensen, S., Lauritsen, J.G., Leyssac, P.P., Rasmussen, A. and Wohlert, M. (1983). Pre-eclampsia — a state of prostaglandin deficiency? Urinary prostaglandin excretion, the renin-aldosterone system, and circulating catecholamines in pre-eclampsia. *Hypertension*, **5**, 105—111

8. Gant, N.F., Daley, G.L., Chand, S., Whalley, P.J. and MacDonald, P.C. (1973). A study of angiotensin II pressor responses throughout primigravid pregnancy. *J. Clin. Invest.*, **52**, 2682—2689

9. Everett, R.B., Worley, R.J., MacDonald, P.C. and Gant, N.F. (1978). Effect of prostaglandin synthetase inhibitors on pressor response to angiotensin II in human pregnancy. *J. Clin. Endocrinol. Metab.*, **46**, 1007—1010

10. Speroff, L. (1973). Toxemia of Pregnancy. Mechanism and therapeutic management. *Am. J. Cardiol.*, **32**, 582—591

11. Demers, L.M. and Gabbe, S.G. (1976). Placental prostaglandin levels in pre-eclampsia. *Am. J. Obstet. Gynecol.*, **126**, 137—139

12. Robinson, J.S., Redman, C.W.G., Clover, L. and Mitchell, M.D. (1979). The concentrations of the prostaglandins E and F, 13,14-dihydro-15-oxo-prostaglandin F and thromboxane B_2 in tissues obtained from women with and without pre-eclampsia. *Prostagl. Med.*, **3**, 223—234

13. Hillier, K. and Smith, M.D. (1981). Prostaglandin E and F concentrations in placentae of normal, hypertensive and pre-eclamptic patients. *Br. J. Obstet. Gynaecol.*, **88**, 274—277

14. Valenzuela, G., Harper, M.J.K. and Hayashi, R.H. (1983). Uterine venous, peripheral venous and radial arterial levels of prostaglandins E and F in women with pregnancy-induced hypertension. *Am. J. Obstet. Gynecol.*, **145**, 11—14

15. Moncada, S. and Vane, J.R. (1979). Pharmacology and endogenous roles of prostaglandin endoperoxides, thromboxane A_2, and prostacyclin. *Pharmacol. Rev.*, **30**, 293—331

16. Moncada, S. and Vane, J.R. (1979). Arachidonic acid metabolites and the interactions between platelets and blood-vessel walls. *N. Engl. J. Med.*, **300**, 1142—1147

17. Moncada, S. and Vane, J.R. (1979). The role of prostacyclin in vascular tissue. *Fed. Proc.*, **38**, 66—71

18. Omini, C., Folco, G.C., Pasargiklian, R., Fano, M. and Berti, F. (1979). Prostacyclin (PGI_2) in pregnant human uterus. *Prostaglandins*, **17**, 113—120

19. Wilhelmsson, L., Wikland, M. and Wiqvist, N. (1981). PGH_2, TxA_2 and PGI_2 have potent and differentiated actions on human uterine contractility. *Prostaglandins*, **21**, 277—286

20. Lye, S.J. and Challis, J.R.G. (1982). Inhibition by PGI_2 of myometrial activity *in vivo* in non-pregnant ovariectomized sheep. *J. Reprod. Fertil.*, **66**, 311—315

21. Lewis, P.J., Moncada, S. and O'Grady, J. (eds.) (1983). *Prostacyclin in Pregnancy*. (New York: Raven Press)

22. Lewis, P.J., Boylan, P., Friedman, L.A., Hensby, C.N. and Downing, I. (1980). Prostacyclin in pregnancy. *Br. Med. J.*, **280**, 1581—1582

23. Goodman, R.P., Killam, A.P., Brash, A.R. and Branch, R.A. (1982). Prostacyclin production during pregnancy: Comparison of production during normal pregnancy and pregnancy complicated by hypertension. *Am. J. Obstet. Gynecol.*, **142**, 817—822

24. Barrow, S.E., Blair, I.A., Waddell, K.A., Shepherd, G.L., Lewis, P.J. and Dollery, C.T. (1983). Prostacyclin in late pregnancy: analysis of 6-oxo-prostaglandin $F_{1\alpha}$ in maternal plasma. In Lewis, P.J., Moncada, S. and O'Grady, J. (eds.) *Prostacyclin in Pregnancy*, pp. 79—85. (New York: Raven Press)

25. Myatt, L. and Elder, M.G. (1977). Inhibition of platelet aggregation by a placental substance with prostacyclin-like activity. *Nature*, **268**, 159—160

26. Mitchell, M.D., Bibby, J.G., Hicks, B.R. and Turnbull, A.C. (1978). Possible role for prostacyclin in human parturition. *Prostaglandins*, **16**, 931—937

27. Jogee, M., Myatt, L., Moore, P. and Elder, M.G. (1983). Prostacyclin production by human placental cells in short-term culture. *Placenta*, **4**, 219—230

28. Rakoczi, I., Tihanyi, K., Falkay, G., Rozsa, I., Demeter, J. and Gati, I. (1983). Prostacyclin

production in trophoblast. In Lewis, P.J., Moncada, S. and O'Grady, J. (eds.) *Prostacyclin in Pregnancy*, pp. 15–23. (New York: Raven Press)

29. Nicolaides, K.H., Craven, D.J., Kirby, D.S., Filshie, G.M. and Symonds, E.M. (1983). Production of prostacyclin by tissues from human fetoplacental unit. In Lewis, P.J., Moncada, S. and O'Grady, J. (eds.) *Prostacyclin in Pregnancy*, pp. 25–30. (New York: Raven Press)

30. Makila, U.-M., Viinikka, L. and Ylikorkala, O. (1984). Increased thromboxane A$_2$ production but normal prostacyclin by the placenta in hypertensive pregnancies. *Prostaglandins*, **27**, 87–95

31. Jeremy, J.Y., Barradas, M.A., Craft, I.L., Mikhailidis, D.P. and Dandona, P. (1985). Does human placenta produce prostacyclin? *Placenta*, **6**, 45–52

32. Walsh, S.W., Behr, M.J. and Allen, N.H. (1985). Placental prostacyclin production in normal and toxemic pregnancies. *Am. J. Obstet. Gynecol.*, **151**, 110–115

33. Walsh, S.W. (1985). Pre-eclampsia: An imbalance in placental prostacyclin and thromboxane production. *Am. J. Obstet. Gynecol.*, **152**, 335–340

34. Remuzzi, G., Misiani, R., Muratore, D., Marchesi, D., Livio, M., Schieppati, A., Mecca, G., de Gaetano, G. and Donati, M.B. (1979). Prostacyclin and human foetal circulation. *Prostaglandins*, **18**, 341–348

35. Terragno, N.A., Terragno, A. and McGiff, J.C. (1980). Role of prostaglandins in blood vessels. *Semin. Perinatol.*, **4**, 85–90

36. Kawano, M. and Mori, N. (1983). Prostacyclin producing activity of human umbilical, placental and uterine vessels. *Prostaglandins*, **26**, 645–662

37. Balconi, G., Pietra, A., Olivieri, S., Vergara-Dauden, M., Busacca, M., Gementi, P., Pangrazzi, J., Recchia, M., Dejana, E. and de Gaetano, G. (1983). Prostacyclin production by umbilical arteries and cultured endothelial cells from umbilical veins: a methodological approach. In Lewis, P.J., Moncada, S. and O'Grady, J. (eds.) *Prostacyclin in Pregnancy*, pp. 37–45. (New York: Raven Press)

38. Seed, M.P., Williams, K.I. and Bamford, D.S. (1983). Influence of gestation on prostacyclin synthesis by the human pregnant myometrium. In Lewis, P.J., Moncada, S., and O'Grady, J. (eds.) *Prostacyclin in Pregnancy*, pp. 31–36. (New York: Raven Press)

39. Remuzzi, G., Marchesi, D., Zoja, C., Muratore, D., Mecca, G., Misiani, R., Rossi, E., Barbato, M., Capetta, P., Donati, M.B. and DeGaetano, G. (1980). Reduced umbilical and placental vascular prostacyclin in severe pre-eclampsia. *Prostaglandins*, **20**, 105–110

40. Bussolino, F., Benedetto, C., Massobrio, M. and Camussi, G. (1980). Maternal vascular prostacyclin activity in pre-eclampsia. *Lancet*, **2**, 702

41. Downing, I., Shepherd, G.L. and Lewis, P.J. (1980). Reduced prostacyclin production in pre-eclampsia. *Lancet*, **2**, 1374

42. Carreras, L.O., Defreyn, G., Van Houtte, E., Vermylen, J. and Van Assche, A. (1981). Prostacyclin and pre-eclampsia. *Lancet*, **1**, 442

43. Stuart, M.J., Clark, D.A., Sunderji, S.G., Allen, J.B., Yambo, T., Elrad, H. and Slott, J.H. (1981). Decreased prostacyclin production: A characteristic of chronic placental insufficiency syndromes. *Lancet*, **1**, 1126–1128

44. Makila, U.-M., Viinikka, L. and Ylikorkala, O. (1984). Evidence that prostacyclin deficiency is a specific feature in pre-eclampsia. *Am. J. Obstet. Gynecol.*, **148**, 772–774

45. Ylikorkala, O., Makila, U.-M. and Viinikka, L. (1981). Amniotic fluid prostacyclin and thromboxane in normal, pre-eclamptic, and some other complicated pregnancies. *Am. J. Obstet. Gynecol.*, **141**, 487–490

46. Bodzenta, A., Thomson, J.M. and Poller, L. (1980). Prostacyclin activity in amniotic fluid in pre-eclampsia. *Lancet*, **2**, 650

47. Lewis, P.J., Shepherd, G.L., Ritter, J., Chan, S.M.T., Bolton, P.J., Jogee, M., Myatt, L. and Elder, M.G. (1981). Prostacyclin and pre-eclampsia. *Lancet*, **1**, 559

48. Yamaguchi, M. and Mori, N. (1985). 6-keto prostaglandin F$_1$, thromboxane B$_2$, and 13,14-dihydro-15-keto prostaglandin F concentrations of normotensive and pre-eclamptic patients during pregnancy, delivery, and the postpartum period. *Am. J. Obstet. Gynecol.*, **151**, 121–127

49. Ylikorkala, O., Kirkinen, P. and Viinikka, L. (1981). Maternal plasma prostacyclin concentration in pre-eclampsia and other pregnancy complications. *Br. J. Obstet. Gynaecol.*, **88**, 968–972

50. Strickland, D.M., Cox, K., McCubbin, J.H., Whalley, P.J., MacDonald, P.C. and Mitchell, M.D. (1984). Plasma prostaglandins during the intravenous infusion of angiotensin II in pregnant women. *Am. J. Obstet. Gynecol.*, **150**, 952–955

51. Moncada, S., Korbut, R., Bunting, S. and Vane, J.R. (1978). Prostacyclin is a circulating hormone. *Nature*, **273**, 767–768
52. Gryglewski, R.J., Korbut, R. and Ocetkiewicz, A. (1978). Generation of prostacyclin by lungs *in vivo* and its release into the arterial circulation. *Nature*, **273**, 765–767
53. Gryglewski, R.J. (1979). Prostacyclin as a circulating hormone. *Biochem. Pharmacol.*, **28**, 3161–66
54. Hensby, C.N., Barnes, P.J., Dollery, C.T. and Dargie, H. (1979). Production of 6-oxo-PGF$_{1\alpha}$ by human lung *in vivo*. *Lancet*, **2**, 1162–1163
55. Christ-Hazelhof, E. and Nugteren, D.H. (1981). Prostacyclin is not a circulating hormone. *Prostaglandins*, **22**, 739–746
56. Masotti, G., Poggesi, L., Galanti, G., Trotta, F. and Neri-Serneri, G.G. (1981). Prostacyclin production in man. In Lewis, P.J. and O'Grady, J. (eds.) *Clinical Pharmacology of Prostacyclin*, pp. 9–19. (New York: Raven Press)
57. Blair, I.A., Barrow, S.E., Waddell, K.A., Lewis, P.J. and Dollery, C.T. (1982). Prostacyclin is not a circulating hormone in man. *Prostaglandins*, **23**, 579–589
58. Ritter, J.M., Blair, I.A., Barrow, S.E. and Dollery, C.T. (1983). Release of prostacyclin *in vivo* and its role in man. *Lancet*, **1**, 317–319
59. Behr, M.J., Walsh, S.W. and Allen, N.H. (1983). Placental prostacyclin production in normal and toxemic pregnancies. Presented at the *Thirtieth Annual Meeting of the Society for Gynecologic Investigation*, March 17–20, Washington, DC (Abstract #342)
60. Jogee, M., Elder, M.G. and Myatt, L. (1983). Decreased prostacyclin production by placental cells in culture from pregnancies complicated by fetal growth retardation. In Lewis, P.J., Moncada, S., and O'Grady, J. (eds.) *Prostacyclin in Pregnancy*, pp. 115–118 (New York: Raven Press)
61. Jogee, M., Myatt, L. and Elder, M.G. (1983). Decreased prostacyclin production by placental cells in culture from pregnancies complicated by fetal growth retardation. *Br. J. Obstet. Gynecol.*, **90**, 247–250
62. Miyamori, I., FitzGerald, G.A., Brown, M.J. and Lewis, P.J. (1979). Prostacyclin stimulates the renin angiotensin aldosterone system in man. *J. Clin. Endocrinol. Metab.*, **49**, 943–944
63. Oates, J.A., Whorton, A.R., Gerber, J., Lazar, J., Branch, R.A. and Hollifield, J.W. (1979). Prostacyclin and the kidney. In Vane, J.R. and Bergstrom, S. (eds.) *Prostacyclin*, pp. 195–199. (New York: Raven Press)
64. Mitchell, M.D., Bibby, J.G., Hicks, B.R., Redman, C.W.G., Anderson, A.B.M. and Turnbull, A.C. (1978). Thromboxane B$_2$ and human parturition: Concentrations in the plasma and production *in vitro*. *J. Endocrinol.*, **78**, 435–441
65. Ylikorkala, O. and Viinikka, L. (1980). Thromboxane A$_2$ in pregnancy and puerperium. *Br. Med. J.*, **281**, 1601–1602
66. Dusting, G.J., Moncada, S. and Vane, J.R. (1982). Prostacyclin: Its biosynthesis, actions and clinical potential. In Oates, J.A. (ed.) *Prostaglandins and the Cardiovascular System. Adv. Prostagl. Thrombox. Leukotr. Res.*, **10**, 59–106
67. Walsh, S.W. and Fenner, P.C. (1984). Toxemia: an imbalance in placental prostacyclin (PGI) and thromboxane (TxA) production. Presented at the *31st Annual Meeting of the Society for Gynecologic Investigation*, March 21–24, San Francisco, (Abstract #414)
68. Makarainen, L. and Ylikorkala, O. (1984). Amniotic fluid 6-keto-prostaglandin F$_{1\alpha}$ and thromboxane B$_2$ during labor. *Am. J. Obstet. Gynecol.*, **150**, 765–768
69. Martensson, L. and Wallenburg, H.C.S. (1984). Uterine venous concentrations of 6-keto-PGF$_{1\alpha}$ (6-K) in normal pregnant (NP) and pregnancy-induced hypertension (PIH) women. Presented at the *31st Annual Meeting of the Society for Gynecologic Investigation*, March 21–25, San Francisco, (Abstract #410)
70. Takagi, S. and Den, K. (1985). Prostacyclin and thromboxane A$_2$ in pre-eclamptic umbilical circulation. In Hayaishi, O. and Yamamoto, S. (eds.) *Adv. Prostagl. Thrombox. Leuktr. Res.*, **15**, 619–621. (New York: Raven Press)
71. Wallenburg, H.C.S. and Rotmans, N. (1982). Enhanced reactivity of the platelet thromboxane pathway in normotensive and hypertensive pregnancies with insufficient fetal growth. *Am. J. Obstet. Gynecol.*, **144**, 523–528
72. Glance, D.G., Elder, M.G. and Myatt, L. (1986). The actions of prostaglandins and their

interactions with angiotensin II in the isolated perfused human placental cotyledon. *Br. J. Obstet. Gynaecol.*, **93**, 488–494.

73. Tulenko, T.N. (1981). The actions of prostaglandins and cyclo-oxygenase inhibition on the resistance vessels supplying the human fetal placenta. *Prostaglandins*, **21**, 1033–1043

74. Myatt, L., Glance, D.G. and Elder, M.G. (1985). Transfer and metabolism of prostaglandins in the isolated perfused human placental cotyledon. Presented at the *32nd Annual Meeting of the Society for Gynecologic Investigation*, March 20–23, Phoenix (Abstract #157)

75. Jouppila, P., Kirkinen, P., Koivula, A. and Ylikorkala, O. (1985). Failure of exogenous prostacyclin to change placental and fetal blood flow in pre-eclampsia. *Am. J. Obstet. Gynecol.*, **151**, 661–665

76. Fidler, J., Bennett, M.J., De Swiet, M., Ellis, C. and Lewis, P.J. (1980). Treatment of pregnancy hypertension with prostacyclin. *Lancet*, **2**, 31–32

77. Belch, J.J.F., Thorburn, J., Greer, I.A., Sarfo, S. and Prentice, C.R.M. (1985). Intravenous prostacyclin in the management of pregnancies complicated by severe hypertension. *Clin. Exp. Hypertens.- Hypertens. Preg.*, **B4**, 75–86

78. Parisi, V.M. and Rankin, J.H.G. (1985). The effect of prostacyclin on angiotensin II-induced placental vasoconstriction. *Am. J. Obstet. Gynecol.*, **151**, 444–449

79. Landauer, M., Phernetton, T.M., Parisi, V.M., Clark, K.E. and Rankin, J.H.G. (1985) Ovine placental vascular response to the local application of prostacyclin. *Am. J. Obstet. Gynecol.*, **151**, 460–464

80. Ramsey, E.M. and Donner, M.W. (1980). *Placental Vasculature and Circulation.* (Philadelphia: W. B. Saunders Company)

81. Faber, J.J. and Thornburg, K.L. (1983). *Placental Physiology, Structure and Function of Fetomaternal Exchange.* (New York: Raven Press)

82. Rankin, J.H.G., Phernetton, T.M., Anderson, D.F. and Berssenbrugge, A.D. (1979). Effect of prostaglandin I_2 on ovine placental vasculature. *J. Dev. Physiol.*, **1**, 151–160

83. De Wolf, F., Robertson, W.B. and Brosens, I. (1975). The ultrastructure of acute atherosis in hypertensive pregnancy. *Am. J. Obstet. Gynecol.*, **123**, 164–174

84. Speroff, L., Glass, R.H. and Kase, N.G. (1983). *Clinical Gynecologic Endocrinology and Infertility.* 3rd Edn. (Baltimore: Williams and Wilkins)

85. Tuvemo, T. (1978). Action of prostaglandins and blockers of prostaglandin synthesis on the isolated human umbilical artery. *Adv. Prostagl. Thrombox. Res.*, **4**, 271–274

86. Tuvemo T. (1980). Role of prostaglandins, prostacyclin and thromboxanes in the control of the umbilical-placental circulation. *Semin. Perinatol.*, **4**, 91–95

87. Cassin, S. (1980). Role of prostaglandins and thromboxanes in the control of the pulmonary circulation in the fetus and newborn. *Semin. Perinatol.*, **4**, 101–107

88. Coceani, F. and Olley, P.M. (1980). Role of prostaglandins, prostacyclin, and thromboxanes in the control of prenatal patency and postnatal closure of the ductus arteriosus. *Semin. Perinatol.*, **4**, 109–113

89. Terragno, N.A., Terragno, A. and McGiff, J.C. (1980). Role of prostaglandins in blood vessels. *Semin. Perinatol.*, **4**, 85–90

90. Samuelsson, B. (1982). The leukotrienes: An Introduction, In Samuelsson, B. and Paoletti, R. (eds.) *Leukotrienes and Other Lipoxygenase Products*, pp. 1–17. (New York: Raven Press)

91. Samuelsson, B. (1983). Leukotrienes: Mediators of immediate hypersensitivity reactions and inflammation. *Science*, **220**, 568–575

92. Saeed, S.A. and Mitchell, M.D. (1982). Formation of arachidonate lipoxygenase metabolites by human fetal membranes, uterine decidua vera and placenta. *Prostagl. Leuktr. Med.*, **8**, 635–640

93. Myatt, L., Rose, M.P. and Elder, M.G. (1985). Lipoxygenase products of arachidonic acid in human fetal membranes. Presented at the *32nd Annual Meeting of the Society for Gynecologic Investigation*, March 20–23, Phoenix (Abstract #160)

94. Fenner, P.C. and Walsh, S.W. (1985). Pre-eclampsia: an imbalance in placental production of hydroxyeicosatraenoic acids (HETE), prostacyclin (PGI) and thromboxane (TxA). Presented at the *32nd Annual Meeting of the Society for Gynecologic Investigation*, March 20–23, Phoenix (Abstract #172)

95. Walsh, S.W., Fenner, P.C., Walsh, J.A. and Salisbury, F. (1985). Placental interactions of hydroxyeicosatetraenoic acids (HETE), prostaglandins (PG) and thromboxane (TxA). Presented at the *32nd Annual Meeting of the Society for Gynecologic Investigation*, March 20–23, Phoenix (Abstract #209P)

96. Bailey, J.M., Bryant, R.W., Low, C.E., Pupillo, M.B. and Vanderhoek, J.Y. (1982). Role of lipoxygenases in regulation of PHA and phorbol ester-induced mitogenesis, In Samuelsson, B. and Paoletti, R. (eds.) *Leukotrienes and Other Lipoxygenase Products*, pp. 341–353. (New York: Raven Press)

97. Goetzl, E.J., Goldman, D.W., Naccache, P.H., Sha'afi, R.I. and Pickett, W.C. (1982). Mediation of leukocyte components of inflammatory reactions by lipoxygenase products of arachidonic acid. In Samuelsson, B. and Paoletti, R. (eds.) *Leukotrienes and Other Lipoxygenase Products*, pp. 273–282. (New York: Raven Press)

98. Piper, P.J. (1984). Formation and actions of leukotrienes. *Physiol. Rev.*, **64**, 744–761

99. Kaijser, L. (1982). Cardiovascular and pulmonary effects of leukotriene C_4 in man. *Eur. J. Respir. Dis.*, **63**, (Suppl. 124), 76

100. Walsh, S.W. and Young, S.R. (1986). Deficient placental 5-lipoxygenase may cause hypertension in pregnancy. Presented at the *33rd Annual Meeting of the Society for Gynecologic Investigation*, March 19–22, Toronto, (Abstract #288P)

101. Cramer, E.B., Pologe, L., Pawlowski, N.A., Cohn, Z.A. and Scott, W.A. (1983). Leukotriene C promotes prostacyclin synthesis by human endothelial cells. *Proc. Natl. Acad. Sci. USA*, **80**, 4109–4113

102. Clark, M.A., Littlejohn, D., Mong, S. and Crooke, S.T. (1986). Effect of leukotrienes, bradykinin and calcium ionophore (A 23187) on bovine endothelial cells: release of prostacyclin. *Prostaglandins*, **31**, 157–166

103. Marx, J.L. (1982). The leukotrienes in allergy and inflammation. *Science*, **215**, 1380–1383

104. Bach, M.K. (1983). *Current Concepts. The Leukotrienes: Their Structure, Actions, and Role in Diseases*. (Kalamazoo: Scope Publication, Upjohn Company)

105. Williams, T.J. (1983). Interactions between prostaglandins, leukotrienes and other mediators of inflammation. *Br. Med. Bull.*, **39**, 239–242

106. Letts, L.G. and Cirino, M. (1985). Vascular actions of leukotrienes. In Lefer, A.M., and Gee, M.H. (eds.) *Leukotrienes in Cardiovascular and Pulmonary Function*, pp. 47–58. (New York: Alan R. Liss, Inc.)

107. Smedegard, G., Hedqvist, P., Dahlen, S-E, Revenas, B., Hammarstrom, S. and Samuelsson, B. (1982). Leukotriene C_4 affects pulmonary and cardiovascular dynamics in monkey. *Nature*, **295**, 327–329

108. Yokocki, K., Olley, P.M., Sideris, E., Hamilton, F., Huhtanen, D. and Coceani, F. (1982). Leukotriene D_4: a potent vasoconstrictor of the pulmonary and systemic circulations in the newborn lamb. In Samuelsson, B., Paoletti, R. (eds.) *Leukotrienes and Other Lipoxygenase Products*, pp. 211–214. (New York: Raven Press)

109. Leffler, C.W., Mitchell, J.A. and Green, R.S. (1984). Cardiovascular effects of leukotrienes in neonatal piglets – Role in hypoxic pulmonary vasoconstriction? *Circ. Res.*, **55**, 780–787

110. Soifer, S.J., Loitz, R.D., Roman, C. and Heymann, M.A. (1985). Leukotriene end organ antagonists increase pulmonary blood flow in fetal lambs. *Am. J. Physiol.*, **249**, H570–H576

111. Stenmark, K.R., James, S.L., Voelkel, N.F., Toews, W.H., Reeves, J.T. and Murphy, R.C. (1983). Leukotriene C_4 and D_4 in neonates with hypoxaemia and pulmonary hypertension. *N. Engl. J. Med.*, **309**, 77–80

112. Schreiber, M.D., Heymann, M.A. and Soifer, S.J. (1985). Leukotriene inhibition prevents and reverses hypoxic pulmonary vasoconstriction in newborn lambs. *Pediatr. Res.*, **19**, 437–441

113. Parisi, V.M., Phernetton, T.M. and Rankin, J.H.G. (1985). Placental vascular responses to leukotriene receptor antagonist FPL 55712. *Prostaglandins*, **30**, 125–130

114. Mehta, J. and Roberts, A. (1983). Human vascular tissues produce thromboxane as well as prostacyclin. *Am. J. Physiol.*, **244**, R839–R844

115. Dunham, B., Shepro, D. and Hechtman, H.B. (1984). Leukotriene induction of TxB_2 in cultured bovine aortic endothelial cells. *Inflammation*, **8**, 313–321

116. Engineer, D.M., Jose, P.J., Piper, P.J. and Tippins, J.R. (1978). Modulation of slow-reacting substance of anaphylaxis and histamine release by prostacyclin and thromboxanes. *J. Physiol.*, **281**, 42P

117. Burka, J.F. and Garland, L.G. (1976). A possible modulatory role for prostacyclin (PGI_2) in IgG_α-induced release of slow-reacting substance of anaphylaxis in rats. *Br. J. Pharmacol.*, **61**, 697–699

118. Vanderhoek, J.Y. and Bailey, J.M. (1984). Activation of a 15-lipoxygenase/leukotriene pathway in human polymorphonuclear leukocytes by the anti-inflammatory agent ibuprofen. *J. Biol. Chem.*, **259**, 6752–6756

119. Vane, J.R. (1978). The mode of action of aspirin-like drugs. *Agents Actions*, **8**, 430–431

120. Hansen, H.S. (1974). Inhibition by indomethacin and aspirin of 15-hydroxy-prostaglandin dehydrogenase *in vitro. Prostaglandins*, **8**, 95–105

121. Ramwell, P.W., Leovey, E.M.K. and Sintetos, A.L. (1977). Regulation of the arachidonic acid cascade. *Biol. Reprod.*, **16**, 70–87

122. Fenner, P.C., Walsh, S.W., Wagner, M.A. and Salisbury, F. (1984). Placental estradiol (E2) and progesterone (P4) production and their effects on prostacyclin (PGI) and thromboxane (TxA) in normal and toxemic pregnancies. Presented at the *31st Annual Meeting of the Society for Gynecologic Investigation*, March 21–24, San Francisco, (Abstract #338P)

123. Winkel, C.A., Snyder, J.M., MacDonald, P.C. and Simpson, E.R. (1980). Regulation of cholesterol and progesterone synthesis in human placental cells in culture by serum lipoproteins. *Endocrinology*, **106**, 1054–1060

124. Gant, N.F., Whalley, P.J., Everett, R.B., Worley, R.J. and MacDonald, P.C. (1983). Evidence for a vasodepressor prostaglandin deficiency in pregnancy-induced hypertension. In Lewis, P.J., Moncada, S. and O'Grady, J. (eds.) *Prostacyclin in Pregnancy*, pp. 99–107. (New York: Raven Press)

125. Lindheimer, M.D. and Katz, A.I. (1981). Pathophysiology of pre-eclampsia. *Annu. Rev. Med.*, **32**, 273–289

126. Myatt, L., Jogee, M. and Elder, M.G. (1983). Regulation of prostacyclin metabolism in human placental cells in culture by steroid hormones. In Lewis, P.J., Moncada, S. and O'Grady, J. (eds.) *Prostacyclin in Pregnancy*, pp. 119–129. (New York: Raven Press)

127. Alam, N.A., Russell, P.T., Tabor, M.W. and Moulton, B.C. (1976). Progesterone and estrogen control of uterine prostaglandin dehydrogenase activity during deciduomal growth. *Endocrinology*, **98**, 859–863

128. Hall, A.K. and Behrman, H.R. (1982). Prostaglandins: biosynthesis, metabolism and mechanism of cellular action. In Lee, J.B. (ed.) *Prostaglandins*, pp. 1–38. (New York: Elsevier)

129. Sun, F.F., Taylor, B.M., McGuire, J.C., Wong, P.Y.-K., Malik, K.U. and McGiff, J.C. (1979). Metabolic disposition of prostacyclin, In Vane, J.R. and Bergstrom, S. (eds.) *Prostacyclin*, pp. 119–131. (New York: Raven Press)

130. Schlegel, W., Demers, L.M., Hildebrant-Stark, H.E., Behrman, H.R. and Greep, R.O. (1974). Partial purification of human placental 15-hydroxyprostaglandin dehydrogenase: kinetic properties. *Prostaglandins*, **5**, 417–433

131. Dembele-Duchesne, M.J., Thaler-Dao, H., Chavis, C. and Crastes de Paulet, A. (1981). Some new prospects in the mechanism of control of arachidonate metabolism in human placenta and amnion. *Prostaglandins*, **22**, 979–1002

132. MacDonald, P.C. and Porter, J. (eds.) (1983). *Initiation of Parturition: Prevention of Prematurity*. (Columbus: Ross Laboratories)

133. Rehnstrom, J., Ishikawa, M., Fuchs, F. and Fuchs, A.-R. (1983). Stimulation of myometrial and decidual prostaglandin production by amniotic fluid from term, but not midtrimester pregnancies. *Prostaglandins*, **26**, 973–981

134. Mitchell, M.D., Craig, D.A., Saeed, S.A. and Strickland, D.M. (1985). Endogenous stimulant of prostaglandin endoperoxide synthase activity in human amniotic fluid. *Biochem. Biophys. Acta.*, **833**, 379–385

135. Wilson, T., Liggins, G.C., Aimer, G.P. and Skinner, S.J.M. (1985). Partial purification and characterisation of two compounds from amniotic fluid which inhibit phospholipase activity in human endometrial cells. *Biochem. Biophys. Res. Commun.*, **131**, 22–29

136. Wilson, T., Liggins, G.C., Aimer, G.P. and Watkins, E.J. (1986). The effect of progesterone on the release of arachidonic acid from human endometrial cells stimulated by histamine. *Prostaglandins*, **31**, 343–360

137. Hammarstrom, S. and Falardeau, P. (1977). Resolution of prostaglandin endoperoxide synthase and thromboxane synthase of human platelets. *Proc. Natl. Acad. Sci. USA*, **74**, 3691–3695

138. Alila, H.W., Milvae, R.A. and Hansel, W. (1983). Inhibition of bovine luteal cell progesterone and prostacyclin synthesis by 5 hydroxy-eicosatetraenoic acid (5-HETE). *J. Anim. Sci.*, **57**, (suppl. 1), 316. (Abstract #447)

139. Folco, G.C., Omini, C., Vigano, T., Brunelli, G., Rossoni, G. and Berti, F. (1982). Biological activity of leukotriene C_4 in guinea pigs: *in vitro* and *in vivo* studies. In Samuelsson, B., Paoletti, R. *Leukotrienes and Other Lipoxygenase Products*, pp. 153–167. (New York: Raven Press)

140. Nelson, D.M., Meister, R.K., Ortman-Nabi, J., Sparks, S. and Stevens, V.C. (1986) Differentiation and secretory activities of cultured human placental cytotrophoblast. *Placenta*, 7, 1–16

141. Abitbol, M.M., Ober, W.B., Gallo, G.R., Driscoll, S.G. and Pirani, C.L. (1977). Experimental toxemia of pregnancy in the monkey, with a preliminary report on renin and aldosterone. *Am. J. Pathol.*, 86, 573–583

142. Creasy, R.K., Barrett, C.T., De Swiet, M., Kahanpaa, K.V. and Rudolph, A.M. (1972). Experimental intrauterine growth retardation in the sheep. *Am. J. Obstet. Gynecol.*, 112, 566–573

143. Lee, M.I. and Sokol, R.J. (1986). The pregnant rabbit: a model for inducing hypertension and proteinuria. Presented at the *33rd Annual Meeting of the Society for Gynecologic Investigation*, March 19–22, Toronto (Abstract #57)

144. Gerretsen, G., Huisjes, H.J., Hardonk, M.J. and Elema, J.D. (1983). Trophoblast alterations in the placental bed in relation to physiological changes in spiral arteries. *Br. J. Obstet. Gynaecol.*, 90, 34–39

145. Hustin, J., Foidart, J.M. and Lambotte, R. (1983). Maternal vascular lesions in pre-eclampsia and intrauterine growth retardation: light microscopy and immunofluorescence. *Placenta*, 4, 489–498

146. Althabe, O., Labarrere, C. and Telenta, M. (1985). Maternal vascular lesions in placentae of small-for-gestational-age infants. *Placenta*, 6, 265–276

147. Thorbert, G., Alm, P., Bjorklund, A.B., Owman, C. and Sjoberg, N.-O. (1979). Adrenergic innervation of the human uterus. Disappearance of the transmitter and transmitter-forming enzymes during pregnancy. *Am. J. Obstet. Gynecol.*, 135, 223–226

148. O'Shaughnessy, R.W., O'Toole, R., Tuttle, S. and Zuspan, F.P. (1983). Uterine catecholamines in normal and hypertensive pregnancy. *Clin. Exp. Hypertens.-Hypertens. Preg.*, B2, 447–457

149. Lunell, N.O., Lewander, R., Mamoun, I., Nylund, L., Sarby, S. and Thornstrom, S. (1984). Uteroplacental blood flow in pregnancy-induced hypertension. *Scand. J. Clin. Lab. Invest.*, (Suppl.), 169, 28–35

150. Owman, C.H., Rosengren, E. and Sjoberg, N.-O. (1967). Adrenergic innervation of the human female reproductive organs: a histochemical and chemical investigation. *Obstet. Gynecol.*, 30, 763–773

151. Lewis, P.J. (1983). Does prostacyclin deficiency play a role in pre-eclampsia? In Lewis, P.J., Moncada, S. and O'Grady, J. (eds.) *Prostacyclin in Pregnancy*, pp. 215–220. (New York: Raven Press)

152. Vane, J.R. (1985). The road to prostacyclin. In Hayaishi, O., Yamamoto, S. (eds.) *Adv. Prostagl. Thrombox. Leuktr. Res.*, 15, 11–19. (New York: Raven Press)

153. Moncada, S. and Korbut, R. (1978). Dipyridamole and other phosphodiesterase inhibitors act as antithrombotic agents by potentiating endogenous prostacyclin. *Lancet*, 1, 1286–1289

154. Honn, K.V., Cicone, B. and Skoff, A. (1981). Prostacyclin: a potent antimetastatic agent. *Science*, 212, 1270–1272

155. Chesley, L.C. and Cooper, D.W. (1986). Genetic basis of pre-eclampsia-eclampsia. Presented at the *33rd Annual Meeting of the Society for Gynecologic Investigation*, March 19–22, Toronto (Abstract #7)

156. Van Assche, F.A., Spitz, B., Vermylen, J. and Deckmijn, H. (1984). Preliminary observations on treatment of pregnancy-induced hypertension with a thromboxane synthetase inhibitor. *Am. J. Obstet. Gynecol.*, 148, 216–218

157. Gorman, R.R. (1979). Modulation of human platelet function by prostacyclin and thromboxane A_2. *Fed. Proc.*, 38, 83–88

158. Beaufils, M., Donsimoni, R., Uzan, S. and Colau, J.C. (1985). Prevention of pre-eclampsia by early antiplatelet therapy. *Lancet*, 1, 840–842

159. Mehta, J., Mehta, P., Pepine, C.J. and Conti, C.R. (1981). Platelet function studies in coronary artery disease. X. Effect of dipyridamole. *Am. J. Cardiol.*, 47, 1111–1114

160. Burch, J.W., Stanford, N. and Majerus, P.W. (1978). Inhibition of platelet prostaglandin synthetase by oral aspirin. *J. Clin. Invest.*, **61**, 314–319
161. Masotti, G., Poggesi, L., Galanti, G., Abbate, R. and Neri Serneri, G.G. (1979). Differential inhibition of prostacyclin production and platelet aggregation by aspirin. *Lancet*, **2**, 1213–1216
162. Makila, U.-M., Kokkonen, E., Viinikka, L. and Ylikorkala, O. (1983). Differential inhibition of fetal vascular prostacyclin and platelet thromboxane synthesis by nonsteroidal anti-inflammatory drugs in humans. *Prostaglandins*, **25**, 39–46
163. Wallenburg, H.C.S., Makovitz, J.W., Dekker, G.A., Rotmans, P. (1986). Low-dose aspirin prevents pregnancy-induced hypertension and pre-eclampsia in angiotensin-sensitive primigravidae. *Lancet*, **1**, 1–3

8
The physiological role of eicosanoids in controlling the form and function of the cervix

N. Uldbjerg, U. Ulmsten and G. Ekman

INTRODUCTION

In this chapter we will review the 'ripening process' that takes place in the stroma tissue of the human uterine cervix during pregnancy and labour. Our present knowledge about the role of eicosanoids in controlling this phenomenon will be presented by discussing evidence of a synthesis of eicosanoids in the human uterine cervix and by showing that many of the changes taking place in the uterine cervix during pregnancy can be induced pharmacologically by treatment with eicosanoids or by stimulation of their endogenous secretion. Finally, the delayed cervical ripening induced by inhibition of cylo-oxygenase will be reviewed. Our conclusion is that eicosanoids, together with other hormones most probably are involved in the connective tissue modification of the uterine cervix necessary for normal parturition. It is, however, less obvious if the effect on the scanty smooth muscle component is of physiological importance.

CERVIX: CLINICAL AND BIOMECHANICAL CHARACTERISTICS

Softening of the cervix (Goodell's sign and Hegar's sign) is observed in early pregnancy, whereas, the so called ripening process takes place late in pregnancy. It consists of a marked increase in cervical compliance, effacement and eventually early dilatation of the cervical canal[1]. These changes are necessary for normal dilatation of the cervix during labour. In the daily routine the described changes can be assessed and quantitated according to different scoring systems[2-3] or by ultrasound examination. About 10% of all pregnant women will reach term with an unripe cervix. In these patients induction of labour is hazardous, resulting in a high frequency of instrumental deliveries including caesarean sections[4], thus demonstrating the importance of cervical ripening before the start of labour.

Experimentally, cervical softening or increased compliance can be evaluated by different methods. Cervical dilators attached to a force-sensing handle demonstrate a decreased resistance in early pregnancy[5–6]. This observation harmonizes with the results obtained by Bakke[7] who used a mechanical instrument which determined the deformation of cervical tissue as induced by a 20 g force applied at a well defined small area of the organ. Using this device, steadily decreasing cervical resistance was registered throughout pregnancy.

The biomechanical properties of cervical tissue strips have been tested by Conrad and Ueland[8]. The maximum stress that could be applied to strips taken immediately after delivery was 22 % of that which could be applied to strips from non-pregnant women.

No major change in cervical shape has been observed during the menstrual cycle. During the first trimester of pregnancy, however, inspection of the vaginal part of the cervix gives the impression of some hypertrophy. The length of the cervical canal was unchanged (4.5 cm) during the first half of pregnancy as recorded by a Foley catheter, which was retracted to bring the balloon against the internal os[9]. By ultrasound techniques the transition between the uterine cervix and the uterine body can be defined as the place at which the anterior–posterior diameter of the organ increases. Using this definition the cervical length remains unchanged (3.1 cm) during the first 28 weeks of pregnancy whereas the anterior–posterior diameter increases from 2.7 cm to 3.1 cm (Uldbjerg, Haubek and Klebe, unpublished observations). Shortening, effacement and sometimes early dilatation is observed by ultrasound during the third trimester of pregnancy.

There has been discussion as to whether cervical ripening depends on myometrial activity or if it is due to processes taking place within the organ. In animals it is possible surgically to separate the uterine cervix from the uterine body, thus preventing the spread of forces from uterine contractions to the cervix. In rats such an operation did not affect the spontaneous cervical ripening taking place during the latter half of pregnancy[10]. In sheep both cervical ripening and labour can be induced by injection of dexamethasone into the fetus, even after surgical transection of the cervix from the uterine body[11]. In women cervical ripening can be accomplished by prostaglandin E_2 without induction of significant myometrial activity[12–14]. It is therefore believed that cervical ripening can be due to local processes within the cervix without a direct influence of myometrial activity.

CERVIX: CONNECTIVE TISSUE AND SMOOTH MUSCLE

In most women there is a histologically abrupt transition between the uterine body, rich in smooth muscle, and the uterine cervix, dominated by fibrous connective tissue[15,16] (Figure 8.1). The muscle cells in the cervical stroma are randomly scattered in the tissue[17] and the collagen fibres transverse the tissue in all directions without regular orientation[18]. Between the collagen fibres

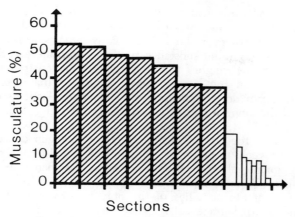

Figure 8.1 The smooth muscle content of a uterus during the seventh month of pregnancy. The fixed uterus was sectioned from the portio vaginalis to the fundus transversely in parallel sections. The smooth muscle contents in each section were determined by planometry. Hatched bars: uterine corpus (fundus to the left); open bars: uterine cervix (portio vaginalis to the right). Modified from Schwalm and Dubrauszky[23]

there is an amorphous substance, called 'ground substance', with small amounts of elastin, fibroblasts, white blood cells and blood vessels[18]. At the end of the first trimester of pregnancy the collagen fibres are less densely packed[19]. At term and immediately after delivery the collagen fibres appear at conventional histological examination to be dissociated into their fibrillar components and often they are separated by spaces representing oedema, amorphous substance or partly degraded collagen[20]. Junqueira et al.[18] have confirmed these findings using the Picrosirius—polarization method by which it is possible to identify the intact collagen fibres. Also electron micrographs of 'intrapartum biopsies' show irregular collagenous fibrils with decreased diameter and frequently granular material between them[18].

During pregnancy, the fibroblasts show several indications of high activity: a well developed rough endoplasmic reticulum, secretory vesicles[19,21], and long dendrites allowing secretion of for example proteolytic enzymes relatively far from the cell body. The vascularization and the number of inflammatory cells are considerably increased in the ripened cervix at term[20,22]. The neutrophilic polymorphonuclear leukocytes may be of importance as they are greatly increased in number at term. In addition they are often surrounded by a halo without collagen fibres suggesting fast degradation of this component[18]. Hyperplasia of the smooth muscle has not been observed[23–24], even though some 'maturation' of the muscle cells may be of importance[17].

The biochemical composition of the cervical stroma is rather similar to that of skin, tendon and other fibrous connective tissues characterized by a high physical strength. Quantitatively, collagen is the dominating protein, constituting about 80 % of the dry weight of the non-pregnant cervix[25–9]. The collagen fibrils are highly important for the biomechanical resistance of the cervix. The proteoglycans, glycosaminoglycans[30–2] and other glycoconjugates together with hyaluronic acid are also important molecules as they modify the collagen fibrils in terms of thickness[33], plasticity and ultimate stress[34-5]. The proteoglycans, however, should not be considered as quantitatively major components of the 'ground substance' as they constitute less than 2.5 % of the cervical dry tissue weight[31-2]. Elastin has been demonstrated in relatively low concentration in the human cervix similar to that found in skin[36]. Therefore, the cervix does not belong to the family of elastic tissues including the aorta and the lung, organs in which this protein gives a high degree of elasticity.

Compared with the non-pregnant cervix the collagen concentration has decreased at 10 weeks of pregnancy (Figure 8.2), and at term it has only 35% of its non-pregnant value[28-29]. We do not know if a change in the synthesis of collagen contributes to this fall in the concentration. It has however been demonstrated that the activities of the only two mammalian extracellular enzymes known to degrade collagen are increased 10-fold at term. These enzymes are collagenase (DNP-peptide hydrolyic activity) and leukocyte elastase[29,37-8] (Figure 8.2). The collagen concentration and the activities of collagenase and leukocyte elastase are similar in biopsies obtained at elective caesarean section from term pregnant women not in labour and in cervical biopsies taken immediately after normal spontaneous deliveries[29]. Thus there are no indications of any major collagen degradation during labour. In addition to a decrease in collagen concentration during pregnancy, the extractability of the collagen into acetic acid with pepsin is increased from 18% in the non-pregnant state to 79% at term of pregnancy, and it is further increased to 89% immediately after delivery[25-9]. Most probably this dramatic increase in collagen extractability reflects a reduced number and a reduced stability of

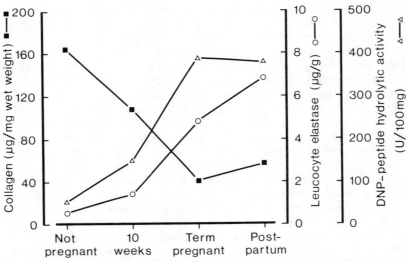

Figure 8.2 Collagen, DNP-peptide hydrolytic activity (collagenase) and leukocyte elastase in cervical biopsies obtained at different gestational ages. Modified from Uldbjerg et al.[29]

the collagen intermolecular 'cross links', which are considered to be of importance for the strength of the individual collagen fibrils.

Even though the cervical glycosaminoglycans/proteoglycans have been described in a number of reports[25-6,30,39-41], little is known of their role in the cervical ripening process. Most probably the major part of the dermatan sulphate proteoglycans are located at the surface of the collagen fibrils[33], where they may affect the collagen as discussed above. It is then not surprising that the concentration of these molecules has been found to decrease at term in a similar way to the collagen[29,30,39]. The heparan sulphate proteoglycans are associated with the cell surface and blood vessel. Accordingly they have been demonstrated in increased concentrations at term[30,39]. Hyaluronic acid has an extreme waterbinding capacity. This glycosaminoglycan could therefore be expected to be responsible for the palpable cervical oedema found at term and measured as an increase in the concentration of water[29]. However, this does not seem to be the case, as hyaluronic acid is unchanged or decreased in concentration at term[29,30,39].

The clinical significance of the decreased concentration of cervical collagen and the increased extractability of the remaining collagen at term has been examined in two reports[29,42]. It was shown that in women with spontaneous, normal deliveries, the cervical dilatation time is proportional to the cervical collagen concentration. For instance, women with four hours dilatation time had a cervical collagen concentration of 35 μg/mg wet tissue weight, whereas women with 10 hours dilatation time had 85 μg/mg wet tissue weight. Women with prolonged duration of labour (on average 18 hours dilatation time) in spite of regular myometrial contractions seem to have both increased collagen concentration and decreased collagen extractability. At this time no such relationship has been demonstrated for the other connective tissue components in the human uterine cervix.

Cervical smooth muscle markers do not suggest increased muscular concentration at term of pregnancy: the concentration of actin is unchanged and the activity of creatinine kinase is unchanged or reduced[43]. Furthermore, Danforth[16] found the cervical muscular contractility in vitro was limited at term of pregnancy. Bryman et al.[44] reported that in 20% of strips from non-pregnant as well as pregnant cervices contractile activity could not be demonstrated, indicating a very low muscle content.

EICOSANOIDS: SYNTHESIS AND RECEPTORS

So far, it has not been possible to study the in vivo synthesis of eicosanoids in the human uterine cervix. However, the cervical venous drainage of ewes in late pregnancy and labour contains increased concentrations of prostaglandin E_2 and the stable degradation product of prostacyclin, 6-keto-prostaglandin $F_{1\alpha}$ (6-keto-PGF$_{1\alpha}$), as pregnancy proceeds[45-7]. The hormonal control of parturition might, however, differ between animal and man.

These authors have also studied the ability of cervical biopsies from pregnant women to produce prostanoids from endogenous arachidonic acid using radioimmunoassay[48]. The biopsies released similar amounts of PGE$_2$,

$PGF_{2\alpha}$ and 6-keto-$PGF_{1\alpha}$, whereas the production of thromboxane B_2 (TxB_2) was minimal.

Recently, a Swedish group[49,50] and a Japanese group[51-2] have studied the ability of whole cell homogenates of cervical tissue to convert exogenous [^{14}C]-arachidonic acid to eicosanoids. Both groups used reliable biochemical techniques including silicic acid chromatography, thin layer chromatography, reverse phase partition chromatography, radio–gas chromatography and gas chromatography–mass spectrometry. Mitsuhashi and Kato[52] obtained material from six patients undergoing hysterectomy and found the homogenates produced equivalent amounts of 6-keto-$PGF_{1\alpha}$, $PGF_{2\alpha}$ and TxB_2. Furthermore, a so far unknown compound which could be a hydroxyacid different from 5-HETE and 12-HETE, was produced in amounts exceeding those of the prostaglandins. Cervices obtained from eight patients undergoing elective caesarian section converted arachidonic acid to 6-keto-$PGF_{1\alpha}$, PGE_2, $PGF_{2\alpha}$ and TxB_2 and mainly to 12-HETE[51]. These authors could not demonstrate any relation between the arachidonic conversion rate and the Bishop score. Christensen et al.[49,50] found the conversion of arachidonic acid into $PGF_{2\alpha}$, PGE_2, TxB_2 and an unknown less polar compound to be significantly higher in homogenates of cervical tissue obtained from women at elective caesarian section compared to that in homogenates from late first trimester patients. These differences were, however, relatively small except for the unknown compound. On the thin-layer radiochromatogram this metabolite had an Rf value similar to a hydroxyacid and at term of pregnancy the production was increased 5- to 10-fold, thus being considerably higher than that of the other eicosanoids. In accordance with Mitsuhashi and Kato[51], Christensen et al.[49] found that there was no correlation between the Bishop score and the conversion of [^{14}C]-arachidonic acid. In contrast with these authors, however, they could only occasionally demonstrate small amounts of 6-keto-$PGF_{1\alpha}$.

Tanaka et al.[53] incubated microsomal fractions of human uterine cervix with [^{14}C]-arachidonic acid. They could only demonstrate limited amounts of material which on thin layer chromatography behaved like PGE_2, $PGF_{2\alpha}$ or TxB_2 whereas a dominating degradation product was observed which might have been 6-keto-$PGF_{1\alpha}$. The production was 7-fold increased at term of pregnancy and was completely inhibited by an inhibitor of prostacyclin synthetase (15-hydroperoxy-5,8,11,13-eicosatetraenoic acid).

Taken together these *in vitro* studies indicate that the human uterine cervix has the machinery necessary to synthesize eicosanoids. Furthermore, the capacity of this machinery seems increased at term of pregnancy. However, it has been shown that in other tissues the amount of prostaglandin formed from exogenous arachidonic acid is sometimes quite different from that formed from endogenous arachidonic acid[54]. In addition, the differences in the techniques used should be considered, when the results are compared. In a preliminary report by Manabe et al.[55] the connective tissue of the human vagina has been found to change during pregnancy in a way similar to that of the cervix. In that study immuno-histochemical examinations demonstrated free prostaglandin E_2 to be present in increasing amounts during pregnancy.

As discussed above, the human uterine cervix at term pregnancy is characterized by an invasion of neutrophilic polymorphonuclear leukocytes[18].

These cells are known to produce several eicosanoids[56] and it has been suggested that they are at least partly responsible for the changes in eicosanoid synthesis observed during pregnancy[49]. Also the increased vascularization described in late pregnancy can be of importance. In particular, PGI_2 and TxB_2 are related to the vascular system.

Due to diffusion and to transport by the venous system, eicosanoids might also reach the cervical stroma from production sites in the cervical mucosa, in the fetal membranes and to some extent from sites in the myometrium and the placenta. Whole cell homogenates of cervical mucosa convert arachidonic acid to $PGF_{2\alpha}$, PGE_2, TxB_2 and a compound which might be a hydroxyacid[49]. Mitsuhashi and Kato[51] who found that 6-keto-$PGF_{1\alpha}$ was produced in the cervical tissue could not demonstrate this metabolite after incubation of arachidonic acid with homogenates of cervical mucosa. The fetal membranes are enriched in phospholipids with arachidonic acid and might be an important source for eicosanoids[57-8]. Furthermore, the enzymes responsible for arachidonic acid release and metabolism, phospholipase A_2 and C and diacylglycerol lipase, as well as cyclo-oxygenase are present in the fetal membranes, decidua, placenta, and the myometrium[59-62]. The activities of phospholipase A_2 and C in amnion are reported to increase with advancing gestation[60]. Whole cell homogenates of fetal membranes convert $[^{14}C]$-arachidonic acid into PGE_2 but not to $PGF_{2\alpha}$[62-4]. Using other determination techniques in combination with radioimmunoassays Mitchell et al.[65] have in addition to PGE measured significant amounts of 6-keto-$PGF_{1\alpha}$ as well as small quantities of PGF and TxB_2[66-8] produced by the fetal membranes in vitro. An increase in the output of prostaglandins by the fetal membranes has been related to labour[62,68]. Also the myometrium produces prostaglandins and hydroxyacids[52,69]. It is therefore not surprising that the concentrations of free arachidonic acid[70-1] and prostaglandins in the amniotic fluid seem to increase markedly during labour[61,71-7].

Prostaglandin receptors or more precisely the binding of prostaglandins to human cervical tissue have been described in only a few reports. Studies have mainly focused on the myometrium, less attention being paid to the cervix. However, it is well established that non-pregnant uterine tissue binds PGE in accordance with that expected by the presence of at least two types of free specific receptors with different affinities[78-81]. The majority of these receptors are located at the plasma membrane as evaluated by fractionation of tissue homogenates on sucrose gradients[79]. The topical distribution within the uterus is similar to that of the smooth muscle cells. Thus the binding capacity in the cervix is from less than 10%[80] to 30%[81] of that in the corpus. Forty eight hours pretreatment of postmenopausal woman with oestrogen seems to reduce the number of free PGE_2 binding sites markedly (one patient)[80]. Equally low levels of free PGE_2 binding sites were found in a uterus obtained at the 20th week of pregnancy. In the fundus as well as in the cervix the $PGF_{2\alpha}$ binding is much less than the PGE_2 binding. It is not clear if a greater affinity of some PGE sites or a greater number of PGE binding sites compared to those for the two specific $PGF_{2\alpha}$ binding sites can account for this difference[81]. Alternatively $PGF_{2\alpha}$ may exhibit low grade binding to PGE receptors[78,80].

EICOSANOIDS: PHARMACOLOGICAL EFFECTS

In this section we will present data on the treatment of the uterine cervix with prostaglandins *in vivo* followed by data obtained from *in vitro* studies.

The pharmacological effect of prostaglandin E_2 applied within the cervical canal or in the vagina is closely related to the state of pregnancy. In non-pregnant women intravaginal suppositories of 20 mg PGE_2 do not give any detectable change in the cervix[82] but are associated with considerable side-effects including heavy gastrointestinal discomfort, chills and severe hypotension. However Lauersen et al.[83], found that 0.5 mg 15(S)-15-methyl-$PGF_{2\alpha}$ administered as a vaginal suppository one hour prior to insertion of IUD caused a 2.1 mm increase in cervical diameter. To illustrate the increasing sensitivity of the cervix to PGE_2 with advancing gestational age, the effect of local treatment with this prostaglandin at various stages of pregnancy can be compared. At 10 weeks gestational age intracervical application of 0.5 mg PGE_2 induces a significant softening and dilatation of the cervix within 12 hours as evaluated by palpation[84] or by the force required to dilate the cervical canal to a diameter of 8 mm[85]. Women with missed abortions or intrauterine fetal death respond with pronounced cervical 'ripening' to such treatment[86]. Despite a low cervical score intracervical application of 0.5 mg PGE_2 at term is usually followed by a dramatic cervical ripening[14,87]. Conrad and Ueland[8] determined the biomechanical properties of biopsies obtained from the region of the external os from patients immediately following delivery. The stress moduli of cervical tissue from spontaneous and oxytocin-induced labour patients were similar and twice that of tissue from women with orally PGE_2-induced labour. Thus these authors confirmed the clinical experience that PGE_2 has the ability to lower the stiffness of cervical tissue at term of pregnancy[88]. It has been suggested that the sensitivity of the cervix to PGE_2 is related to plasma oestrogen. For example, it was found that 43 term pregnant women who went into labour after intravaginal installation of PGE_2 had significantly higher 17β-oestradiol levels (27 ng/ml) than 26 who did not (19 ng/ml)[89]. In these studies it is not obvious if the pharmacological effect of PGE_2 is solely due to local phenomena taking place within the cervix or if a uterotonic prostaglandin effect is involved. However, it still seems well established that the cervical sensitivity to PGE_2 increases with advancing pregnancy.

In the daily routine, induction of cervical ripening by local application of PGE_2 in gel will often involve increased myometrial activity. This is almost certainly due to inappropriate application or leakage of the gel from the cervical canal to the extra-amniotic space or to systemic access of the PGE_2 via the vaginal vascular system. Forman et al.[12] measured the intrauterine pressure in two groups of 10 weeks pregnant women. One group received intravenous infusion of oxytocin and the other 0.5 mg PGE_2 in gel strictly applied within the cervical canal. In the oxytocin treated group, there was a pronounced increase in the uterine activity but no palpable change in cervical state. In the PGE_2 treated group there was a limited and only initial myometrial stimulation but a significant softening of the cervix after six hours. These results that have been confirmed in a double-blind study by Sørensen et al.[90]

and suggest a direct effect of PGE_2 on the cervical tissue[14]. Moreover cervical ripening induced by PGE_2 at term or in early pregnancy before termination of pregnancy by dilatation and evacuation is unaffected by simultaneous treatment with tocolytics like β-receptor stimulating drugs or calcium blockers[13,84]. It is therefore concluded that PGE_2 has a direct cervical ripening potency.

PGE_2 is almost 10 times more potent than $PGF_{2\alpha}$ in its ripening effect on the cervix. MacKenzie and Embrey[91] showed by intrauterine pressure recording that cervical gel containing 25 mg $PGF_{2\alpha}$ had the same uterotonic effect as gel with 5 mg PGE_2 but the $PGF_{2\alpha}$ had much less effect than PGE_2 on cervical ripening. Neilson et al.[92] compared vaginal instillation of gel with 40 mg $PGF_{2\alpha}$ and 5 mg PGE_2 respectively. They also found PGE_2 to be superior to $PGF_{2\alpha}$ as measured by the change in the Bishop score and rate of cervical dilatation at established labour. These clinical results which might reflect the characteristics of the prostaglandin binding sites must be considered when the importance of endogenous synthesis of eicosanoids discussed above are evaluated.

Another consideration is whether treatment with prostaglandins triggers the endogenous secretion of eicosanoids. After studying the plasma levels of 15-methyl-$PGF_{2\alpha}$, and degradation product of PGE_2 and $PGF_{2\alpha}$ Gréen et al.[93] concluded that following administration of vaginal suppositories containing 15-methyl-$PGF_{2\alpha}$ for induction of abortion, the initially induced uterine contractility is due to the effect of the drug itself, but that after several hours there is an increasing, probably intrauterine production of PGE_2 and $PGF_{2\alpha}$ which might contribute to finalization of the abortion process. This hypothesis is supported by the fact that simultaneous inhibition of the biosynthesis of prostaglandins by indomethacin and administration of 15-methyl-$PGF_{2\alpha}$ increases the induction–termination interval and the number of failed cases[94]. As described previously Christensen and Bygdeman[50] have investigated the conversion of [^{14}C]-arachidonic acid by whole cell homogenates from late first trimester cervices. They found that 12 to 14 hours treatment with intracervical PGE_2 or intravaginal 9-deoxo-16,16-dimethyl-9-methylene PGE_2 before sampling does not cause any dramatic change in the bioconversion of exogenous arachidonic acid into prostaglandin compounds, whereas the production of non-prostaglandin eicosanoids might be increased. Five minutes pre-incubation in vitro with PGE_2 (50 μg/ml) did not change the profile of products formed from [^{14}C]-arachidonic acid. Most probably these contradictions between the clinical experience including measurement of plasma concentrations and the eicosanoid production in whole cell homogenates reflects the myometrial activity induced by the treatment, as myometrial activity and myometrial prostaglandin production are related as discussed below. In early pregnancy such an activity does not necessarily involve marked stimulation of the cervix, even though cervical prostaglandin synthesis might be influenced by mechanical stress.

Histological and electron microscopic examination of cervical stroma tissue from 9–14 weeks pregnant women treated with PGE_2 compared with examinations of tissue obtained before application of PGE_2 show changes similar to those observed during the physiological ripening process. After treatment the fibroblasts have distended Golgi apparatus, a rough endoplasmic reticulum and many mitochondria as well as an increased number of cytoplasm vesicles located close to the plasma membrane[21,95]. These signs indicate an activation of the fibroblasts by PGE$_2$. The extracellular matrix is 'oedematous' and the collagen fibres are less densely packed, more spread out, and run in various directions[19,95]. In some areas they disappear and only 'amorphous substance' can be observed[21]. Using histochemical techniques, Joh et al.[95] have shown vesicles in the extracellular matrix after PGE$_2$ application. These vesicles localized between the collagen fibres, showed the reaction product of acid phosphatase and were often surrounded by an electron-lucent halo. Most probably, they represent 'matrix lysosomes' containing proteolytic enzymes of importance for connective tissue degradation. Also a dilatation of small vessels has been observed after treatment (Uldbjerg, N., Ekman, G., Malmström, A. and Ulmsten, U., unpublished observation), whereas invasion of leukocytes has not been described.

Relatively few studies have described biochemical changes in the cervical connective tissue after treatment with prostaglandin in vivo. We have compared the biochemical composition of cervical biopsies taken before and after application of 0.5 mg PGE$_2$ intracervically in late first trimester of pregnancy. Surprisingly, there was a significant decrease (sic) in collagenolytic activity as determined by a synthetic DNP-peptide[96]. The concentration of collagen decreased after PGE$_2$ treatment, but the difference was not statistically significant (three patients). Neither the concentration of water, sulphate glycosaminoglycans nor hyaluronic acid were changed after treatment. Rath et al.[97] compared cervical biopsies from women in whom abortion was induced between the 7th and 12th weeks of pregnancy. Eight hours before sampling one group had intracervical PGF$_{2\alpha}$ and 50 % of these women had 'low' collagen concentrations in their biopsies, whereas this was only the case in 20 % of the women in the untreated control group. Nakanishi[98] reported that four days treatment with PGE$_2$ orally in non-pregnant women caused an increased cervical glycosaminoglycan concentration.

Using a biological assay Szalay et al.[99] determined the collagenolytic activity in cervical tissue of 16 women who had received 1.25 mg PGE$_2$ through a portioadaptor, and another 16 women in whom cervical ripening had occurred spontaneously. The mean lysis of a collagen film was 5.4 mm^2 in the untreated group and 7.8 mm^2 in the PGE$_2$ treated group. This difference was statistically significant. Furthermore, the PGE$_2$ induced collagenolytic activity at term of pregnancy as determined by the DNP-peptide correlates well with the clinical response to the treatment[100]. In four women with prompt response to the treatment, i.e. favourable cervical state combined with established labour within five hours after PGE$_2$ gel application, the DNP-peptide hydrolytic activity was 688 U/100 mg versus 372 U/100 mg in a control untreated group, and only 365 U/100 mg in women in whom the treatment had moderate clinical response. All women had unfavourable cervical states before intracervical application of PGE$_2$ gel. It is therefore likely that they had low initial DNP-peptide hydrolytic activities. Thus a normalization of the activity in the patients with the moderate clinical response is possible. The collagen concentration seems decreased after treatment, most probably as a result of the increased collagenolytic activity[42]. Also in patients with missed abortion it has been possible to demonstrate a similar correlation between the clinical response to prostaglandin treatment and the change in DNP-peptide hydrolytic activity in cervical tissue (Uldbjerg, N., Ekman, G., Malmström, A. and Ulmsten, U., unpublished observation). Women with a diameter of the cervical canal ⩽ 11 mm after treatment showed changes in DNP-peptide hydrolytic activity and in collagen concentration similar to those described in first trimester of pregnancy (decreased DNP-peptide hydrolytic activity and unchanged collagen). Three patients with diameters ⩾ 12 mm after PGE_2 showed increased DNP-peptide hydrolytic activities and decreased collagen. Thus it can be concluded that a degradation of cervical collagen by collagenase and other collagenolytic enzymes is involved in the cervical ripening induced by local application of prostaglandins.

Even though it remains unknown if cervical smooth muscle is of importance for the ripening process a study of the effect of intravenous injection of prostaglandins on the contractility of the non-pregnant uterine cervix has been performed[101]. The intraluminal pressure was recorded through latex balloons. $PGF_{2\alpha}$ was found to stimulate contractility at all phases of the menstrual cycle, whereas PGE_2 was inhibitory. The sensitivity to PGE_2 was most marked during the pre-ovulatory phase. The authors therefore suggested that this effect of PGE_2 which is present in semen may be a prerequisite for sperm penetration.

The following part of this section will be concerned with *in vitro* studies on the effect of arachidonic acid and prostaglandins on different components in the cervix.

The influence of prostaglandins (0.05–2.0 μg/ml) on the contractility of isolated non-pregnant cervical smooth muscle has been studied by Najak *et al.*[102]. They found PGE_2 to cause a marked relaxation whereas the effect of $PGF_{2\alpha}$ was more variable. Bryman *et al.*[44] confirmed these findings (ED_{50} for PGE_2 approximately 300 pg/ml). Furthermore, they found strips from 12 weeks pregnant women to be inhibited by PGE_2 at concentrations down to 0.01 pg/ml (ED_{50} about 20 pg/ml). PGI_2 and 6-keto-$PGF_{1\alpha}$ were much less potent.

Conrad and Ueland[103] tested the biomechanical properties of cervical biopsies taken immediately after delivery. The biopsies were placed in an aerated organ bath and strain–stress curves were obtained. The effect of PGE_2 at a bath concentration of 1–10 μg/ml was to reduce the stiffness of the biopsies within 5–15 minutes. To explain this very interesting observation, which has never been confirmed by other groups, we determined the concentration of collagen and the collagenolytic activity (DNP-peptide hydrolytic activity) in similar biopsies treated under similar conditions (Uldbjerg, N., Malmström, A., Wingerup, L., Ekman, G. and Ulmsten, U., unpublished observation). These parameters were, however, unchanged and could not explain the decreased stiffness described by Conrad and Ueland[103].

Wallis and Hillier[104] incubated explants of non-pregnant human cervices for 10 days. The release of hydroxyproline (collagen and collagen degradation products) to the medium was determined to express the collagen degradation in the explants. Only low levels of hydroxyproline were released to the medium during days 1–4 of culture and increasing amounts appeared through days 4–10. PGE_2 and $PGF_{2\alpha}$ (0.3 pg/ml to 3.5 mg/ml) had no effect on collagen dissolution, whereas arachidonic acid stimulated the dissolution at low concentrations (0.3 pg/ml to 30 ng/ml). Indomethacin inhibited the spontaneous collagen dissolution but did not affect the stimulant effect of arachidonic acid. Furthermore, the synthesis of PGE_2, $PGF_{2\alpha}$ and 6-keto-$PGF_{1\alpha}$ was unaffected by the arachidonic acid. The physiological significance is difficult to evaluate as the explants were taken from non-pregnant women and a five day culture period was needed to demonstrate collagen dissolution. However, there was a significant effect of arachidonic acid which might have been a direct one or could be due to the formation of lipoxygenase products, the synthesis of which is not blocked by indomethacin.

The incorporation of the collagen precursor, proline, and the proteoglycan/hyaluronic acid precursor, glucosamine, into macromolecular material by cervical biopsies seems to be influenced by PGE_2 and $PGF_{2\alpha}$[105-7]. The effect of both prostaglandins were similar but changed during the menstrual cycle and during pregnancy and labour. Thus it was demonstrated that prostaglandins can affect the synthesis of cervical connective tissue components. However, a logical relation to cervical ripening remains to be demonstrated.

The effect of eicosanoids on cervical blood vessels has also been studied. Allen et al.[108] determined the in vitro contractility of small cervical arteries from non-pregnant uteri. PGI_2 and PGE_2 showed relaxant effects in preparations contracted by noradrenaline. Thus, these compounds might provide a mechanism for modulation of the adrenergic vascular control. $PGF_{2\alpha}$ did not show relaxant effects in the cervical arteries but produced minor inconsistent contractions, and slightly increased the tension induced by noradrenaline. Leukotrienes did not show marked effects on these vessels. The findings do not support any idea of major direct effects of $PGF_{2\alpha}$ and leukotrienes on medial smooth muscle in cervical arteries.

EICOSANOIDS: EFFECT OF MODULATION OF SYNTHESIS ON THE CERVIX

The synthesis of prostaglandins in the cervix is enhanced by a number of procedures known to stimulate the ripening process such as intra-amniotic injection of arachidonic acid, digital manipulation of the cervix and stretching the tissue in vivo and in vitro. Furthermore it is possible that oestrogens stimulate the local secretion of prostaglandins in the uterine cervix.

Intra-amniotic injection of arachidonic acid but not placebo in the second trimester of pregnancy causes abortion[70]. In two patients the effect was blocked by oral intake of acetylsalicylic acid thus suggesting a conversion of the injected arachidonic acid into prostaglandins as an essential part of the mechanism. It is, however, uncertain if these prostaglandins have direct effects on the cervical tissue or if they activate the myometrium, the contractions of which might start a local production of eicosanoids in the cervix (see below).

The release of eicosanoids from the fetal membranes and the myometrium seems sensitive to mechanical stress *in vivo*[76-7]. Thus, cervical softening induced by mechanical stretching of the uterus by means of intrauterine application of a rubber balloon is probably mediated by increased $PGF_{2\alpha}$ production. A similar response to mechanical stress might also characterize the cervix. Hillier and Coad[109] suspended strips (1 mm x 1 mm x 1 cm) from non-pregnant cervices in an organ bath. They found that passive stretch with 2 g more than doubled the release of immunoreactive PGE_2 and $PGF_{2\alpha}$ to the Krebs solution. Even though similar experiments have not been performed on cervical tissue material from pregnant women, it was hypothesized that the subclinical uterine contractions occuring well before labour[110] might stretch the cervix to release eicosanoids, thereby inducing cervical ripening. Accordingly, it is possible that hormones, drugs, and clinical handling inducing myometrial contractions can ripen the cervix through the same mechanism. However, as described in the beginning of this chapter, myometrial contractions are not a prerequisite for cervical ripening.

The effect of regular vaginal examination and amniotomy, respectively on the synthesis of eicosanoids have been studied. Erkkola *et al.*[111] found the plasma levels of prostaglandin precursors including arachidonic acid unchanged after plain vaginal examination and after amniotomy at term pregnancy. Mitchell *et al.*[112], however, showed that the concentration of the major circulating metabolite of $PGF_{2\alpha}$, 13,14-dihydro-15-keto-$PGF_{2\alpha}$, was doubled five minutes after vaginal examination which included sweeping of the membranes, as well as after amniotomy. The concentration remains elevated for at least half an hour and is not preceded by a rise in circulating oxytocin concentration[113]. Most probably, the local concentration of eicosanoids is much more increased than that in blood and can almost certainly contribute to the cervical ripening and labour which follow these procedures[114]. To our knowledge the effect of intracervical application of laminaria[115] or Lamicel[116] to stimulate the local synthesis of eicosanoids has not been studied. One could, however, speculate that the mechanical stress induced by the laminaria or an inflammatory reaction caused by the magnesium sulphate in Lamicel would ripen the cervix through stimulation of the local synthesis of eicosanoids.

Oestrogens are likely to be involved in cervical ripening[117]. For example, pregnancies with placental sulphatase deficiency and following low circulating oestrogen levels are in a number of cases characterized by failure of the cervix to ripen properly (for review see Lykkesfeldt[118]). However, in most of these pregnancies vaginal delivery can be accomplished without complications. Pinto[22] found that intravenous infusion of 17β-oestradiol at term produced cervical ripening as judged by clinical and histological examination. Dehydroepiandrosterone sulphate injected intravenously is metabolized in the placenta resulting in increased 17β-oestradiol levels in both serum and cervical tissue. At term of pregnancy this treatment is followed by cervical ripening within four hours and increased cervical collagenolytic activity as determined by a tissue culture method[119]. Furthermore, local application of oestradiol has been reported to ripen the cervix[120-4]. Other investigators, however, did not find oestrogens more effective than placebo[125-6] (Ekman, G., Stenberg, P. and Ulmsten, U., unpublished observation). To explain a possible role for oestrogens in cervical ripening Ellwood *et al.*[45] have hypothesized that these hormones stimulate the synthesis of prostaglandins in the cervix. There are, however, no convincing results in favour of this idea[98]. In fact Wallis and Hillier[127] showed that 17β-oestradiol could inhibit the collagen dissolution in cervical biopsies from non-pregnant women.

Nonsteroidal anti-inflammatory agents like acetylsalicylic acid and indomethacin inhibit cyclo-oxygenase resulting in decreased synthesis of PGE_2, $PGF_{2\alpha}$, PGI_2 and TxA_2. It is interesting therefore to notice that their regular intake seems to prolong the length of gestation as well as the length of labour[128-9]. In a retrospective study pregnancy was found to be lengthened by an average of seven days in women who ingested 3.25 g aspirin or more daily. In 42 % of these women, pregnancy lasted $\geqslant$ 42 weeks. Moreover, labour lasted five hours longer in patients taking aspirin than in controls[128]. Furthermore, these drugs have been used with some success for treatment of premature labour[130-2]. However, from these studies it is impossible to evaluate the effect on the myometrium and the cervix separately. In sheep it has been possible to evaluate this relationship in some detail. In two studies cervical ripening was blocked by treatment with inhibitors of prostaglandin synthesis[133-4].

These observations suggest that during pregnancy an increased synthesis of prostaglandins in the cervix will be followed by softening of the organ and that inhibition of the synthesis will delay cervical ripening.

CONCLUSIONS

(1)   The human uterine body is mainly muscular whereas the uterine cervix is dominated by fibrous connective tissue.

(2)   Cervical ripening is essential for normal vaginal delivery and involves increased collagenolytic activity with concomitant decreased concentration of collagen.

(3)   The human cervix has the machinery necessary to produce eicosanoids. The synthesis of lipoxygenase products might be increased at term of pregnancy. The importance of PGI_2 remains unknown.

(4)   The cervical tissue seems to contain free prostaglandin receptors but there are less compared to the uterine body. The binding of PGE_2 to cervical tissue is several times that of $PGF_{2\alpha}$. There are no indications of increased binding capacity during pregnancy.

(5)   Treatment of the cervix with PGE_2 during pregnancy induces softening of the organ, histological changes like those described during the physiological ripening of the cervix, and increased collagenolytic activity. PGE_2 is almost 10 times more potent that $PGF_{2\alpha}$ in that respect. Myometrial activity is not a prerequisite for the ripening potency of PGE_2.

(6)   Most probably intra-amniotic injection of arachidonic acid, sweeping of the membranes, amniotomy and possibly oestrogens will trigger the synthesis of cervical eicosanoids. The described procedures are also followed by cervical ripening. Non-steroidal anti-inflammatory agents inhibit the synthesis of prostaglandins and delay cervical ripening.

(7)   Taken together, these data indicate a physiological role of eicosanoids in controlling the form and function of the cervix.

ACKNOWLEDGEMENTS

This work was supported by grants from the Danish Medical Research Council, from Institut for Eksperimentiel Forskning, from Aarhus Universitets Forskningsfond, and from Konto for Klassisk Klinisk Forskning, University of Aarhus.

REFERENCES

1. Hendricks, C.H., Brenner, W.E. and Kraus, G. (1970). Normal cervical dilatation pattern in late pregnancy and labor. *Am. J. Obstet. Gynecol.*, **106**, 1065–82
2. Bishop, E.H. (1964). Pelvic scoring for elective induction. *Obstet. Gynecol.*, **24**, 266
3. Lange, A.P., Secher, N.J., Westergaard, J.G. and Skovgård I. (1982). Prelabour evaluation of inducibility. *Obstet. Gynecol.*, **60**, 137–47
4. Embrey, M.P. and Calder, A.A. Induction of labour. In Beard, R., Brudenell, M., Dunn, P., Fairweather, D. (eds.) (1975). *The Management of Labour*, p. 62 (London: Royal College of Obstetricians and Gynaecologists)
5. Hulka, J.F., Lefler, H.T., Anglone, A. and Lachenbruch, P.A. (1974). A new electronic force monitor to measure factors influencing cervical dilation for vacuum curettage. *Am. J. Obstet. Gynecol.*, **120**, 166–173
6. Anthony, G.S., Fisher, J., Coutts, J.R.T. and Calder, A.A. (1982). Forces required for surgical dilatation of the pregnant and non-pregnant human cervix. *Br. J. Obstet. Gynaecol.*, **89**, 913–6
7. Bakke, T. (1974). Cervical consistency in women of fertile age measured with a new mechanical instrument. *Acta Obstet. Gynecol. Scand.*, **53**, 293–302
8. Conrad, J.T. and Ueland, K. (1976). The stretch modulus of human cervical tissue in spontaneous, oxytocin-induced, and prostaglandin E_2-induced labor. *Am. J. Obstet. Gynecol.*, **133**, 11–4
9. Calder, A.A. (1981). The human cervix in pregnancy: a clinical perspective. In: Ellwood, D.A., Anderson, A.B.M. (eds.) *The Cervix in Pregnancy and Labour. Clinical and Biochemical Investigations*, pp. 103–22. (New York: Churchill Livingstone)
10. Hollingsworth, M. and Gallimore, S. (1981). Evidence that cervical softening in the pregnant rat is independent of increasing uterine contractility. *J. Reprod. Fertil.*, **63**, 449–54
11. Ledger, W.L., Webster, M., Harrison, L.P., Anderson, A.B.M. and Turnbull, A.C. (1985). Increase in cervical extensibility during labour-induced after isolation of the cervix from the uterus in pregnant ewes. *Am. J. Obstet. Gynecol.*, **151**, 397–402
12. Forman, A., Ulmsten, U., Banyai, J., Wingerup, L. and Uldbjerg, N. (1982). Evidence for a local effect of intracervical prostaglandin E_2-gel. *Am. J. Obstet. Gynecol.*, **143**, 756–760
13. Goeschen, K., Fuchs, A.-R., Fuchs, F., Rasmussen, A.B., Rehnström, J.V. and Saling, E. (1985). Effect of β-mimetic tocolysis on cervical ripening and plasma prostaglandin $F_{2\alpha}$ metabolite after endocervical application of prostaglandin E_2. *Obstet. Gynecol.*, **65**, 166–71
14. Ekman, G., Forman, A., Marsal, K. and Ulmsten, U. (1983). Intravaginal versus intracervical application of prostaglandin E_2 in viscous gel for cervical priming and induction of labor at term in patients with an unfavourable cervical state. *Am. J. Obstet. Gynecol.*, **147**, 657–61
15. Danforth, D.N. (1947). The fibrous nature of the human cervix, and its relation to the isthmic segment in gravid and nongravid uteri. *Am. J. Obstet. Gynecol.*, **53**, 541–60
16. Danforth, D.N. and Evanston, M.D. (1954). The distribution and functional activity of the cervical musculature. *Am. J. Obstet. Gynecol.*, **68**, 1261–1271

17. Hughesdon, P.E. (1952). The fibromuscular structure of the cervix and its changes during pregnancy and labour. *J. Obstet. Gynaecol. Br. Emp.*, **59**, 763–76
18. Junqueira, L.C.U., Zugaib, M., Montes, G.S., Toledo, O.M.S., Krisztan, R.M. and Shigihara, K.M. (1980). Morphologic and histochemical evidence for the occurrence of collagenolysis and for the role of neutrophilic polymorphonuclear leukocytes during cervical dilation. *Am. J. Obstet. Gynecol.*, **138**, 273–81
19. Theobald, P.W., Rath, W., Kühnle, H. and Kuhn, W. (1983). Histological and electron-microscopic examinations of collagenous connective tissue of the non-pregnant cervix, the pregnant cervix and the pregnant prostaglandin-treated cervix. *Arch. Gynecol.*, **231**, 241–5
20. Danforth, D.N., Buckingham, J.C. and Roddick, J.W. (1960). Connective tissue changes incident to cervical effacement. *Am. J. Obstet. Gynecol.*, **80**, 939–945
21. Uldbjerg, N., Ekman, G., Malmström, A., Sporrong, B., Ulmsten, U. and Wingerup, L. (1981). Biochemical and morphological changes of human cervix after local application of prostaglandin E_2 in pregnancy. *Lancet*, **2**, 267–8
22. Pinto, R.M., Rabow, W. and Votta, R.A. (1965). Uterine cervix ripening in term pregnancy due to the action of estradiol-17β. A histological and histochemical study. *Am. J. Obstet. Gynecol.*, **92**, 319–24
23. Schwalm, H. and Dubrauszky, V. (1966). The structure of the musculature of the human uterus-muscles and connective tissue. *Am. J. Obstet. Gynecol.*, **94**, 391–404
24. Strauss, G. (1969). Funktionsbedingte unterschiede der feinstruktur des kollagenen bindegewebes menschlicher Uteri. *Arch. Gynäk*, **208**, 147–77
25. von Maillot, K.V. and Zimmermann, B.K. (1976). The solubility of collagen of the uterine cervix during pregnancy and labour. *Arch. Gynäk*, **220**, 275–80
26. Danforth, D.N., Veis, A., Breen, M., Weinstein, H.G., Buckingham, J.C. and Manalo, P. (1974). The effect of pregnancy and labour on the human cervix: Changes in collagen, glycoproteins, and glycosaminoglycans. *Am. J. Obstet. Gynecol.*, **120**, 641–651
27. Kleissl, H.P., van der Rest, M., Naftolin, F., Glorieux, F.H. and De Leon, A. (1978). Collagen changes in the human cervix at parturition. *Am. J. Obstet. Gynecol.*, **130**, 748–753
28. Ito, A., Kitamura, K., Mori, V. and Hirakawa, S. (1979). The change in solubility of type I collagen in human uterine cervix in pregnancy at term. *Biochem. Med.*, **21**, 262–70
29. Uldbjerg, N., Ekman, G., Malmström, A., Olsson, K. and Ulmsten, U. (1983). Ripening of the human uterine cervix related to changes in collagen, glycosaminoglycans, and collagenolytic activity. *Am. J. Obstet. Gynecol.*, **147**, 662–6
30. Kitamura, K., Ito, A., Mori, Y. and Hirakawa, S. (1980). Glycosaminoglycans of human uterine cervix: Heparan sulfate increase with reference to cervical ripening. *Biochem. Med.*, **23**, 159–66
31. Uldbjerg, N., Carlstedt, I., Ekman, G., Malmström, A., Ulmsten, U. and Wingerup, L. (1983). Dermatan sulphate and mucin glycopeptides from the human uterine cervix. *Gynecol. Obstet. Invest.*, **16**, 199–209
32. Uldbjerg, N., Malmström, A., Ekman, G., Sheehan, J., Ulmsten, U. and Wingerup, L. (1983). Isolation and characterization of dermatan sulphate proteoglycan from human uterine cervix. *Biochem. J.*, **209**, 497–503
33. Scott, E. (1984). The periphery of the developing collagen fibril. *Biochem. J.*, **218**, 229–33
34. Danielsen, C.C. (1982). Mechanical properties of reconstituted collagen fibrils. Influence of a glycosaminoglycan: dermatan sulfate. *Conn. Tissue. Res.*, **9**, 219–25
35. Hukins, D.W.L. and Aspden, R.M. (1985). Composition and properties of connective tissues. *Trends Biochem. Sci.*, 260–4
36. Leppert, P.C., Keller, S., Cerreta, J., Hosannah, Y. and Mandl, I. (1983). The content of elastin in the uterine cervix. *Arch. Biochem. Biophys.*, **222**, 53–8
37. Kitamura, K., Ito, A., Mori, Y. and Hirakawa, S. (1979). Changes in the human uterine cervical collagenase with special reference to cervical ripening. *Biochem. Med.*, **22**, 332–8
38. Kitamura, K., Ito, A. and Mori, Y. (1980). The existing forms of collagenase in the human uterine cervix. *J. Biochem.*, **87**, 753–60
39. Cabrol, D., Breton, M., Berrou, E., Visser, A., Sureau, C. and Picard, J. (1980). Variations in the distribution of glycosaminoglycans in the uterine cervix of the pregnant woman. *Eur. J. Obstet. Gynecol. Reprod. Biol.*, **10**, 281–7

40. Shimizu, T., Endo, M. and Yosizawa, Z. (1980). Glycoconjugates (Glycosaminoglycans and Glycoproteins) and glycogen in the human cervix uteri. *Tohoku J. Exp. Med.*, **131**, 289–299

41. Nakaya, T. (1973). Studies on acid mucopolysaccharides in the human cervix uteri. *Nagoya Med. J.*, **18**, 295–319

42. Ekman, G., Malmström, A., Uldbjerg, N. and Ulmsten, U. Cervical collagen an important regulator of cervical function in term labour. *Gynecol. Obstet.*, (in press)

43. Martin, A., Fara, J.F., Alallon, W., Thoulon, J.M., Dumont, M. and Louisot, P. (1983). Enzymatic screening of human uterine cervical biopsies in non-pregnant and pregnant women at parturition. *Am. J. Obstet. Gynecol.*, **145**, 44–50

44. Bryman, I., Sahni, S., Norström, A. and Lindblom B. (1984). Influence of prostaglandins on contractility of the isolated human cervical muscle. *Obstet. Gynecol.*, **63**, 280–4

45. Ellwood, D.A., Mitchell, M.D., Anderson, A.B.M. and Turnbull, A.C. (1979). Prostaglandin production by the cervix. Observations in vitro and in vivo. *Br. J. Obstet. Gynaecol.*, **86**, 826

46. Ellwood, D.A., Mitchell, M.D., Anderson, A.B.M. and Turnbull, A.C. (1979). Prostacyclin may be involved in cervical ripening. *Fourth International Prostaglandins Conference*, Washington.

47. Ellwood, D.A., Mitchell, M.D., Anderson, A.B.M. and Turnbull, A.C. (1979). A significant increase in the in vitro production of prostaglandin E by ovine cervical tissue at delivery. *J. Endocrinol.*, **81**, 133 P

48. Ellwood, D.A., Mitchell, M.D., Anderson, A.B.M. and Turnbull, A.C. (1980). The in vitro production of prostanoids by the human cervix during pregnancy: preliminary observations. *Br. J. Obstet. Gynaecol.*, **87**, 210–4

49. Christensen, N.J., Belfrage, P., Bygdeman, M., Floberg, J., Miszuhashi, N. and Gréen, K. (1985). Bioconversion of arachidonic acid in human pregnant uterine cervix. *Acta Obstet. Gynecol. Scand.*, **64**, 259–65

50. Christensen, N.J. and Bygdeman, M. (1985). The effect of prostaglandins on the bioconversion of arachidonic acid in cervical tissue in early human pregnancy. *Prostaglandins*, **29**, 291–302

51. Mitsuhashi, N. and Kato, J. (1984). Bioconversion of arachidonic acid by human uterine cervical tissue and endocervix in late pregnancy. *Endocrinol. Jpn.*, **31**, 533–8

52. Mitsuhashi, N. and Kato, J. (1984). Bioconversion of arachidonic acid to prostaglandins and related compounds in human myometrium and uterine cervix. *Endocrinol. Jpn.*, **31**, 815–20

53. Tanaka, M., Morita, I., Hirakawa, S. and Murota, S.I. (1981). Increased prostacyclin synthesizing activity in human ripening uterine cervix. *Prostaglandins*, **21**, 83–6

54. Dimov, V., Christensen, N.J. and Gréen, K. (1983). Analysis of prostaglandins formed from endogenous and exogenous arachidonic acid in homogenates of human reproductive tissues. *Biochem. Biophys. Acta*, **754**, 38–43

55. Manabe, Y., Yoshida, Y., Kasai, K. and Kawanami, D. (1985). Collagenolysis in human vaginal tissue during delivery: A light and electron microscopic, and immunofluorescent study. *Arch. Gynecol.*, **237**, 347

56. Hansson G., Malmsten, C. and Rådmark, O. (1983). The leukotrienes and other lipoxygenase products. In Pace-Asciak, C.R., Granström, E. (eds.) *Prostaglandins and Related Substances*, pp. 127–69. (Holland: Elsevier Science Publishers B.V.)

57. Schwarz, B.E., Schultz, F.M., MacDonald, P.C. and Johnston, J.M. (1975). Initiation of human parturition. III. Fetal membrane content of prostaglandin E_2 and $F_{2\alpha}$ precursor. *Obstet. Gynecol.*, **46**, 564–8

58. Curbelo, V., Bejar, R., Benirschke, K. and Gluck, L. (1981). Premature labour. I. Prostaglandin precursors in human placental membranes. *Obstet. Gynecol.*, **57**, 473–8

59. Grieves, S.A. and Liggins, G.C. (1976). Phospholipase A activity in human and ovine uterine tissues. *Prostaglandins*, **12**, 229–41

60. Okazaki, T., Sagawa, N., Bleasdale, J.E., Okita, J.R., MacDonald, P.C. and Johnston, J.M. (1981). Initiation of human parturition: XIII. Phospholipase C, phospholipase A_2, and diacylglycerol lipase activities in fetal membranes and decidua vera tissues from early and late gestation. *Biol. Reprod.*, **25**, 103–9

61. Salmon, J.A. and Amy, J.-J. (1973). Levels of prostaglandin $F_{2\alpha}$ in amniotic fluid during pregnancy and labour. *Prostaglandins*, **4**, 523–33

62. Okazaki, T., Casey, M.L., Okita, J.R., MacDonald, P.C. and Johnston, J.M. (1981). Initiation of human parturition. XII. Biosynthesis and metabolism of prostaglandins in human fetal membranes and uterine decidua. *Am. J. Obstet. Gynecol.*, **139**, 373–81

63. Kinoshita, K., Satoh, K. and Sakamoto, S. (1977). Biosynthesis of prostaglandin in human decidua, amnion, chorion and villi. *Endocrinol. Jpn.*, **24**, 343–50

64. Kinoshita, K. and Gréen, K. (1980). Bioconversion of arachidonic acid to prostaglandins and related compounds in human amnion. *Biochem. Med.*, **23**, 185–97

65. Mitchell, M.D., Bibby, J., Hicks, B.R. and Turnbull, A.C. (1978). Specific production of prostaglandin E by human amnion in vitro. *Prostaglandins*, **15**, 377–82

66. Mitchell, M.D., Bibby, J., Hicks, B.R. and Turnbull, A.C. (1978). Possible role for prostacyclin in human parturition. *Prostaglandins*, **16**, 931

67. Mitchell, M.D., Bibby, J.G., Hicks, B.R., Redman, C.W.G., Anderson, A.B.M. and Turnbull, A.C. (1978). Thromboxane B_2 and human parturition: Concentrations in the plasma and production in vitro. *J. Endocrinol.*, **78**, 435

68. Olson, D.M., Skinner, K. and Challis, J.R.G. (1983). Prostaglandin output in relation to parturition by cells dispersed from human intrauterine tissues. *J. Clin. Endocrinol. Metab.*, **57**, 694–9

69. Saeed, S.A. and Mitchell, M.D. (1983). Lipoxygenase activity in human uterine and intrauterine tissues: new prospects for control of prostacyclin production in pre-eclampsia. *Clin. Exp. Hypert. Pregnan.*, **B2**, 103–11

70. MacDonald, P.C., Schultz, F.M., Duenhoelter, J.H., et al. (1974). Initiation of human parturition. I. Mechanism of action of arachidonic acid. *Obstet. Gynecol.*, **44**, 629–36

71. Keirse, M.J.N.C., Mitchell, M.D. and Turnbull, A.C. (1977). Changes in prostaglandin F and 13,14-dehydro-15-keto-prostaglandin F concentrations in amniotic fluid at the onset of and during labor. *Br. J. Obstet. Gynaecol.*, **84**, 743–6

72. Karim, S.M.M. and Devlin, J. (1967). Prostaglandin content of amniotic fluid during pregnancy and labour. *J. Obstet. Gynecol. Br. Commonw.*, **74**, 230–4

73. Dray, F. and Frydman, R. (1976). Primary prostaglandins in amniotic fluid in pregnancy and spontaneous labour. *Am. J. Obstet. Gynecol.*, **126**, 13–9

74. Willman, E.A. and Collins, W.P. (1976). Distribution of prostaglandin E_2 and $F_{2\alpha}$ within the foetoplacental unit throughout human pregnancy. *J. Endocrinol.*, **69**, 413–9

75. Nieder, J. and Augustin, W. (1983). Increase of prostaglandin E and F equivalents in amniotic fluid during late pregnancy and rapid PGF elevation after cervical dilatation. *Prostagl. Leukotr. Med.*, **12**, 289–97

76. Manabe, Y., Manabe, A. and Takahashi, A. (1982). F prostaglandin levels in amniotic fluid during balloon-induced cervical softening and labour at term. *Prostaglandins*, **23**, 247–56

77. Manabe, Y., Okazaki, T. and Takahashi, A. (1983). Prostaglandins E and F in amniotic fluid during stretch-induced cervical softening and labour at term. *Gynecol. Obstet. Invest.*, **15**, 343–50

78. Schillinger, E. and Prior, G. (1976). Characteristics of prostaglandin receptor sites in human uterine tissue. In Samuelsson, B., Paoletti, R. (eds.) *Advances in Prostaglandin and Thromboxane Research*, Vol. 1. pp. 259–63. (New York: Raven Press)

79. Crankshaw, D.J., Crankshaw, J., Branda, L.A. and Daniel, E.E. (1979). Receptors for E type prostaglandins in the plasma membrane of non-pregnant human myometrium. *Arch. Biochem. Biophys.*, **198**, 70–7

80. Bauknecht, T., Krahe, B., Rechenbach, U., Zahradnik, H.P. and Breckwoldt, M. (1981). Distribution of prostaglandin E_2 and prostaglandin $F_{2\alpha}$ receptors in human myometrium. *Acta Endocrinol.*, **98**, 446–50

81. Hofmann, G.E., Rao, C.V., Barrows, G.H. and Sanfilippo, J.S. (1983). Topography of human uterine prostaglandin E and $F_{2\alpha}$ receptors and their profiles during pathological states. *J. Clin. Endocrinol. Metab.*, **57**, 360–6

82. Ostergard, D.R. (1973). The cervical relaxant properties of prostaglandin E_2 in non-pregnant subjects. *Prostaglandins*, **4**, 701–2

83. Lauersen, N.H., Kurkulos, M., Graves, Z.R. and Leeds, L. (1982). A new IUD insertion technique utilizing cervical priming with prostaglandin. *Contraception*, **26**, 59–63

84. Wingerup, L., Ulmsten, U. and Andersson, K.E. (1979). Ripening of the cervix by intracervical application of PGE_2-gel before termination of pregnancy with dilatation and evacuation. *Acta Obstet. Gynecol. Scand. Suppl.*, **84**, 15–8

85. Anthony, G.S., Fisher, J., Coutts, J.R.T. and Calder, A.A. (1984). The effect of exogenous hormones on the resistance of the early pregnant human cervix. *Br. J. Obstet. Gynaecol.*, **91**, 1249–53

86. Ekman, G., Uldbjerg, N., Wingerup, L. and Ulmsten, U. (1983). Intracervical instillation of PGE$_2$-gel in patients with missed abortion or intrauterine fetal death. *Arch. Gynecol.*, **233**, 241–5

87. Wingerup, L., Andersson, K.E. and Ulmsten, U. (1979). Ripening of the cervix and induction of labour in patients at term by single intracervical application of prostaglandin E$_2$ in viscous gel. *Acta Obstet. Gynecol. Scand. Suppl.*, **84**, 11–4

88. MacKenzie, I.Z. and Embrey, M.P. (1977). Cervical ripening with intravaginal prostaglandin E$_2$ gel. *Br. Med. J.*, **2**, 1381–4

89. MacKenzie, I.Z., Jenkin, G. and Bradley, S. (1979). The relation between plasma oestrogen, progesterone and prolactin concentrations and the efficacy of vaginal prostaglandin E$_2$ gel in initiating labour. *Br. J. Obstet. Gynaecol.*, **86**, 171–4

90. Sørensen, S.S., Brocks, V. and Lenstrup, C. (1985). Induction of labour and cervical ripening by intracervical prostaglandin E$_2$. *Obstet. Gynecol.*, **65**, 110–4

91. MacKenzie, I. and Embrey, M. (1979). A comparison of PGE$_2$ and PGF$_{2\alpha}$ vaginal gel for ripening of the cervix before induction of labour. *Br. J. Obstet. Gynaecol.*, **86**, 167

92. Neilson, D.R., Prind, R.P., Bolton, R.N. Mark, C. and Watson, P. (1983). A comparison of prostaglandin E$_2$ gel and prostaglandin F$_{2\alpha}$ gel for preinduction cervical ripening. *Am. J. Obstet. Gynecol.*, **146**, 526–32

93. Gréen, K., Christensen, N.J. and Bygdeman, M. (1981). The chemistry and pharmacology of prostaglandins, with reference to human reproduction. *J. Reprod. Fertil.*, **62**, 269–81

94. Souka, A.R., Karsoon, O., Shams, A. and Toppozada, M. (1983). Role of endogenous prostaglandins in pregnancy termination by 15-methyl PGF$_{2\alpha}$. *Prostaglandins*, **25**, 711–4

95. Joh, K., Riede, U.N. and Zahradnik, H.P. (1983). The effect of prostaglandins on the lysosomal function in the cervix uteri. *Arch. Gynecol.*, **234**, 1–16

96. Uldbjerg, N., Ekman, G., Malmström, A., Ulmsten, U. and Wingerup, L. (1983). Biochemical changes in human cervical connective tissue after local application of prostaglandin E$_2$. *Gynecol. Obstet. Invest.*, **15**, 291–9

97. Rath, W., Theobald, P., Kühnle, H., Kuhn, W., Hilglers, H. and Weber, L. (1982). Changes in collagen content of the first trimester cervix uteri after treatment with prostaglandin F$_{2\alpha}$ gel. *Arch. Gynecol.*, **107**, 84–5

98. Nakanishi, M. (1980). Effects of prostaglandin E$_2$ and various hormones on acid mucopolysaccharides in the tissue of the human cervix uteri. *Jpn. J. Fertil. Steril.*, **25**, 432–7

99. von Szalay, S., Husslein, P. and Grünberger, W. (1981). Die kollagenolytische aktivität von menschlicher zervixgewebe nach lokaler applikation von prostaglandin E$_2$ (PGE$_2$) mit einem portioadaptor. *Zbl. Gynäkol.*, **103**, 1107–12

100. Ekman, G., Uldbjerg, N., Malmström, A. and Ulmsten, U. (1983). Increased postpartum collagenolytic activity in cervical connective tissue from women treated with prostaglandin E$_2$. *Gynecol. Obstet. Invest.*, **16**, 292–8

101. Coutinho, E.M. and Darzé, E. (1976). Spontaneous contractility and the response of the human uterine cervix to prostaglandins F$_{2\alpha}$ and E$_2$ during the menstrual cycle. *Am. J. Obstet. Gynecol.*, **126**, 224–5

102. Najak, Z., Hillier, K. and Karim, S.M.M. (1970). The action of prostaglandins on the human isolated non-pregnant cervix. *J. Obstet. Gynecol. Br. Commonw.*, **77**, 701–9

103. Conrad, J.T., and Ueland, K. (1976). Reduction of the stretch modulus of human cervical tissue by prostaglandin E$_2$. *Am. J. Obstet. Gynecol.*, **126**, 218–23

104. Wallis, R.M. and Hillier, K. (1982). The effect of arachidonic acid and prostanoids on collagen dissolution in human uterine cervix in vitro. *Prostaglandins*, **24**, 377–85

105. Norström, A. (1982). Influence of prostaglandin E$_2$ on the biosynthesis of connective tissue constituents in the pregnant human cervix. *Prostaglandins*, **23**, 361–7

106. Norström, A. (1983). Effects of endocervical administration of prostaglandin E$_2$ on cervical dilatation and connective tissue biosynthesis in the first trimester of pregnancy. In Samuelsson, B., Paoletti, R., Ramwell, P. (eds.) *Advances in Prostaglandin, Thromboxane and Leukotriene Research*, Vol. 12, pp. 461–4. (New York: Raven Press)

107. Norström, A. (1984). Acute effects of prostaglandins on the biosynthesis of connective

tissue constituents in the non-pregnant human cervix uteri. *Acta Obstet. Gynecol. Scand.*, **63**, 169–73

108. Allen, J., Maigaard, S., Forman, A. and Anderson, K.E. (1986). Effects of some neurotransmitters and prostanoids on isolated human intracervical arteries. *Am. J. Obstet. Gynecol.*, (submitted)

109. Hillier, K. and Coad, N. (1982). Synthesis of prostaglandins by the human uterine cervix in vitro during passive mechanical stretch. *J. Pharm. Pharmacol.*, **34**, 262–3

110. Anderson, A.B.M. and Turnbull, A.C. (1969). Relationship between length of gestation and cervical dilatation, uterine contractility, and other factors during pregnancy. *Am. J. Obstet. Gynecol.*, **105**, 1207–14

111. Erkkola, R., Grönroos, M., Ekblad, U., Haataja, M. and Nieminen, A.L. (1984). Serum prostaglandin precursors after vaginal examination and amniotomy. *Prostagl. Leukotr. Med.*, **13**, 307–10

112. Mitchell, M.D., Flint, A.P.F., Bibby, J., Brunt, J., Arnold, J.M., Anderson, A.B.M. and Turnbull, A.C. (1977). Rapid increase in plasma prostaglandin concentrations after vaginal examination and amniotomy. *Br. Med. J.*, **2**, 1183–5

113. Sellers, S.M., Hodgson, H.T., Mitchell, M.D., Anderson, A.B.M. and Turnbull, A.C. (1980). Release of prostaglandins after amniotomy is not mediated by oxytocin. *Br. J. Obstet. Gynaecol.*, **87**, 43–6

114. Sellers, S.M., Mitchell, M.D., Anderson, A.B.M. and Turnbull, A.C. (1984). The influence of spontaneous and induced labour on the rise in prostaglandins at amniotomy. *Br. J. Obstet. Gynaecol.*, **91**, 849–52

115. Killick, S.R., Williams, C.A.V. and Elstein, M. (1985). A comparison of prostaglandin E_2 pessaries and laminaria tents for ripening the cervix before termination of pregnancy. *Br. J. Obstet. Gynaecol.*, **92**, 518–21

116. Johnson, I.R., Macpherson, M.B.A., Welch, C.C. and Filshie, G.M. (1985). A comparison of lamicel and prostaglandin E_2 vaginal gel for cervical ripening before induction of labor. *Am. J. Obstet. Gynecol.*, **151**, 604–7

117. Lerner, U. (1980). The uterine cervix and the initiation of labor: action of estradiol-17β. In Naftolin, F., Stubblefield, P.G. (eds.) *Dilatation of the Uterine Cervix*, pp. 301–16. (New York: Raven Press)

118. Lykkesfeldt, G., Nielsen, M.D. and Lykkesfeldt, A.E. (1984). Placental steroid sulfatase deficiency: biochemical diagnosis and clinical review. *Obstet. Gynecol.*, **64**, 49–54

119. Mochizuki, M., Honda, T. and Tojo, S. (1978). Collagenolytic activity and steroid levels after administration of dehydroepiandrosterone sulfate. *Int. J. Gynaecol. Obstet.*, **16**, 248

120. Gordon, A.J. and Calder, A.A. (1977). Oestradiol applied locally to ripen the unfavourable cervix. *Lancet*, **2**, 1319–21

121. Craft, I. and Yovich, J. (1978). Oestradiol and induction of labour. *Lancet*, **2**, 208

122. Tromans, P.M., Beazley, J.M. and Shenouda, P.I. (1981). Comparative study of oestradiol and prostaglandin E_2 vaginal gel for ripening the unfavourable cervix before induction of labour. *Br. Med. J.*, **282**, 679–81

123. MacLennan, A.H., Green, R.C., Bryant-Greenwood, G.D., Greenwood, F.C. and Seamark, R.F. (1981). Cervical ripening with combinations of vaginal prostaglandin $F_{2\alpha}$, estradiol, and relaxin. *Obstet. Gynecol.*, **58**, 601–4

124. Quinn, M.A., Murphy, A.J., Kuhn, R.J.P., Robinson, H.P. and Brown, J.B. (1981). A double blind trial of extra-amniotic oestradiol and prostaglandin $F_{2\alpha}$ gels in cervical ripening. *Br. J. Obstet. Gynaecol.*, **88**, 644–9

125. Thiery, M., De Gezelle, H., Van Kets, H. et al. (1979). The effect of local administered oestrogens on the human cervix. *Geburtsch. Perinat.*, **183**, 448

126. Luther, E.R., Roux, J., Popat, R., Gardner, A., Gray, J., Soubiran, E. and Korcaz, Y. (1980). The effect of oestrogen priming on induction of labour with prostaglandins. *Am. J. Obstet. Gynecol.*, **137**, 351–7

127. Wallis, R.M. and Hillier, K. (1981). Regulation of collagen dissolution in the human cervix by oestradiol-17β and progesterone. *J. Reprod. Fertil.*, **62**, 55

128. Lewis, R.B. and Schulman, J.D. (1973). Influence of acetylsalicylic acid, an inhibitor of prostaglandin synthesis, on the duration of human gestation and labour. *Lancet*, **2**, 1159–61

129. Collins, E. and Turner, G. (1975). Maternal effects of regular salicyclate ingestion in pregnancy. *Lancet*, **2**, 335–7

130. Wiqvist, N. (1979). The use of inhibitors of prostaglandin synthesis in obstetrics. In Keirse, M.J.N.C., Anderson, A.B.M., Gravenhorst, J.B. (eds.) *Human Parturition, New Concepts and Developments*, pp. 189–200. (Leiden: Leiden University Press)
131. Niebyl, J.R., Blake, D.A., White, R.D. *et al.* (1980). The inhibition of premature labor with indomethacin. *Am. J. Obstet. Gynecol.*, **136**, 1014–9
132. Amy, J.J. and Thiery, M. (1985). The prevention of preterm labour. *Prostagl. Perspect.*, **1**, 9–11
133. Mitchell, M.D. and Flint, A.P.F. (1978). Use of meclofenamic acid to investigate the role of prostaglandin biosynthesis during induced parturition in sheep. *J. Endocrinol.*, **76**, 101–9
134. Ledger, W.L., Webster, M.A., Anderson, A.B.M. and Turnbull, A.C. (1985). Effect of inhibition of prostaglandin synthesis on cervical softening and uterine activity during ovine parturition resulting from progesterone withdrawal induced by epostane. *J. Endocrinol.*, **105**, 227–33

9
The clinical use of prostaglandins for early and late abortion

A. Calder

In the eyes of many the prostaglandins are immediately and most often associated with therapeutic abortion. Although the biological roles and clinical uses of these substances are many and varied they first made their impact fifteen to twenty years ago as abortifacients. Indeed progress in prostaglandin research, dramatic and exciting as it has been, may have been hampered in some quarters by this association. In countries with repressive abortion legislation and in pharmaceutical companies in which the management have held anti-abortion views, the climate has been restrictive and has sometimes hindered advances in aspects of prostaglandin capabilities quite unrelated to abortion. While this may be unfortunate it reflects the status prostaglandins of the E and F series have attained as the pre-eminent abortifacients. No other agent has yet been identified which has the capacity to interrupt human pregnancy so consistently and so effectively regardless of the stage of gestation.

The value of PGE_2 and $PGF_{2\alpha}$ as well as a variety of synthetic analogues lies in their ability to induce the uterus to expel its contents in a manner which closely reproduces the process of spontaneous abortion. The principal mechanisms whereby this occurs are (a) stimulation of myometrial contractions and (b) modification of the cervical stroma to facilitate dilatation. The ways in which these occur will be discussed presently but first the clinical place of the prostaglandins should be put in perspective by reviewing the historical development of techniques of abortion.

HISTORICAL BACKGROUND

Since the dawn of history women (and men) have had occasion to seek to interrupt unwanted pregnancies. The commonest reason was the stigma and disgrace associated with a pregnancy conceived outside the approved social framework of marriage. Before the rise of female emancipation it was the woman who almost invariably reaped the consequences of such a pregnancy and was often driven in desperation to interfere with the pregnancy. In a society which viewed such a thing as legally, morally and socially unacceptable criminal abortion was an inevitable development. The growth of this particular science was advanced by 'criminals', untrained individuals or members of the medical profession who were driven as often by compassion as by financial concerns.

While attitudes and legal provisions have varied widely and altered from time to time it is broadly true that the nineteenth century saw the position at its most restrictive while the latter half of the twentieth century has seen an almost universal move towards more liberal conditions. Thus David[1] could claim in 1981 that two-thirds of the world's population lived under conditions which provided for therapeutic abortion on social as well as medical grounds and only 8% lived in countries with strictly enforced prohibitions of abortion.

This changing tapestry of attitudes has been paralleled by rapidly improving knowledge and methods, leading in turn to increased safety for the woman. It is interesting to review the methods available for performing (mostly criminal) abortions prior to the introduction of the 1967 Abortion Act in the United Kingdom.

A leading authority on medical jurisprudence at that time[2] divided the methods into two main classes, namely drugs and instruments. In discussing the former it is of interest to read "It is impossible to assert that any given drug in any given dose will produce abortion". Even in 1967 Jeffcoate[3] could still write "medical induction of abortion is always ineffective unless the foetus is dead". The end of the 1960s marks the watershed for two quite different but equally significant reasons: the introduction of sensible legislation and the discovery of the abortifacient potential of the prostaglandins.

Nevertheless, in spite of their lack of efficacy, drugs were widely employed because of the difficulty of detection. In some instances women even died of poisoning from so-called abortifacients before they achieved their object. Agents such as cathartics, aloes, savin, pennyroyal and tansy were employed with little rational basis. More rational, if little more effective, were ergot alkaloids, quinine and preparations containing lead or mercury. To combat legislation preventing the advertisement or sale of preparations for this purpose the enterprising exploiters of these unfortunate women resorted to disguising their products under names such as 'female remedies'.

The use of instruments was more effective and more dangerous. Not only was the risk of detection much greater but the dangers to the woman were profound. Knitting and crochet needles, skewers, sounds, syringes and catheters were all employed, sometimes by the woman herself, more often by a second party. Rupture of the amniotic membranes inevitably led to abortion but at considerable risk to the woman.

Other techniques included injection of fluids such as carbolic acid or lysol into the uterus by means of a Higginson's syringe. Tents made of material such as laminaria or slippery elm bark and placed in the cervical canal would absorb fluid and swell to dilate the cervix. The most compelling arguments for Abortion Law Reform were the death and morbidity which resulted from criminal abortions. Sepsis and haemorrhage were then, and remain, the two prime complications of abortion although uterine or cervical trauma and embolic phenomena were by no means rare. By bringing abortion within the control and supervision of the medical profession its safety has increased immeasurably and much of this change can be attributed to the new scope which has been given by prostaglandin research.

THERAPEUTIC ABORTION

The term 'therapeutic' is generally employed to distinguish abortions performed by doctors under properly regulated conditions from spontaneous miscarriages on the one hand and criminal abortions on the other.

As statutory provisions for abortion have been established so there have grown up a variety of clinical techniques which have increased the safety and acceptability of such procedures. Although much has been learned from the experience of criminal abortionists down the years, the altered circumstances of recent times have made study and research into methods of abortion a legitimate and important scientific pursuit.

No single method of abortion is well suited to all types of case, the most important variable being the gestational age. Thus a distinction is immediately drawn between abortion in the first and second trimesters. Even so, gynaecologists may yet differ in their views of the best technique for a particular woman.

THE PRE-PROSTAGLANDIN ERA

In the years immediately preceding the availability of prostaglandins as abortifacients the methods used were predominantly surgical. It was even more true in those days that the earlier an abortion was performed the safer it would be and that the end of the first trimester marked the passage into more dangerous territory. In the first trimester the more or less standard approach was to carry out surgical dilatation of the cervix followed by suction curettage of the uterine contents under general anaesthesia.

Cases in the second trimester presented greater difficulty and anxiety. The most reliable technique was to carry out abdominal hysterotomy. This surgical approach, representing a kind of mini-caesarian section, could certainly be regarded as efficient but was not without its drawbacks, the most important of which was the scar left on the uterus which might lead to rupture during a subsequent pregnancy. Consequently abdominal hysterotomy was associated with a significant mortality and morbidity both in the short and in the long term.

The only reliable alternative was to perform an amniocentesis and inject hypertonic solutions of substances such as saline, glucose or urea into the amniotic cavity. This approach led to death of the foetus and eventually to its expulsion and the process could be enhanced by intravenous infusion of oxytocin. Although these techniques had the advantage of avoiding a permanent uterine scar they were not without risks, and maternal deaths occurred from complications such as hypernatraemia and convulsions when saline was used or coagulopathies and intrauterine infections in association with glucose solutions[4,5]. Another disadvantage lay in the fact that amniocentesis could not be reliably performed much before 16 weeks gestation and consequently if the pregnancy in question had passed beyond the safe limit for suction curettage a further delay might be required before intraamniotic techniques could be employed. It is of interest to reflect that the main biological effect of hypertonic techniques is the release of endogenous prostaglandins from the decidua[6].

The arrival and availability of prostaglandins as abortifacients quickly transformed the clinical picture and these agents soon established a place as the agents of choice for therapeutic abortion in the second trimester. Since that time they have also had a considerable impact in the first trimester.

MODE OF ACTION OF PROSTAGLANDINS

Uterine contractility has long been known to be influenced by prostaglandins. Indeed the late Arpad Csapo described $PGF_{2\alpha}$ as "the ultimate uterine stimulant"[7]. This referred not only to its pre-eminence as an agent for uterine stimulation but also to the concept that while a wide variety of substances and stimuli may provoke uterine contractility the ultimate link in the chain, the final common pathway, is probably local release of prostaglandins.

The pregnant myometrium is sensitive to other prostaglandins besides $PGF_{2\alpha}$. Thus PGE_2[8], as well as a wide variety of prostaglandin analogues (including 15-methyl-$PGF_{2\alpha}$[9] and 16-phenoxy-PGE_2 methyl sulphonylamide)[10] have been successfully employed as abortifacients. Indeed PGE_2 (although in some conditions an inhibitor of the non-pregnant myometrium[11]) is a potent stimulant of the pregnant myometrium and its potency as well as its relative freedom from side-effects compared to $PGF_{2\alpha}$ make it an admirable abortifacient[8].

In one other regard PGE_2 is especially suited. The uterine cervix, whose principal function in early pregnancy is to remain firmly closed[12], can be induced to soften by the action of PGE_2, thus facilitating dilatation[13]. This phenomenon, which is physiologically normal when it occurs in association with parturition, is an important consideration in the context of induced abortion. Such softening facilitates dilatation whether surgical or in response to uterine contractility. If either type of dilatation is attempted when the cervix remains rigid the result may be permanent damage to the cervix or uterus[14].

It is now widely accepted that PGE_2 is a central participant in the process of cervical softening. This change is the result of modification of the connective tissue which constitutes the cervix so that the bio-mechanical properties of the stromal tissue are altered[15,16]. The site of production of PGE_2 for this physiological purpose would seem to be the cervical tissue itself[17].

CLINICAL APPLICATIONS OF PROSTAGLANDINS

The use of prostaglandins as abortifacient agents will now be considered and the most convenient way of doing this is to discuss their use in relation to different stages of gestation. For the purpose of this discussion I will consider four distinct categories as follows:

In the first trimester   (a) up to 8 weeks
                                   (b) 8–12 weeks

In the second trimester   (c) 12–16 weeks
                                   (d) beyond 16 weeks

Before considering these categories individually it is apposite to mention the five main determinants of the choice of technique for each particular clinical indication. These are:

(i) choice of agent
(ii) vehicle
(iii) route of administration
(iv) dosage regimen
(v) potential side effects

It must be remembered that prostaglandins are by their very nature unlike most other naturally occurring substances (especially hormones) used in clinical practice. They are essentially unspecific with numerous biological actions. Such biological specificity as they display results from their local site of synthesis and action and their rapid degradation thereafter rather than from any degree of chemical specificity. Prostaglandin E_2 for instance is capable of having effects on the contractility of smooth muscle in blood vessels, bronchi, gut and uterus and may also influence gastric secretion, brain and kidney function[18]. Thus systemic administration may well provoke unwanted side-effects and the nearest the clinician can get to mimicking the biological situation is to employ local routes of administration where these are feasible. Thus, for abortion, although systemic routes (especially intravenous and intramuscular) have been employed, local routes (vaginal, intra-cervical, intra-amniotic and extra-amniotic) have generally met with greater success and fewer side-effects. Interruption of pregnancy at its various stages of gestation will now be considered.

(a) Early first trimester (up to 8 weeks)

During this phase the successful continuation of pregnancy depends on the production of progesterone by the corpus luteum[19]. Destruction of the corpus luteum at this stage results in abortion. The discovery in the early 1970s that in some mammals $PGF_{2\alpha}$ is responsible for regression of the corpus luteum (luteolysis) and a decline in progesterone secretion[20] excited speculation that prostaglandins might offer a radical new approach to fertility control. It was thought possible that administration of prostaglandins might induce luteolysis in the human and that if this were achieved in the early weeks of pregnancy then abortion or 'menstrual induction' might result. It was even proposed that such therapy might be employed as soon as a menstrual period was noted to be late, or even on a regular monthly basis at the time the period was expected.

The attraction of this approach lay in the fact that spontaneous miscarriage occurring in these early weeks is often little different from (perhaps only a little heavier than) a normal menstrual period, warranting no intervention such as admission to hospital or surgical evacuation of the uterus.

In the event these prospects have not been realized. Although there is some evidence that $PGF_{2\alpha}$ is luteolytic in the human, its site of production for this purpose would seem to lie wholly within the ovary itself[21,22] in contrast to other species in which its source is the uterus. Even accepting the possibility that $PGF_{2\alpha}$ may indeed be luteolytic in the human, attempts to exploit this have been frustrated. It is not possible to target prostaglandin therapy directly to the corpus luteum without at the same time stimulating other organs, notably the uterus. All attempts at such 'menstrual induction' with natural prostaglandins have provoked unacceptable side-effects especially in the form of severe uterine cramping pains[23]. The approach which has most nearly achieved acceptability in this regard has been the intrauterine instillation of 50 mg sulprostone[24].

A more logical approach has more recently explored the use of the antiprogesterones such as Epostane (Winthrop Laboratories)[25] and RU486 (Roussel Laboratories)[26]. Although differing in their mode of action, both of these agents have the effect of reducing the influence of progesterone. This may be sufficient to provoke abortion either alone or in combination with prostaglandin therapy[27,28].

The effectiveness of this approach, both proven and potential, raises some questions of a legal and logistic nature relating to matters such as the definition of "treatment" and "an approved place" in respect to the 1967 Abortion Act. The Act was framed at a time when effective medical abortifacients of this sort were not envisaged and it is becoming necessary to re-examine the precise terms of the Act in the light of recent scientific and therapeutic advances. Strict interpretation of the law would require that all patients undergoing this form of management would be admitted to hospital for the entire duration of treatment from first administration of the agent or agents employed until the abortion process was complete. It might well become clear that the safest approach to this technique would be to extend the programme of treatment over several days beginning with antiprogesterone therapy and culminating with prostaglandin therapy. To remain in hospital throughout this time would almost certainly be unnecessary from a medical standpoint (indeed it might not be necessary to admit such women to hospital at all) and so a re-interpretation of the requirements of the Act in the light of these altered circumstances is now required.

For the meantime, the majority of early abortions will continue to be performed by surgical means. The prostaglandins may however have a useful role in such cases as a preliminary therapy to promote softening and dilatation of the uterine cervix to reduce the resistance to and potential damage resulting from surgical dilatation. This use of prostaglandins will be discussed more fully in the following section.

(b) Late first trimester (8–12 weeks)

At this stage of pregnancy the prostaglandins, although capable of acting as primary abortifacients, are not well suited to this purpose. There are two main reasons for this – pain and bleeding. The degree of uterine contractility necessary to produce abortion is considerable and there may also be profuse haemorrhage. Spontaneous abortion occurring at this stage of gestation is often associated with severe pain and bleeding so that the woman may be profoundly shocked.

Therapeutic abortion at this stage is more appropriately performed by surgical means but that is not to say that the prostaglandins may not yet have a valuable role to play. The cervical softening or 'priming' effect referred to above may be very useful in preventing or reducing the trauma associated with surgical abortion.

Although vaginal administration of the primary prostaglandins (PGE$_2$, PGF$_{2\alpha}$) in large doses has been shown to reduce the cervical resistance[29], side-effects have been troublesome. The analogues 15-methyl-PGF$_{2\alpha}$ methyl ester and 16,16-dimethyl-*trans*-Δ^2-PGE$_1$ methyl ester seem to be superior in this regard, producing convincing cervical softening and dilatation within a few hours of vaginal administration[30,31]. Side-effects do not appear to be troublesome and the benefit in reducing both the risk of surgical trauma and the blood loss associated with the procedure commend this approach[32].

(c) Early second trimester abortion (12–16 weeks)

At this stage of pregnancy, many gynaecologists consider that it is dangerous to dilate the cervix surgically to the degree necessary to allow evacuation of the uterus[33]. Equally, abdominal hysterotomy has the major disadvantages referred to earlier. On the other hand the uterus is not yet large enough for amniocentesis to be carried out with consistent reliability for intra-amniotic therapy.

For all these reasons it is at this stage of pregnancy that the prostaglandins have probably had their greatest impact as abortifacients. Since many of the patients presenting with requests for abortion at this gestation are young girls at the start of their reproductive years, it is doubly valuable to have a technique of abortion which is associated with increased safety and this reflects the fact that prostaglandin techniques are much more physiological than are surgical techniques.

Systemic administration, either intravenous or intramuscular, may be associated with high success rates but this is generally bought at the cost of troublesome side-effects[34] and this seems true with prostaglandin analogues as well as with the primary prostaglandins[35]. Nevertheless, such routes may be favoured in some centres and on some programmes depending on the facilities and clinical staff available.

In general, however, the most satisfactory technique at this stage of gestation is extra-amniotic administration of prostaglandins either in solution as a continuous infusion[8] or as a bolus in gel[36]. The agent of choice for this purpose is prostaglandin E$_2$ and the usual method of administration is via a Foley catheter passed through the endocervical canal and retained beyond the internal os by inflating the balloon with 20 ml of fluid. Expulsion of the catheter usually occurs within 10 to 16 hours of the start of such therapy and this is usually followed soon after by abortion of the uterine contents. If abortion is delayed longer than this it may be accelerated by the additional use of intravenous oxytocin. Side-effects associated with this technique have generally been found to be minimal. Opinions differ[8,36] as to the need for routine surgical evacuation of the uterus after such abortion.

(d) Late second trimester abortion (beyond 16 weeks)

At this stage of pregnancy the techniques described in the preceding section are also highly effective but the options are now extended to include intra-amniotic therapy and this is favoured in many units. It may be desirable to ensure that the fetus shows no signs of activity at the time of abortion, which may be distressing for the medical and nursing attendants, and this can be achieved by the use of hypertonic intra-amniotic instillations for which purpose urea represents the agent of choice. Since an amniocentesis will be required for this purpose it is often found convenient to combine this with intra-uterine instillation of prostaglandins. This is generally successful in achieving abortion within 24 hours and it is commoner in these later second trimester terminations to find that the process is complete because the placenta then separates more efficiently.

The applications of prostaglandins at these four different stages of gestation are summarized in Table 9.1.

HAZARDS AND PRECAUTIONS

The natural prostaglandins and their analogues are highly potent substances and while this makes them very effective as clinical weapons they also carry grave potential dangers. The common side-effects resulting from the use of prostaglandins as abortifacients are nausea, vomiting and diarrhoea. While these may be extremely disagreeable they are hardly life-threatening. In contrast, however, haemorrhage, sepsis and trauma to the genital tract may threaten the patient's life and her reproductive future. There is no substitute for close clinical supervision and the greatest hazards are associated with prolongation of the process of induced abortion. The clinician should not be afraid to abandon the procedure and resort to abdominal hysterotomy if induction of second trimester abortion does not follow the expected course. The alternative of uterine rupture may lead to loss of the uterus, thereby rendering the patient incapable of further pregnancy.

Strict asepsis is essential as is rigorous removal of any retained products of conception within the uterus. With these provisos the prostaglandins represent a very safe and valuable agent for therapeutic abortion.

Table 9.1 Summary of recommended techniques of applying prostaglandins at varying stages of gestation

Gestation	Choice of prostaglandin	Route, dose vehicle etc.	Additional therapy or procedure	Side-effects	Ref.
Less than 8 weeks	16-phenoxy-tetranor-PGE$_2$ methyl sulphonylamide	0.25 mg i.m.	RU486 25 mg b.d. for preceding 4 days	Nausea Uterine cramps	27
	16,16-dimethyl-trans- Δ^2-PGE$_1$ methyl ester	1 mg p.v.	RU486 150 mg/day for preceding 4 days		28
8–12 weeks	15-methyl-PGF$_{2\alpha}$ methyl ester	1 mg p.v.	Followed 3–12 h later by suction curettage	Moderate pain, bleeding and nausea	30
	16,16-dimethyl-trans- Δ^2-PGE$_1$ methyl ester	1 mg p.v.			31
12–16 weeks	PGE$_2$	Continuous extra-amniotic infusion via Foley catheter (100 μg/ml in normal saline). Dose range 100–250 μg/h	i.v. Oxytocin 80 mu/min after 18 hours if required. Surgical evacuation if retained products	Uterine cramps, nausea, occasional vomiting	8
	or				
	PGE$_2$	Extra-amniotic dose 2 mg in viscous gel	As above		36
Beyond 16 weeks	As for 12–16 weeks or				
	PGE$_2$	10 mg intra-amniotic plus 80 g urea	As above		37

192

REFERENCES

1. David, H. P. (1981). Abortion policies. In Hodgson, J. E. (ed.) *Abortion and Sterilisation*, pp. 1–40. (London: Academic Press)
2. Glaister, J. (1953). *Medical Jurisprudence and Toxicology*, (Edinburgh: Livingstone)
3. Jeffcoate, T. N. A. (1967). *Principles of Gynaecology*. (3rd Edn.) (London: Butterworth)
4. Cameron, J. M. and Dayan, A. D. (1966). Association of brain damage with therapeutic abortion induced by amniotic fluid replacement. *Br. Med. J.*, **1**, 1010–1014
5. Briggs, D. W. (1964). Induction of labour with hypertonic glucose. *Br. Med. J.*, **1**, 701–702
6. Brunk, U. and Gustavii, B. (1973). Lability of human decidual cells: In vitro effect of autolysis and osmotic stress. *Am. J. Obstet. Gynecol.*, **115**, 811–816
7. Csapo, A. I. and Pulkkinen, M. G. (1979). The mechanism of prostaglandin action on the pregnant human uterus. *Prostaglandins*, **17**, 283–299
8. Miller, A. W. F., Calder, A. A. and Macnaughton, M. C. (1972). Termination of pregnancy by continuous intrauterine infusion of prostaglandins. *Lancet*, **2**, 5–7
9. Tejuja, S., Choudhury, S. D. and Manchanda, P. K. (1978). Use of intra- and extra-amniotic prostaglandins for the termination of pregnancies – Report of multicentre trial in India. *Contraception*, **18**, 641
10. Karim, S. M. M., Illancheran, A., Wun, W., Ho, T. H. and Ratnam, S. S. (1978). Intramuscular administration of 16-phenoxy-ω-17,18,19,20-tetranor-PGE$_2$ methylsulfonylamide for preoperative cervical dilatation in first trimester nulliparae. *Prostgl. Med.*, **1**, 71–75
11. Lundstrom, V. (1977). The myometrial response to intra-uterine administration of PGF$_{2\alpha}$ and PGE$_2$ in dysomenorrheic women. *Acta Obstet. Gynecol. Scand.*, **56**, 167–172
12. Calder, A. A. (1981). The human cervix in pregnancy – a clinical perspective. In Ellwood, D. A. and Anderson, A. B. M. (eds.) *The Cervix in Pregnancy and Labour*, pp. 103–122. (Edinburgh: Churchill Livingstone)
13. Calder, A. A. (1979). Prostaglandins for pre-induction cervical ripening. In Karim, S. M. M. (ed.) *Practical Applications of Prostaglandins and their Synthesis Inhibitors*, pp. 301–318. (Lancaster: MTP Press)
14. Karim, S. M. M. (1979). Termination of second trimester pregnancy with prostaglandins. In Karim, S. M. M. (ed.) *Practical Applications of Prostaglandins and their Synthesis Inhibitors*, pp. 375–409. (Lancaster: MTP Press)
15. Liggins, G. C. (1978). Ripening of the cervix. *Semin Perinatol.*, **2**, 261–271
16. Calder, A. A. (1979). Management of the unripe cervix. In Keirse, M. J. N. C., Anderson, A. B. M. (eds.) *Human Parturition*, pp. 201–217. (Leiden University Press)
17. Ellwood, D. A., Anderson, A. B. M., Mitchell, M. D., Murphy, G. and Turnbull, A. C. (1981). Prostanoids, collagenase and cervical softening in the sheep. In Ellwood, D. A. and Anderson, A. B. M. (eds.) *The Cervix in Pregnancy and Labour*, pp. 57–73. (Edinburgh: Churchill Livingstone)
18. Hillier, K. and Karim, S. M. M. (1979). General introduction and practical implications of some pharmacological actions of prostaglandins, thromboxanes and their synthesis inhibitors. In Karim, S. M. M. (ed.), *Practical Applications of Prostaglandins and their Synthesis Inhibitors*. (Lancaster: MTP Press)
19. Csapo, A. I. and Pulkkinen, M. (1978). Indispensibility of the human corpus luteum in the maintenance of early pregnancy. *Obstet. Gynecol. Surv.*, **33**, 69–81
20. Horton, E. W. and Poyser, N. L. (1976). Uterine luteolytic hormone: a physiological role for prostaglandin F$_{2\alpha}$. *Physiol. Rev.*, **56**, 595–651
21. Henderson, K. M. and McNatty, K. P. (1975). A biochemical hypothesis to explain the mechanism of luteal regression. *Prostaglandins*, **9**, 779–797
22. Challis, J. R. G., Calder, A. A., Dilley, S., Forster, C. S., Hillier, K., Hunter, D. J. S., MacKenzie, I. Z. and Thorburn, G. S. (1976). Production of prostaglandins E and F$_{2\alpha}$ by corpora lutea, corpora albicantes and stroma from the human ovary. *J. Endocrinol.*, **68**, 401–408
23. Karim, S. M. M. and Amy, J. J. (1975). Interruption of pregnancy with prostaglandins. In Karim, S. M. M. (ed.), *Prostaglandins and Reproduction*, pp. 77–148. (Lancaster: MTP Press)
24. Bygdeman, M. (1979). Menstrual regulation with prostaglandins. In Karim, S. M. M. (ed.), *Practical Applications of Prostaglandins and their Synthesis Inhibitors*, pp. 267–282. (Lancaster: MTP Press)

25. Webster, M. A., Phipps, S. L. and Gillmer, M. D. G. (1985). Interruption of first trimester human pregnancy following Epostane therapy. *Br. J. Obstet. Gynaecol.*, **92**, 963–968

26. Couzinet, B., Le Strat, N., Ulmann, A., Baulieu, E. E. and Schaison, G. (1986). Termination of early pregnancy by the progesterone antagonist RU 486 (mifepristone). *N. Engl. J. Med.*, **315**, 1565–1570

27. Bygdeman, M. and Swahn, M. L. (1985). Progesterone receptor blockage – effect on uterine contractility and early pregnancy. *Contraception*, **32**, 42–49

28. Cameron, I. T., Michie, A. F. and Baird, D. T. (1986). Therapeutic abortion in early pregnancy with antiprogestogen RU 486 alone or in combination with prostaglandin analogue (Gemeprost). *Contraception*, **34**, 459–468

29. Dingfelder, J. R., Brenner, W. E., Hendricks, C. H. and Staurovsky, L. G. (1975). Reduction of cervical resistance by prostaglandin suppositories prior to dilatation for induced abortion. *Am. J. Obstet. Gynecol.*, **122**, 25–30

30. Lauersen, N. H., Seidman, S. and Wilson, K. H. (1979). Cervical priming prior to first-trimester suction abortion with a single 15-methyl-prostaglandin $F_{2\alpha}$ vaginal suppository. *Am. J. Obstet. Gynecol.*, **135**, 1116–1118

31. Welch, C. and Elder, M. G. (1982). Cervical dilatation with 16,16-dimethyl-*trans*-Δ^2-PGE_1 methyl ester vaginal pessaries before surgical termination of first trimester pregnancies. *Br. J. Obstet. Gynaecol.*, **89**, 849

32. Lauersen, N. H. and Graves, Z. R. (1964). Preabortion cervical dilatation with a low-dose prostaglandin suppository. *J. Reprod. Med.*, **29**, 133–135

33. Wright, C. W. S., Campbell, S. and Beasley, J. (1972). Second trimester abortion after vaginal termination of pregnancy. *Lancet*, **1**, 1278–1279

34. Hendricks, C. H., Brenner, W. E., Ekbladh, L., Brotanek, V. and Fishburne, J. I. Jr. (1971). Efficacy and tolerance of intravenous prostaglandins $F_{2\alpha}$ and E_2. *Am. J. Obstet. Gynecol.*, **111**, 564–578

35. Karim, S. M. M., Choo, H. T., Lim, A. L., Yeo, K. C. and Ratnam, S. S. (1978). Termination of second trimester pregnancy with intramuscular administration of 16-phenoxy-ω-17,18,19,20-tetranor-PGE_2 methyl sulfonylamide. *Prostaglandins*, **15**, 1063–1068

36. MacKenzie, I. Z. and Embrey, M. P. (1976). Single injection of prostaglandins in viscous gel to induce abortion. *Br. J. Obstet. Gynaecol.*, **83**, 505–507

37. Craft, I. (1973). Induction of abortion by combined intra-amniotic urea and prostaglandin E or prostaglandin E alone. *Lancet*, **1**, 1344

10
The clinical use of prostaglandins for cervical ripening and induction of labour

I. Z. MacKenzie

HISTORICAL DEVELOPMENT

By the end of the 1960s there was good evidence for the high rate of success in inducing labour with oxytocin by intravenous infusion. Given as buccal pitocin it had not found favour due to uncertain absorption and uterine response with serious questions over the safety of the method. The obvious benefits of titrated infusions of oxytocin promoted by Turnbull and Anderson[1] led to the ready adoption of this principle by many obstetric units. It is very probable that the success generally achieved with intravenous oxytocin when combined with low amniotomy contributed to the enthusiasm shown for induction of labour with very high rates being reported in many centres by the mid 1970s. When the prostaglandins were introduced into clinical practice towards the end of the 1960s the potential of these newly-discovered oxytocics for labour management was soon explored. Early studies[2,3], indicated that of the two naturally occurring prostaglandins PGE_2 and $PGF_{2\alpha}$, both would successfully induce term labour if given by intravenous infusion. PGE_2 was found to be approximately five times more potent than $PGF_{2\alpha}$ in stimulating myometrial contractions and if infused intravenously in increasing dose rates, the range required to establish labour was found to be 0.5–2.0 μg/min for PGE_2 and 5–20 μg/min for $PGF_{2\alpha}$. Subsequent series confirmed these initial reports but when observations were controlled comparing results with patients whose labours were induced by the then well-established method of low amniotomy and intravenous oxytocin titration, there appeared little obvious benefit in using prostaglandins; indeed, gastrointestinal side-effects were commonly provoked with both prostaglandins thus detracting from these agents. Two possible advantages with the prostaglandins compared with oxytocin were however observed. Labour resulting from prostaglandin stimulation was considered more physiological than that provoked by

195

oxytocin and likened to the contractions evolving with spontaneous labour and also success was more readily achieved when the uterine cervix was very unripe at the start of induction[3].

Alternative routes of prostaglandin administration were tried during the early years of clinical trials with the object of providing less invasive techniques, and reducing the gastrointestinal side-effects associated with the relatively large dosages required intravenously to successfully induce labour, particularly in those patients with an unfavourable cervix: Fig. 10.1 illustrates the various routes that have been explored. Oral ingestion of draughts of PGE_2 or $PGF_{2\alpha}$[4] and vaginal insertion of pessaries of PGE_2 or $PGF_{2\alpha}$[5] were both tried in small series. The oral route was investigated further by many groups, some comparing outcome with intravenous oxytocin, and the general conclusion reached was that PGE_2 0.5–2.0 mg hourly, was effective if the cervix was ripe, but the frequency of gastrointestinal side-effects was a disadvantage. $PGF_{2\alpha}$ 5 mg–40 mg as a draught or capsule was found to cause even higher incidences of side-effects and subsequently received no further attention. PGE_2 2 mg or $PGF_{2\alpha}$ 5 mg as a vaginal pessary, although capable of inducing labour, was not investigated further until the late 1970s. Sublingual[6,7] and rectal[8] application has also been studied but the results obtained by the researching groups did not encourage others to investigate

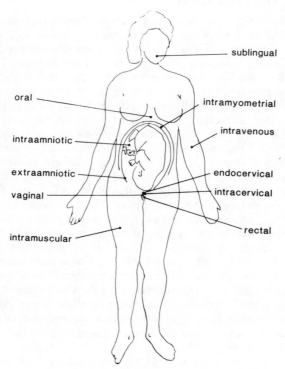

Figure 10.1 Routes of prostaglandin administration that have been explored

these routes further.

Following the initial optimism over the potential of the prostaglandins for labour induction, there followed a lean period with general disenchantment, largely due to the distressing side-effects reported with all the explored routes. Since gastrointestinal side-effects were directly correlated with the relatively high dosages required with routes relying upon systemic absorption particularly when induction was needed in the presence of an unfavourable cervix, local administration by extra-amniotic injection, previously developed so successfully for mid-trimester therapeutic abortion, was explored. In the difficult induction cases Calder *et al.*[9] showed that an extra-amniotic infusion of PGE$_2$ via an indwelling transcervical Foley catheter was successful and subsequently spawned the concept of prostaglandin priming or induction pretreatment for the unfavourable cervix. Later modifications with single extra-amniotic prostaglandin injections, intracervical instillation and vaginal protocols all followed, endeavouring to improve induced labour outcome while searching for acceptable, effective regimens. It is in this area that much of the effort has been directed over the past ten years and this has resulted in a reassessment of labour induction methods in general with a much greater awareness by obstetricians of the importance of cervical state at the time of labour induction.

Although considerable attention was directed to the area of the unripe cervix, a reappraisal of oral and vaginal administration for routine induction followed and protocols were explored which have resulted in a dramatic change in labour induction management in many obstetric units. Possible further refinements of administration methods and wider applications in specific pregnancy situations have followed (Fig. 10.2). Throughout the past twenty years, many of the innovations and advances in the stimulation of

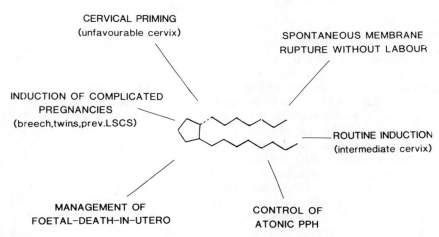

Prostaglandins and labour induction

CERVICAL PRIMING
(unfavourable cervix)

SPONTANEOUS MEMBRANE
RUPTURE WITHOUT LABOUR

INDUCTION OF COMPLICATED
PREGNANCIES
(breech,twins,prev.LSCS)

ROUTINE INDUCTION
(intermediate cervix)

MANAGEMENT OF
FOETAL–DEATH–IN–UTERO

CONTROL OF
ATONIC PPH

Figure 10.2 Current uses of prostaglandins in clinical obstetric practice

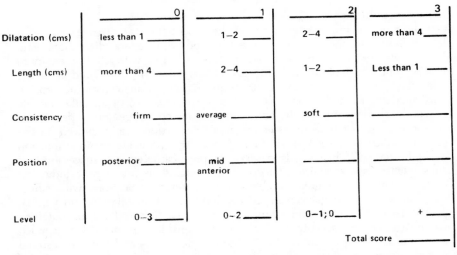

Figure 10.3 Cervical assessment using a modification of Bishop's pelvic scoring system (Calder and Embrey[11])

labour have resulted from the clinical needs of obstetricians, disenchanted with current unsatisfactory management methods, seeking to improve results. As with much research, unexpected observations have heralded newer developments and progress. To some extent, the application of prostaglandins for labour management has been impeded by the lack of suitable administration vehicles and the impetus to search for an acceptable, reliable carrier into which the prostaglandins could be incorporated has provided an additional dimension to the use of prostaglandins for labour induction. Progress, on occasions, has been serendipitous.

CERVICAL RIPENING

The influence that the state of the cervix has upon the outcome of induced labour has been recognised for many years but it was not until the past 15 years with the introduction of the prostaglandins into clinical practice that the appropriate attention has been paid to this factor. Bishop's pelvic scoring system[10] or a modification thereof[11], which takes account of cervix length, consistency, dilatation and position, as well as the level of the presenting part within the pelvis has now been adopted by most clinicians involved in assessing cervical ripening methods and induced labour outcomes (Fig. 10.3). Furthermore, it is recognised by many that the unripe cervix is a state that can seriously influence labour outcome in primiparae, but rarely presents a problem in multiparae unless previously delivered by caesarean section. Assessments of treatment methods for ripening the unfavourable cervix are of greatest value when primiparae and multiparae are analysed separately; this has often not been the case in many published trials. As illustrated in

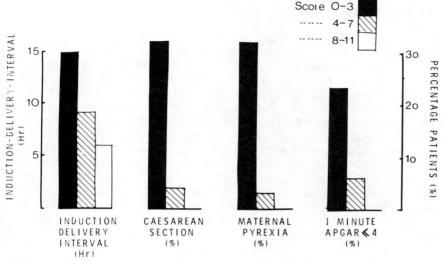

Figure 10.4 Influence of cervical state upon the outcome of induced labour in primiparae (Calder *et al.*[9])

Fig. 10.4, both fetal and maternal morbidity are increased when the cervix is very unripe at the time of induction compared with patients with a moderately favourable or ripe cervix. It had been suggested that any management which would enhance cervical ripeness could also improve labour outcome and this has been found to be especially true with the prostaglandins.

As described in the preceding chapter by Uldbjerg, there is good evidence that prostaglandins are involved in the physiological maturation of the cervix during the latter part of gestation in the human. Since the mid 1970s there has been a growing number of reports indicating that exogenously administered prostaglandins can induce the same maturing effect upon the cervix. The mechanism is presumed to be similar to the normal physiological process but speeded into a short 'latent' phase of a matter of hours rather than many days and weeks as occurs spontaneously in the latter weeks of pregnancy. While most clinicians administering prostaglandins have reported that myometrial activity commonly accompanies their use when given for this purpose, there is mounting evidence that the prostaglandins can produce their effect upon the cervix in the absence of any direct myometrial involvement. Hillier and Wallis[12] conducting controlled *in vitro* experiments found that the addition of arachidonic acid, the precursor of PGE_2 and $PGF_{2\alpha}$ to the culture medium of explants of human cervical tissue resulted in significantly increased collagen dissolution over a ten day observation period compared with control cultures. Interestingly, however, PGE_2 and $PGF_{2\alpha}$ when added to the culture medium did not enhance collagenolysis.

Direct observational studies in humans are difficult to design and researchers have therefore resorted to using the sheep model. Infusions of PGE_2 directly into the cervical artery cause cervical softening, and dilatation without any marked changes in intrauterine pressure being recorded via intrauterine catheters[13]. Using an even more sophisticated preparation Ledger et al.[14] has shown that, in vivo in the sheep, cervical softening can be induced with a local infusion of PGE_2 into the cervical artery, the cervix having been surgically sectioned from the body of the uterus; the possibility of an influence from myometrial contraction was thus totally excluded as well as any direct vascular connection between uterine body and cervix. An indirect in vivo approach in the human has been used in a small number of patients by Goeschen et al.[15]. They administered oral tocolytic agents immediately prior to the intracervical application of PGE_2 0.4 mg gel to ripen the unfavourable cervix and induce labour in women of varying parity and some with ruptured membranes. Compared with a control group not given any tocolysis, increased uterine activity following prostaglandin treatment was suppressed in the study patients, but similar degrees of cervical ripening were observed in both groups. They thus concluded that in vivo in the human pharmacologically induced cervical ripening need not depend upon uterine contraction; this study does however require to be confirmed.

When the cervix is unfavourable, prostaglandin doses required are high if given by administration routes relying upon systemic absorption, but local application provides a reasonably reliable acceptable method using much lower dosages. The extra-amniotic route was proposed by Calder et al.[9] and is relatively simple. The original proposal was to give PGE_2 as a continuous infusion in the range $60-180\mu g/min$, the rate increasing at $30\ \mu g/h$ till labour was established. The technique was subsequently modified to a single injection of PGE_2 0.4 mg in 10 ml of a viscous cellulose gel[16]. Other publications examining the method have followed over the past eight years and all have confirmed the efficacy of the technique. In many instances, the method has been compared with other subsequently developed techniques and generally it has been found that the extra-amniotic route is at least as good and possibly better than other techniques. However, a distinct disadvantage of extra-amniotic instillation is the inadvertent perforation of the fetal membranes[17]; also there is a risk of provoking haemorrhage with insertion of the catheter into a previously unsuspected placenta praevia[16].

Direct instillation of a viscous prostaglandin gel into the endocervical canal was proposed by Wingerup et al.[18]. This approach appears logical since the prostaglandins seem to exert a direct effect upon cervical form and function thus allowing direct application to the target organ. The doses required with endocervical instillation of the gel are similar to those with extra-amniotic instillation and the results in general appear to be the same. However, like the extra-amniotic method aseptic considerations are required and care and skill are necessary to ensure that the prostaglandin preparation is placed precisely into the endocervical canal rather than the extra-amniotic space and that leakage into the vagina does not occur. An even more intricate technique involving perfusion of the cervix using a needle inserted into the anterior cervix and infusing $PGF_{2\alpha}$ 20 $\mu g/min$ has been suggested by Boemi et al.[19]; although seemingly effective, the technique represents an even more invasive concept than either extra-amniotic or endocervical instillation and is thus unlikely readily to attract patients or staff.

For simplicity, application into the posterior vaginal fornix was introduced in the mid-1970s and has become widely accepted in the UK[20]. Compared with the extra-amniotic and intracervical routes, aseptic precautions are minimal, and usually PGE_2 2–5 mg is required. Table 10.1 lists some of the protocols that have been used for patients with an unripe cervix. Most importantly, gastrointestinal side-effects very rarely occur with vaginal, extra-amniotic and endocervical prostaglandin treatment.

It is evident, however, from most published series, that failed induction with little or no cervical dilatation, leading to poor progress in labour disassociated from any mechanical obstruction and requiring delivery by caesarean section occurs in up to 5% of primigravidae treated irrespective of which local administration route is used. The precise explanation for such failures is still not established and doubtless varies between cases. While an adequate dose of PGE_2 is necessary this dose has not been firmly established. From published series, examining different doses given vaginally as a pessary or gel PGE_2 1.5 mg through to 7.5 mg appears to result in similar clinical efficacy, the larger doses not seeming to offer any added improvement as shown in Table 10.2. Possible variations in release and absorption of prostaglandins from the many preparations that have been tried in clinical practice has not received much attention but must be considered a possible explanation. There has been difficulty in performing kinetic studies *in vivo* since the measurement of PGE_2 in peripheral plasma is extremely unreliable due to its rapid degradation with one circulation through the lungs. There have also been problems in establishing a reliable assay for 15-keto-13,14-dihydro-PGE_2, the primary metabolite of PGE_2 but some advance has been made measuring the stable PGE_2 metabolite 11-deoxy-13,14-dihydro-15-keto-11β,16-cyclo PGE_2 (bicyclo PGEM)[32]. Gordon-Wright and Elder[33] assaying 15-keto PGE_2 found very variable concentrations in peripheral plasma after intravaginal PGE_2 gel and tablets had been administered. Castle et al.[34] using the more reliable bicyclo PGEM assay also found a similar variable picture with vaginal tablets, gels and lipid pessaries; in all groups relatively quick increases in concentration were observed. In contrast, Husslein et al.[35] using the bicyclo PGEM assay failed to observe any change in concentration following vaginal, endocervical or extra-amniotic instillation of PGE_2 which is particularly surprising with the latter administration route. A more recent study looked at the increase in PGEM using the bicyclo assay in peripheral plasma three hours after vaginal PGE_2 administration compared with pretreatment values in women with an unfavourable cervix. This failed to produce any good correlation with improvement in cervical score and onset of 'spontaneous labour' although there was an association with the subsequent duration of labour[36].

It seems probable that sufficient time must be allowed for the exogenously administered prostaglandins to exert their effect upon the cervix or to act as an intermediary in the maturation process. It is the author's opinion that this probably is in the region of 6–16 hours, an opinion that has not been fully substantiated. However, in unpublished observations, attempts to induce labour with shorter prostaglandin treatment times is more frequently associated with unsuccessful inductions and failed progress of labour, while Walker and

Table 10.1 Cervical ripening with PGE$_2$

Reference	n	parity	protocol	interval before further treatment	maximum Cx score	mean score increase	augmented %	L.O.L. (h)	failed induction (%)
Extra-amniotic									
Calder et al.[15]	121	P	240–480 μg	overnight	3	4.0	80	10.7	0.8
Thiery et al.[17]	68	P	250–500 μg	8 h	4	3.6	NS	NS	4.4
Stewart et al.[21]	21	P	450 μg	18 h	4	NS	69	9.1	0
Toplis and Sims[22]	20	P & M	500 μg	9½ h	3	2.4	40	10.3	5.0
Endocervical									
Wingerup et al.[23]	115	P & M	500–1000 μg	overnight	5	3.2	34	NS	5.2
Eckman et al.[24]	27	P	500 μg	24 h	5	3.4	34	NS	3.7
Ulmsten et al.[25]	35	P	500 μg	24 h	5	3.3	57	NS	6.3
Vaginal									
MacKenzie and Embrey[20]	102	P	2 mg gel	overnight	3	3.2	76	10.5 ⎱	3.0
	68	P	5 mg gel	overnight	3	3.6	52	10.6 ⎰	
O'Herlihy and MacDonald[26]	54	P	2 mg gel	overnight	3	6.6	52	8.5	1.5
Shepherd et al.[27]	110	P	3 mg pessary	12 h	4	NS	40	16.0	5.5
Embrey and MacKenzie[28]	32	P	5 or 7.5 polymer	overnight	3	NS	72	10.6	NS
Wilson[29]	15	P	2 mg tablets	overnight	3	2.3	70	NS	13.3

P = Primiparae   M = Multiparae   L.O.L. = Length of labour   NS = not started

Table 10.2 Influence of PGE$_2$ dosage upon cervical ripening (cervical score 0–3 before treatment)

	n	cervical score increase	score < 5 after treatment (%)	augmentation (%)	failed induction (%)
1.0 mg pessary*	77	NS	49[a]	95	NS
1.5 mg pessary*	56	NS	21[a]	91	NS
2.0 mg pessary[c]	102	3.2	28	77	3.9
5.0 mg pessary[c]	120	5.2	21	67	4.2
7.5 mg pessary[c]	60	5.2	13	76	3.3
10.0 mg pessary[d]	32	NS	NS	72	NS

[a] 6 h after treatment; * from Read and Mattock[31]; [c] from MacKenzie[30]; [d] from Embrey and MacKenzie[28]

Gordon[37] found no added benefit in ripening the cervix by waiting 24 hours rather than 12 hours. An alternative approach to single treatments has been tried by some workers[38,39] using PGE$_2$ 0.5 mg pessaries repeated at 2–3 hour intervals for variable periods. This approach does not appear to offer any advantage but results in prolonged treatment to delivery times. It seems with this regime, tachyphylaxis may well develop in some cases leading to a resistant cervix. Management of the woman whose cervix remains very unfavourable 12–18 hours after a single prostaglandin treatment is debatable; while many would treat the patient with a further dose of prostaglandins, there is no evidence that this leads to an improved outcome in labour compared with immediate oxytocin titration and amniotomy when possible[30].

The relative merits of PGE$_2$ compared with PGF$_{2\alpha}$ have surprisingly received little attention. While the majority of studies concerning cervical ripening or priming have involved the administration of PGE$_2$ in many different forms and regimens, it cannot be concluded that PGE$_2$ alone is useful. PGF$_{2\alpha}$ was reported to be effective in one study when given as an intravaginal gel compared with placebo treated controls[40]; in that study, patients of mixed parity and many with a relatively favourable cervix at the start of treatment were treated. This work is thus inconclusive. There is little reported data assessing both prostaglandins. MacKenzie and Embrey[41] treating primiparae with cervical scores of three or less in a double-blind trial comparing PGE$_2$ 5 mg and PGF$_{2\alpha}$ 25 mg reported that the former had greater cervical ripening properties than PGF$_{2\alpha}$. However the outcome of the subsequent induced labour was similar in the two groups: in this study it was emphasized that the PGF$_{2\alpha}$ dose may have been inappropriately low compared with the PGE$_2$ dose. However, Neilsen et al.[42] compared PGE$_2$ 5 mg and PGF$_{2\alpha}$ 50 mg by vaginal instillation using a double-blind, randomized allocation. Unfortunately, they studied both primips and multips and concluded that PGE$_2$ resulted in a greater degree of cervical ripening and shorter induced labour, lower oxytocin requirement and fewer failed inductions than occurred with PGF$_{2\alpha}$. Owing to the heterogeneity of the patients studied, the conclusions must be accepted with reservation and the comparison between PGE$_2$ and PGF$_{2\alpha}$ still needs to be more thoroughly assessed.

The pre-existing hormonal milieu within the mother and possibly even the fetus may well represent the most important regulating factor in cervical response to the exogenous prostaglandins. Low circulating oestradiol levels have been found in women in whom cervical ripening was not achieved with prostaglandins and the resulting induction failed with poor cervical dilatation and the need to deliver by caesarean section[43]. Therapies with high doses of oestrogens have been used in the past for inducing late abortion or premature labour and there has been renewed enthusiasm for exploring the possibility of treatment with oestradiol or oestriol to provoke cervical ripening and improve labour outcome. Small series have been reported indicating that cervical ripening can be produced with a local application of high doses of both into the extra-amniotic space. In a double-blind trial involving 50 primiparae with an unfavourable cervix, Calder and Gordon[44] found oestradiol valerate (150 mg) produced significant cervical changes and a better induced labour outcome compared to placebo. Craft and Yovich[45] using oestradiol 300 mg extra-amniotically reported that 11 of 15 patients proceeded into labour following treatment, while Thiery et al.[46] reported that oestriol 250 mg was more effective than oestradiol-17β 180 mg in enhancing cervical favourability.

Comparing extra-amniotically injected oestradiol 150 mg and PGE_2 450 μg Stewart et al.[47] found that the effect upon the cervix was similar with both agents but that PGE_2 stimulated labour in more patients and overall the outcome for labour was better with PGE_2 with fewer failed inductions than oestradiol. Tromans et al.[48] with a similar study design reported similar results. Quinn et al.[49] in their double-blind study of nulliparae with cervical scores of three or less found that extra-amniotically only 15 mg oestriol gel produced similar results to those produced with the massive dose of $PGF_{2\alpha}$ 10 mg extra-amniotically, with regard to ripening the cervix and the length of subsequent induced labour: both were significantly better than placebo treatment. Whether this study indicates that oestriol is more effective in enhancing labour outcome when the cervix is unfavourable compared with oestradiol, or merely supports the view that $PGF_{2\alpha}$ is less effective than PGE_2 cannot be known for certain. Oestradiol valerate given intramuscularly prior to oral PG induction was not found to enhance the outcome of labour induction[50]. However, in this study, as in some others, primiparae and multiparae were not analyzed separately.

It appears therefore that cervical ripening can be produced with little or no myometrial activity using oestrogens thus offering the possibility of a technique unlikely to lead to fetal compromise, particularly when placental function is impaired. However, although cervical state can be modified by oestrogen treatment, there is often little improvement in the outcome of the subsequent induced labour, the prime objective of any cervical ripening exercise. Whether a combined approach using prostaglandins and oestrogens, both in reduced dosages can produce better results avoiding the 3–5 % failure rate currently experienced, has yet to be determined. With the introduction into clinical practice of the anti-progesterone such as the 3β-hydroxy-steroid dehydrogenase enzyme blocker or the progestogen norethindrone derivative, a competitive progesterone receptor blocker, an alternative strategy for cervical ripening may be available. Progesterone is known to inhibit the net loss of collagen from the human cervix in vitro, and thus a block to endogenous progesterone production or receptor availability could modify cervical state and enhance labour progress. Clinical observations using this approach to cervical maturation at present must rely upon studies of cases of fetal death *in utero* until the appropriate maternal and fetal toxicology studies have been completed.

ROUTINE INDUCTION

Largely due to patient demands in the UK, less invasive, more 'natural' methods of labour induction were explored during the mid-1970s. With greater awareness of the influence of cervical state at induction upon labour success, a more rational approach to prostaglandin administration evolved. While the early studies of the intravenous, oral and vaginal administration all indicated that gastrointestinal side-effects were a problem, side-effects could be largely avoided if doses were kept down with oral and vaginal use. Although combined infusions of PGE_2 and oxytocin have been attempted, a move away from continuous infusions has meant that this approach has never been fully explored.

Repeated one to two hourly ingestion of PGE_2 0.5 mg or 1 mg doses in the form of dry tablets have been found to induce progressive labour in virtually all women so treated, especially if multiparous with a favourable cervix (Table 10.3). Nausea, vomiting and diarrhoea are infrequent occurrences and for many women and their attendants this method of induction is very acceptable and attractive. The alternative approach which is equally attractive to all parties is the intravaginal insertion of prostaglandins when success is similarly high and gastrointestinal side-effects extremely uncommon. With the latter regimen, much less agreement exists as to optimum prostaglandin dosage and treatment intervals. Most reports assessing the use of vaginal prostaglandins for labour induction have involved the use of hospital pharmacy produced preparations since commercially produced supplies have generally not been available. Lipid based pessaries, a variety of viscous gels of cellulose and dextran, as well as tablets marketed for oral and vaginal use have all been used vaginally, each producing similar results (Table 10.4). PGE_2 dosages have mostly been in the same range as that used for cervical ripening 2–5 mg.

Since part of the drive to use vaginal instillation has been the desire to avoid intravenous infusions, many workers have devised protocols using repeated pessary or gel treatments at four to six hour intervals with low amniotomy performed once labour is established. Where observations have been controlled, the outcome compared with conventional induction by low amniotomy and immediate oxytocin titration is of a generally longer induction–delivery interval with prostaglandins but similar lengths of labour (Fig. 10.5) and neonatal condition for each group; analgesia requirements and postpartum haemorrhage are usually reduced in prostaglandin treated patients[60,63]. The need for additional oxytocin augmentation to reach full dilatation is generally 34–62 % in primigravidae and 8–23 % for multigravidae whose labours are initiated with prostaglandins[39,59–63]. While there is little

Table 10.3 Routine induction with oral PGE_2

Reference	n	Bishop's score	protocol	side-effects V (%)	D (%)	'success' (%)	definition of 'success'
Craft[51]	P 50	2–10	0.5–3.0 mg 2 hrly	34	0	84	satisfactory progress
	M 30	2–10	0.5–3.0 mg 2 hrly			93	
Thiery[52]	P 46	4–9	0.5–2.0 mg 2 hrly	20	2	96	fully dilated ≤ 24 hours
Thiery[53]	M 51	4–9	0.5–2.0 mg 2 hrly			98	
Yip[54]	P 36	NS	0.5 mg 1–2 hrly	3	0	75	6 cm < 12 hours
	M 21	NS				90	delivery ≤ 24 hours
Ang and Firth[55]	Mixed 37	7.3 mean	0.5–2.0 mg 2 hrly	24	3	95	delivery ≤ 24 hours
Matthews[56]	P 25	favourable	0.5–2.0 mg 2–4 hrly	12	8	76	delivery ≤ 24 hours
	M 25	favourable	0.5–2.0 mg 2–4 hrly	4	0	88	delivery ≤ 24 hours
Mundow[57]	M 82	6+	0.5–1.5 mg 1–2 hrly	4	1	100	NS
	P 18	6+	0.5–1.5 mg 1–2 hrly	4	1	100	NS

V = Vomiting, D = Diarrhoea, NS = not stated

Table 10.4 Routine induction with vaginal prostaglandins

Reference	n	cervical score at treatment	protocol	augmentation (%)	L.O.L. (h)	CS (%)
MacKenzie and Embrey[58]	72 P	6+	2–5 mg gel overnight	34.7	7.0	9.2
	53 M	6+	2–5 mg gel overnight	17.0	3.8	0
Clarke et al.[59]	29 P	6+	2 mg gel 20 h	62.0	NS	NS
	40 M	6+	2 mg gel 20 h	15.0	NS	NS
MacKenzie et al.[60]	96 P	5+	5.0 mg pessary 7 h	37.5	8.1	NS
	167 M	5+	2.5 mg pessary 7 h	19.1	4.8	NS
Khoo et al.[61]	25 P	5.9*	5 mg tablet 24 h	42.0	NS	16
	22 M	6.5*	3 mg tablet 24 h	23.0	NS	0
Shepherd et al.[62]	226 P	5+	3 mg pessary 4–6 h	33.6	8.7	7.1
	253 M	5+	3 mg pessary 4–6 h	9.9	5.1	2.4
Kennedy et al.[63]	50 M	5+	3 mg tablet 6 h	8	NS	2
Embrey and MacKenzie[28]	37 P	6+	10–15 mg polymer 12 h	±38	7.3	3
	52 M	6+	7.0–7.5 mg polymer 12 h	±11	4.3	0

*Mean cervical score; L.O.L. = Length of labour; CS = caesarean section, NS = not started

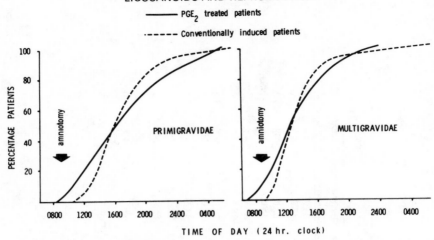

Figure 10.5 Time of delivery through the day following induction by low amniotomy and immediate intravenous oxytocin titration at 09.00 hours or PGE$_2$ vaginal pessary at 06.00 hours, amniotomy at 09.00 hours and oxytocin augmentation when necessary at 14.00 hours (MacKenzie *et al.*[60])

doubt that PGF$_{2\alpha}$ can be used for inducing labour when the cervix is ripe most work has involved intravenous infusions. With few series reported with local administration it is difficult to comment on the value of PGF$_{2\alpha}$ compared with PGE$_2$.

Although labour can be reliably induced in most cases, there remains a degree of unpredictability about the speed with which the myometrium responds, if it responds at all, to the administered prostaglandins. Despite the introduction of commercially produced PGE$_2$ 3 mg vaginal tablets, and a newer triacetin gel, presently undergoing clinical trials, uncertainty remains. An analysis of a possible circadian effect, as reported for mid-trimester prostaglandin injection for therapeutic abortion[64], on lengths of labour following a single vaginal instillation of prostaglandins during the hours of 09.00 and 21.00 resulted in no apparent influence for primigravidae and a marginally foreshortened length of labour in multiparae treated in the evening compared to the morning (Fig. 10.6). Whether there is a more obvious influence if the prostaglandins are given between the hours of 21.00 and 09.00 remains speculative. There appear to be advantages in labour and delivery occurring overnight and thus some preference for treating patients with prostaglandins in the afternoon or evening[58]. Whether this is a true reflection of the influence of prostaglandins on subsequent labour or merely a result of less obstetric intervention during the night with consequent reduced iatrogenic morbidity is not known for certain.

Of particular concern are those patients who respond quickly to the administered prostaglandins resulting in very painful labours with an increased risk of fetal distress. The characteristic prostaglandin induced contractions are of low amplitude, less than 40 mmHg, and at 1–3 minute intervals[20,65]. Uterine

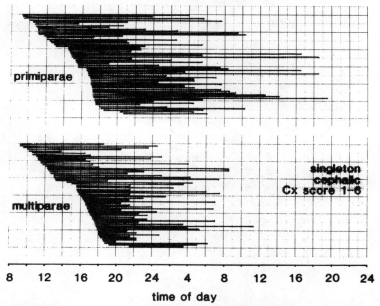

Figure 10.6 Influence of time of day of vaginal PGE$_2$ treatment and length of subsequent 'spontaneous' labour (primiparae $p = 0.36$; multiparae $p = 0.01$)

overstimulation, however, may occur either in the form of overfrequent or excessive amplitude contractions with little respite between (hypersystole) or as a sustained tetany (hypertonus) (Fig. 10.7); both may lead to acute fetal distress. Immediate delivery by caesarean section is one course of action but alternatively intravenous infusion of a potent tocolytic has been shown to suppress prostaglandin induced overstimulation[66] (Fig. 10.8), and has been used with success in clinical practice[25,61,62]. Experience has led most workers to recommend either very cautious use in highly parous patients in whom the cervix is effaced and partly dilated or avoiding prostaglandins in these patients altogether since this group is most likely to be overstimulated.

Efforts at developing a more predictable release system for the prostaglandins have been made by some investigators[67,68]. By incorporating the prostaglandins into a non-biodegradable polymer with predetermined release characteristics, it was hoped that a more predictable release of prostaglandins could be produced with consequent improved results. *In vivo* kinetic observations[34] have substantiated *in vitro* findings[67,69]; absorption across the vaginal skin probably accounts for some of the variation seen between patients. Initial clinical studies using such a release system have yielded encouraging results[28]. It appears however that further attention needs to be given to the optimum release profile for the prostaglandins and it seems possible that a quick release of prostaglandins may be more effective than a slow sustained release, both for induction of labour when the cervix is ripe and for cervical priming.

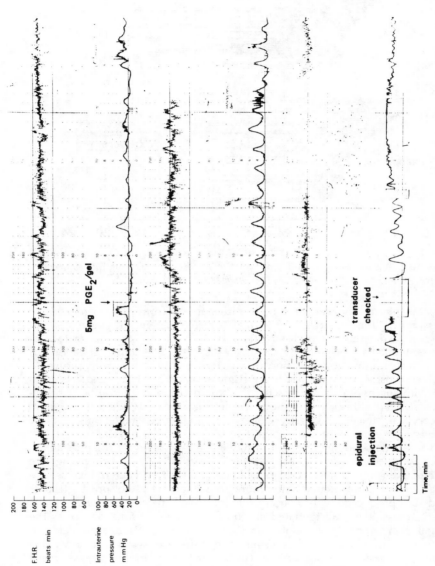

Figure 10.7 Uterine hypertonia recorded via a transcervical extra-amniotic catheter inserted prior to intravaginal administration of PGE₂ 5 mg. Patient delivered by emergency caesarean section

210

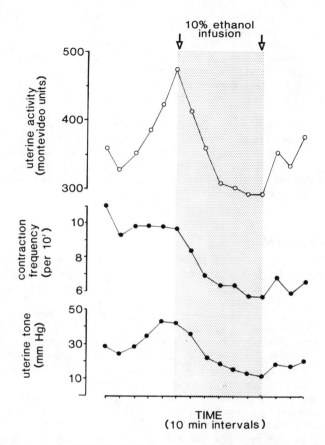

Figure 10.8 The tocolytic effect of an intravenous infusion of 10% ethanol upon the uterine activity induced with PGE_2 2.5 mg injected extra-amniotically in six patients undergoing mid-trimester abortion (Maclean and MacKenzie, unpublished data)

INDUCTION IN COMPLICATED CIRCUMSTANCES

Previous caesarean section

In many countries, deliveries by caesarean section have become much more common with rates up to 25% of all deliveries. Views on the management of women previously delivered by lower segment caesarean section vary considerably and range between electively repeating the caesarean section in all cases to inducing labour at 38 weeks gestation in appropriate cases or awaiting the spontaneous onset of labour anticipating a successful vaginal delivery. There still remains some debate over the wisdom of stimulating uterine activity with oxytocin when a caesarean scar is present although there are little objective data assessing its role. A similar reservation exists about the use of prostaglandins in this situation. One large series using PGE_2 2–2.5 mg administered vaginally as a gel or pessary has been reported; the outcome in 143 patients, 77 of whom had an unfavourable cervix at the time of induction was detailed[70]. A vaginal delivery was successfully achieved in 76% of the total group; 68% of these had an unfavourable cervix, and might have been managed by an elective repeat section by many obstetricians without any attempt at labour. In only two of the 143 patients was there anxiety of possible scar rupture, but in all cases the scar remained intact. Similar optimism has been expressed by Shepherd et al.[62] reporting 16 vaginal deliveries in 19 patients previously delivered by caesarean section and all had an intact scar.

It is the author's belief that the low amplitude contractions provoked by prostaglandins render them potentially more safe than oxytocin for stimulating uterine activity. There is little doubt however that the use of prostaglandins in these women with an unfavourable cervix considerably increases the chances of a delivery vaginally and that in all cases appropriate observations and care are required to ensure that an obstructed labour is not developing.

Fetal breech presentation

As with the management of patients previously delivered by caesarean section, there is much discussion as to the most appropriate method of delivering the baby when presenting by the breech. If labour is to be induced, there seems to be no reason why the prostaglandins should not be used. O'Herlihy[71] managed 13 primigravidae all with an unripe cervix with PGE_2 2 mg in gel and succeeded in inducing labour in all of them but delivered 23% by caesarean section because of poor progress. Shepherd et al.[62] using PGE_2 3 mg pessaries managed 54 patients of mixed parity with varying cervical scores and all were successfully induced. Of 13% requiring delivery by caesarean section, almost all were during the second stage of labour. A personal series of 177 patients including primiparae and multiparae and all degrees of cervical favourability have been treated with vaginal PGE_2 with an overall caesarean section rate of 22% without obvious detriment to mother or neonate from the induction procedure (Table 10.5). Unfortunately, there have been no randomized studies comparing prostaglandins with either oxytocin to induce labour or spontaneous onset labour. The apparent advantage of inducing labour with local prostaglandins as opposed to intravenous oxytocin titration and low amniotomy is the delay possible in rupturing the forewaters until the breech has descended well into the maternal pelvis. Randomized controlled trials are however required before any definite conclusions can be reached.

Multiple pregnancy

There are very little reported data of the use of prostaglandins in the induction of labour in multiple pregnancy. Personal experience indicates that the prostaglandins are as effective in twin pregnancies as in other situations. Since primary postpartum haemorrhage due to uterine hypotonia occurs in

Table 10.5   Vaginal prostaglandin E_2 and labour induction with singleton fetal breech presentation (all degrees of cervical favourability)

Total no. of patients	177
of which:	
primiparae	117
multiparae	60
method of delivery:	
vaginal delivery	137
caesarean section	40
of caesarean sections:	
persistently unfavourable cervix	7
failed induction	12
cord presentation/prolapse	2
fetal distress 1st stage labour	4
2nd stage labour	3
failed descent 2nd stage labour	12

approximately 12% of twin labours, the use of prostaglandins as part of the induction method would seem to be more than justified. (See later section).

Ruptured membranes without ensuing labour

When the membranes rupture spontaneously around term, labour generally follows within a few hours. When there is a delay in labour starting, there are concerns about intrauterine infection occurring and many obstetricians favour stimulating contractions with an oxytocic. Prostaglandins have been used for this purpose in a variety of ways. Thiery et al.[72] have used low dose (0.1 μg/h) intravenous infusions of PGE_2 increasing the rate until labour is stimulated. Treating 38 patients of mixed parity and all with a cervical score of five or less, they successfully delivered 37 vaginally and reported a low incidence of side-effects. Oral administration has been used and compared with intravenous oxytocin by Hauth et al.[73] and Lange et al.[74]. Both conducted a randomized prospective trial and both found that oral PGE_2 0.5–1.5 mg/h was safe and efficient compared with intravenous oxytocin. Furthermore oxytocin tended to result in shorter treatment-to-delivery intervals according to Lange et al.[74]. The design used by Hauth et al.[73] does not allow any worthwhile comparison unfortunately since PGE_2 was instilled three hours after membranes ruptured while oxytocin was given after 12 hours. Vaginal administration as a PGE_2 4 mg gel[75], or as a PGE_2 3 mg pessary[76,77] has been used generally with favourable conclusions. Augmentation with further prostaglandins or intravenous oxytocin appears necessary in about 40% of primiparae and 20% multiparae treated with vaginal prostaglandins.

However, despite the data from these six series there remains considerable uncertainty over the place for prostaglandins in this situation. Apart from the different routes and protocols used, there are large discrepancies over the recommended time to start to stimulate labour after the membranes have ruptured and how long treatment should continue before resorting to other augmentation methods. Further, while appropriate attention has been paid to differences with parity and from cervical state in some of the studies, the total numbers in any one group are very small and worthwhile conclusions comparing prostaglandins with intravenous oxytocin are not possible. It seems reasonable however to state that the prostaglandins are effective in stimulating labour when the membranes have ruptured and given vaginally, appear to be safe. Large, well-designed prospective trials are still required before it will be possible to be sure of any advantage or disadvantage when compared with intravenous oxytocin or even awaiting the spontaneous onset of labour.

PROSTAGLANDINS AND FETAL CONSIDERATIONS

Any method of labour induction requires a careful appraisal of the risks and benefits of the method over other alternative methods with regard to the various indices of labour outcome; critical assessment of possible fetal benefits and potential morbidity is also necessary. Observational data[65,78] have suggested that labour induced with prostaglandins, in these instances by extra-amniotic injections, is no more likely to result in fetal or neonatal acidosis and asphyxia than during labour induced with oxytocin or following spontaneous onset. The low amplitude contractions characteristically stimulated by the prostaglandins should theoretically cause little disturbance to placental bed blood flow with a consequent small risk of fetal distress developing. However the possibility of fetal distress occurring once labour is established is presumably similar to that following induction with oxytocin. Whether continuous electronic fetal monitoring should be instituted before and following prostaglandin treatment remains controversial. The place for routine continuous monitoring of the fetal heart in labour, induced or spontaneous, has still to be proven with virtually all controlled studies showing no advantage. Since the development of vaginal prostaglandin treatment was in part the consequence of a desire to move away from invasive mechanized labour management, then the case for continuous electronic fetal monitoring needs to be proven before being widely recommended. In cases of cervical ripening, any other assessment of fetal wellbeing, notably fetal scalp blood pH measurements, is not tenable, since negotiation of the unripe cervix is generally not possible. Continuous monitoring would seem appropriate in women in whom placental function is thought to be reduced but there is as yet no evidence that such management improves the outcome. One retrospective study comparing continuous electronic monitoring with intermittent auscultation found no obvious benefits for fetal wellbeing from continuous monitoring but the diagnosis of suspected fetal distress was made in 48% of the monitored cases, of which all were delivered by caesarean section, compared with 4% in the intermittent auscultation group[79]. There would seem to be little doubt however that it would be wise for all patients to be carefully watched for the first 4–5 hours after prostaglandin treatment by intermittent fetal auscultation at 15–30 minute intervals as a minimum to ensure that an unexpected response to the exogenous prostaglandins with

214

fetal distress has not occurred.

While the measurement of the natural prostaglandins, PGE_2 and $PGF_{2\alpha}$ in peripheral blood in the adult has been found to be unhelpful, concentrations in the fetal circulation have been found to be much higher. Cord blood levels have been measured following delivery to assess possible differences consequent upon the nature of the preceding labour, whether spontaneous, oxytocin-induced or prostaglandin-induced[80]. Labour induced with PGE_2 given as a vaginal gel or pessary results in a significantly higher level of PGE in cord venous plasma at delivery compared with spontaneous onset and oxytocin induced labour; in all three groups the levels were significantly higher than those found following delivery by elective caesarean section. $PGF_{2\alpha}$ concentrations were similar in all the labouring groups which were significantly higher than those found following elective caesarean section. A more recent study[36] showed a positive correlation between the concentration of 13, 14-dihydro-15-keto-PGE_2 using the bicyclo PGEM assay[32] in cord artery (Fig. 10.9) and vein at delivery and the interval from vaginal administration of PGE_2 3 mg as a pessary or tablet to delivery of the baby. The above evidence supports the view that exogenously administered prostaglandins reach the fetal circulation and on occasions in large amounts. Since the prostaglandins are known to be involved in fetal and neonatal cardiovascular physiology, as well as other systems there may be a risk that high doses of PGE_2 or $PGF_{2\alpha}$ given to the mother to induce labour could interfere with these physiological processes. At present, however, no

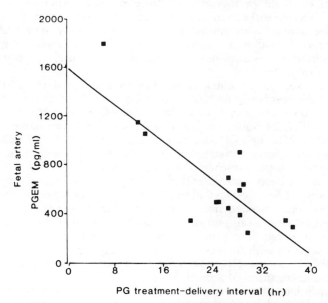

Figure 10.9 PGEM concentrations in cord artery plasma in relation to the interval between maternal treatment with PGE_2 3 mg intravaginally and delivery ($r = 0.817$; $p = 0.0002$) (Sellers and MacKenzie[36])

215

detrimental influence upon neonatal cardio-pulmonary function and ductus arteriosus physiology has been reported. One proven advantage of prostaglandins over oxytocin for labour induction is the reduction in neonatal hyperbilirubinaemia[81-83]; the incidence following PGE$_2$ induced labour is similar to that for spontaneous onset labour. The explanation for the low incidence of hyperbilirubinaemia following prostaglandin treatment compared with oxytocin has not been fully explored but could be explained by the apparent steroidogenic properties of prostaglandins[84,85]. There thus may be particular benefits if very preterm induction is planned. The incidence of maternal water intoxication due to hypernatraemia is a rare hazard of oxytocin-induced labour and is generally the result of high dose infusion over a long period. In such instances, electrolyte imbalance of the neonate has also been recorded and the use of prostaglandins in such cases should avoid such a potentially dangerous condition.

MANAGEMENT OF FETAL DEATH *IN UTERO*

Of all the possible roles for prostaglandins in obstetric practice, the place in the management of fetal death retained *in utero* is probably the most widely acknowledged. Prior to the introduction of the prostaglandins, such cases were either managed expectantly with spontaneous abortion or labour resulting usually within three weeks of death or by repeated high dose infusions of oxytocin or ingestion of large doses of oestrogen. As with induction of labour, most administration routes have been explored and results obtained are similar with regard to treatment–delivery and treatment–abortion intervals, although gastrointestinal side-effect rates vary. While intravenous infusion is successful, local administration has again provided the best results (Table 10.6).

The prime objective in the management of cases of fetal death is to achieve expulsion of the pregnancy within a reasonably short interval after treatment with minimal disturbance and unnecessary distress to the patient. Abortion or delivery within 24 hours has been the goal and extra-amniotic infusions or injections of PGE$_2$ or PGF$_{2\alpha}$ are successful in the majority of cases. Since the introduction of foreign material into the uterus could result in intrauterine sepsis, especially in the presence of a dead fetus with ruptured membranes, this route has not been received enthusiastically; no evidence to support this fear has however been presented in the literature. Similar anxieties exist about intra-amniotic injections and since amniotic fluid embolism is a complication associated with fetal death *in utero*, breaching the fetal membranes may theoretically increase this potential hazard. Further, the injection of a hypertonic solution with the prostaglandins intra-amniotically could increase the possibility of a consumptive coagulopathy, another complication associated with prolonged retention of a dead fetus[93].

Vaginal administration causes minimal inconvenience and distress to the patient and permits delaying the rupturing of fetal membranes until delivery or abortion seems inevitable. Protocols favoured by workers in the United States have involved repeated 3–6 hourly insertions of PGE$_2$ 20 mg pessaries.

Table 10.6 Prostaglandins and fetal death

Reference	n	protocol	expulsion in <24 hrs (%)	mean induction–expulsion interval (h)	side-effects vomiting (%)	diarrhoea (%)
Extra-amniotic						
Calder et al.[86]	50	PGE$_2$ 0.2–3.9 mg PGF$_{2\alpha}$ 3.9–5.7 mg	NR NR	IUD 7.8 Missed abortion 17.2	40	0
Lippert and Luthi[87]	20	PGE$_2$ 0.5–1.0 mg gel 3 mg	90	12.0	NR	
Vaginal						
Rutland and Ballard[88]	50	PGE$_2$ 20 mg 3 hrly	86	11.3	60	60
El-Demarawy[89]	31	PGF$_{2\alpha}$ 20 mg 3–6 hrly	80 approx.	14.6	87	70
MacKenzie et al.[90]	50	PGE$_2$ 5 or 15 mg × 1 + i.v. oxytocin for 18 h	NR	15.0	← 15 →	
Intramuscular						
Toppozada et al.[91]	27	16-phenoxy-PGE$_2$ 500 µg 4–6 hrly	93	12.4	← 48 →	
Wallenburg et al.[92]	97	15-methyl-PGF$_{2\alpha}$ 125–250 µg 2 hrly	94	8.6	52	59

Expulsion times within 24 hours are achieved in the majority but with relatively high rates of vomiting and diarrhoea. An approach using a single instillation of PGE_2 as a gel or pessary combined with an intravenous infusion of oxytocin after 12—18 hours produces very similar treatment to expulsion times but with much lower incidences of side effects[90]. When the fetus is not a consideration, prostaglandin analogues can be explored with relative safety. To date there have been few studies published and at present none have suggested a significant improvement over the results currently provided with the natural prostaglandins. It is a reasonable hope, however, that this model can be used to provide information for the newer prostaglandins to allow subsequent study in viable pregnancies. Further, closer analysis of the endogenous hormonal milieu comparing the profiles in cases readily stimulated into labour with those resistant to oxytocic stimulation might help to elaborate upon the mechanisms involved in the evolution of parturition and successful labour induction.

PROSTAGLANDINS IN POSTPARTUM HAEMORRHAGE

Since the prostaglandins are known to be capable of stimulating myometrial contractions at all stages of gestation, and in particular can provoke strong, prolonged, sustained tetanic contractions, a potential use in uterine hypotonia following delivery has been exploited. Further, it has been observed that women whose labours have been induced with prostaglandins as part of the induction procedure have lower rates of primary postpartum haemorrhage compared with those whose labours have been induced with oxytocin; spontaneous labour results in even lower postpartum haemorrhage rates[60,63,94].

There have been specific reports by various workers using prostaglandins to control the torrential haemorrhage of uterine atonia following delivery. A number of different regimens have been tried and recommended. $PGF_{2\alpha}$ 250—1000 μg by intramyometrial injection have been used by Takagi et al.[95] and 15-methyl-$PGF_{2\alpha}$ 500 μg by intra-muscular injection by Corson & Bolognese[96]. PGE_2 20 mg pessaries repeated as necessary were proposed by Hertz et al.[97] and Henson et al.[98], reported a dramatic response with an infusion of PGE_2 5—10 μg per minute in this situation. For general emergencies, only the natural prostaglandins are available and administration by intravenous infusion of PGE_2 10 μg per minute or $PGF_{2\alpha}$ 50 μg per minute would seem to be the most appropriate protocol; the intramyometrial injection of PGE_2 100 μg or $PGF_{2\alpha}$ 500 μg is a suitable alternative. The use of vaginal pessaries would not seem to be an obvious method since the excess blood loss is likely to wash the administered prostaglandins out of the vagina. Also, with this latter approach, kinetic studies of vaginally instilled prostaglandins indicate that absorption is too slow for effective uterine stimulation in such an urgent potentially lethal situation. Heyl et al.[99] have suggested that all obstetric units should have supplies of 15-methyl-$PGF_{2\alpha}$ 250 μg for intramuscular injection to be given in cases of recurrent uterine inversion, having successfully managed a patient with this condition. Somewhat surprisingly, prostaglandins have also been advocated in the management of severe secondary postpartum haemorrhage[100].

Whether the use of prostaglandins as a third stage oxytocic should be considered as a routine has not been well explored, but there could be some merit in adopting such an approach since ergometrine which is given as a routine is under some question with its recognised effects upon maternal cardiopulmonary function and hypertensive tendencies. Kerekes and Domokos[101] found that $PGF_{2\alpha}$ 1–2 mg intramyometrially resulted in less blood loss than intramuscular ergometrine or no treatment at all. Whether the routine transabdominal intramyometrial injection of prostaglandins would become an acceptable routine, however, is doubtful.

THE FUTURE

Although considerable advantages have accrued from the use of prostaglandins in the management of labour induction there remain some uncertainties.

With the obvious attractions of local administration, vaginal instillation of tablets, gels or pessaries for cervical ripening and routine induction has become widely accepted. However, it is evident that many, if not all, of the preparations used can result in unpredictable prostaglandin release and subsequent uterine response. Moves to produce vehicles with more reliable release profiles have been very encouraging but further work is required to establish the optimum dosages and precise release rates for the different circumstances encountered in clinical practice. The benefits of priming the unfavourable cervix prior to labour induction are now well established and confirmed in a number of prospective randomized trials. Apart from the management of fetal death, where the results are dramatically better than previously achieved, the case for the prostaglandins for routine induction is as yet unproven: labour outcomes are essentially very similar to those following low amniotomy and intravenous oxytocin titration but subjective benefits which are more difficult to quantify including patient acceptability are probably achieved. Whether there are advantages in management with prostaglandins when induction is required in patients who have previously been delivered by caesarean section or when the fetus presents by the breech remains speculative. Augmentation or stimulation of labour in the presence of spontaneously ruptured membranes with prostaglandins as opposed to intravenous infusions of oxytocin also remain uncertain. Large scale randomized trials of such situations need to be designed if these uncertainties are to be answered.

Clinical research involving labour induction has tended to be confined to investigating the natural prostaglandins administered alone and in conjunction with intravenous oxytocin. While the principle of single drug therapies is to be preferred to polypharmacy, it is possible that greater consideration to the presumed physiology of parturition could lead to improved results requiring lower prostaglandin dosages and a reduction in some of the unpredictable post-therapy responses. Further studies assessing the possible benefits of exogenous oestrogen treatment prior to or with prostaglandin administration might enhance the outcome of labour in those women with a very unfavourable cervix. The anti-progesterones have already been found to enhance induced abortion results[102] and could have a role in induction of labour especially in difficult circumstances, providing disturbances to fetal physiology can be excluded and other maternal morbidity does not occur. The alternative approach, exploring some of the newer prostaglandin analogues which have greater propensities towards enhancing cervical collagenolysis could lead to a prostaglandin capable of causing total cervical effacement and dilatation without any demonstrable myometrial activity. Such a concept would permit labour with little risk to the fetus. Similar possibilities exist using one of the recently developed hygroscopic polymers inserted into the cervix when induction is required.

Enormous advantages have been obtained with the use of prostaglandins for labour induction over the past fifteen years and it is to be hoped that further advances will be developed over the next fifteen years.

REFERENCES

1. Turnbull, A.C. and Anderson, A.B.M. (1968). Induction of labour. *J. Obstet. Gynaecol. Br. Commonw.*, **75**, 32–40
2. Karim, S.M.M., Trussell, R.R., Patel, R.C. and Hillier, K. (1968). Response of pregnant human uterus to prostaglandin $F_{2\alpha}$ – induction of labour. *Br. Med. J.*, **4**, 621–623
3. Embrey, M.P. (1969). The effect of prostaglandins on the human pregnant uterus. *J. Obstet. Gynaecol. Br. Commonw.*, **76**, 783–789
4. Karim, S.M.M. and Sharma, S.D. (1971). Oral administration of prostaglandins for the induction of labour. *Br. Med. J.*, **1**, 260–262
5. Karim, S.M.M. and Sharma, S.D. (1971). Therapeutic abortion and induction of labour by the intravaginal administration of prostaglandin E_2 and $F_{2\alpha}$. *J. Obstet. Gynaecol. Br. Commonw.*, **78**, 294–300
6. Scott, J.W. and Craft, I. (1976). Buccal prostaglandin E_2. *Br. J. Obstet. Gynaecol.*, **83**, 729–730
7. Thiery, M., Benijts, G., Martens, G., Sian, A.Y.L., Amy, J.J. and Derom, R. (1977). A comparison of buccal (oromucosal) and prostaglandin E_2 for elective induction of labour. *Prostaglandins*, **14**, 371–379
8. Dommisse, J., Davey, D.A., Martin, B. and Cohen, M. (1981). An evaluation of prostaglandin E_2 administered intrarectally to induce labour. *S. Afr. Med. J.*, **59**, 817–818
9. Calder, A.A., Embrey, M.P. and Hillier, K. (1974). Extra-amniotic prostaglandin E_2 for induction of labour at term. *Br. J. Obstet. Gynaecol.*, **81**, 39–46
10. Bishop, E.H. (1964). Pelvic scoring for elective induction. *Obstet. Gynecol.*, **24**, 266–268
11. Calder, A.A. and Embrey, M.P. (1975). Induction of labour. In Beard, R., Brudenell, M., Dunn, P. and Fairweather, D. (eds.) *The Management of Labour. Proceedings of Third Study Group of RCOG*, pp. 62–91. (London: RCOG)
12. Hillier, K. and Wallis, R.M. (1981). Prostaglandins, steroids and the human cervix. In Ellwood, D.A. and Anderson, A.B.M. (eds.) *The Cervix in Pregnancy and Labour*, pp. 144–162. (London: Churchill Livingstone)
13. Ellwood, D.A., Anderson, A.B.M., Mitchell, M.D., Murphy, G. and Turnbull, A.C. (1981). Prostanoids, collagenase and cervical softening in the sheep. In Ellwood, D.A. and Anderson, A.B.M. (eds.) *The Cervix in Pregnancy and Labour*, pp. 57–73. (London: Churchill Livingstone)
14. Ledger, W.L., Ellwood, D.A. and Taylor, M.J. (1983). Cervical softening in late pregnant sheep by infusion of prostaglandin E_2 into a cervical artery. *J. Reprod. Fertil.*, **69**, 511–515
15. Goeschen, K., Fuchs, F., Rasmussen, A.B., Rehnstrom, J.V. and Saling, E. (1985). Effect of β-mimetic tocolysis in cervical ripening and plasma prostaglandin $F_{2\alpha}$ metabolite after endocervical application of prostaglandin E_2. *Obstet. Gynecol.*, **65**, 166–171

16. Calder, A.A., Embrey, M.P. and Tait, T. (1977). Ripening of the cervix with extra-amniotic prostaglandin E₂ in viscous gel before induction of labour. *Br. J. Obstet. Gynaecol.*, **84**, 264–268

17. Thiery, M., Defoort, P., Bennis, G., van Eyck, J., Hennay, T., van Kets, H. and Martens, C. (1977). Effectiveness of extra-ovular injection of prostaglandin E₂ in tylose gel to ripen the cervix prior to elective induction of labour at term. *Prostaglandins*, **14**, 381–388

18. Wingerup, L., Anderson, K.-E. and Ulmsten, V. (1978). Ripening of the uterine cervix and induction of labour at term with prostaglandin E₂ in viscous gel. *Acta Obstet. Gynecol. Scand.*, **57**, 403–406

19. Boemi, P., Reitano, S. and Cianci, S. (1982). A new cervical perfusion method for induction of labour with prostaglandins. *Am. J. Obstet. Gynecol.*, **144**, 476–479

20. MacKenzie, I.Z. and Embrey, M.P. (1977). Cervical ripening with intravaginal prostaglandin E₂ gel. *Br. Med. J.*, **2**, 1381–1384

21. Stewart, P., Kennedy, J.H., Hillan, E. and Calder, A.A. (1983). The unripe cervix: Management with vaginal or extra-amniotic prostaglandin E₂. *J. Obstet. Gynecol.* **4**, 90–93.

22. Toplis, P.J. and Sims, L.D. (1979). Prospective study of different methods and routes of administration of prostaglandin E₂ to improve the unripe cervix. *Prostaglandins*, **18**, 127–136

23. Wingerup, L., Anderson, K.-E. and Ulmsten, U. (1979). Ripening of the cervix and induction of labour in patients at term by single intracervical application of prostaglandin E₂ in viscous gel. *Acta Obstet. Gynecol. Scand.*, **84**, (Suppl.), 11–14

24. Ekman, G., Persson, P.H., Ulmsten, U. and Wingerup, L. (1983). The impact on labor induction of intracervically applied PGE₂ gel related to gestational age in patients with an unripe cervix. *Acta Obstet. Gynecol. Scand.*, **113**, (Suppl.) 173–175

25. Ulmsten, U., Wingerup, L., Belfrage, P., Ekman, G. and Wiqvist, N. (1982). Intracervical application of prostaglandin gel for induction of term labor. *Obstet. Gynecol.*, **59**, 336–339

26. O'Herlihy, C. and McDonald, H.N. (1979). Influence of pre-induction prostaglandin E₂ gel on cervical ripening and labor. *Obstet. Gynecol.*, **54**, 708–710

27. Shepherd, J., Pearce, J.M.F. and Sims, C. (1979). Induction of labour using prostaglandin E₂ pessaries. *Br. Med. J.*, **2**, 108–110

28. Embrey, M.P. and MacKenzie, I.Z. (1985). Labour induction with a sustained release prostaglandin E₂ polymer vaginal pessary. *J. Obstet. Gynecol.*, **6**, 38–41

29. Wilson, P.D. (1978). A comparison of four methods of ripening the unfavourable cervix. *Br. J. Obstet. Gynaecol.*, **85**, 941–944

30. MacKenzie, I.Z. (1981). Clinical studies on cervical ripening. In Ellwood, D.A. and Anderson, A.B.M. (eds.) *The Cervix in Pregnancy and Labour*, pp. 161–186. (London: Churchill Livingstone)

31. Reed, M.D. and Mattock, E.J. (1982). Cervical ripening with prostaglandin E₂ pessaries – a question of dose. *J. Obstet. Gynecol.*, **3**, 71–74

32. Demers, L.M., Brennecke, S.P., Mountford, L.A., Brunt, J.D. and Turnbull, A.C. (1983). Development and validation of a radioimmunoassay for prostaglandin E metabolite levels in plasma. *J. Clin. Endocrinol. Metab.*, **57**, 101–106

33. Gordon-Wright, A.P. and Elder, M.G. (1979). The systemic absorption from the vagina of prostaglandin E₂ administered for the induction of labour. *Prostaglandins*, **18**, 153–160

34. Castle, B.M., Bellinger, J., Brennecke, S.P., Embrey, M.P. and MacKenzie, I.Z. (1983). In vivo studies using the bicyclo PGEM assay to assess release of PGE₂ from vaginal preparations used for labour induction. *Abstr. Br. Congr. Obstet. Gynaecol.*, July, Birmingham

35. Husslein, P., Reiche, L.R., Goeschen, K., Rasche, M. and Sinzinger, H. (1984). Plasma concentrations of 13,14-dihydro-15-keto PGE₂ (PGEM) after various ways of cervix ripening with PGE₂. *Prostaglandins*, **28**, 209–215.

36. Sellers, S.M. and MacKenzie, I.Z. (1985). Prostaglandin release following vaginal prostaglandin treatment for labour induction. In Wood, C. (ed.) *The Role of Prostaglandins in Labour*, pp. 77–84. Royal Society of Medicine Services Symposium No. 92

37. Walker, E. and Gordon, A.J. (1983). Lengths of exposure to prostaglandin E₂ and cervical ripening in primigravidae. *J. Obstet. Gynecol.*, **4**, 88–89

38. Liggins, G.C. (1979). Controlled trial of induction of labour by vaginal suppositories containing prostaglandin E₂. *Prostaglandins*, **18**, 167–172

39. Hunter, I.W.E., Cato, E. and Ritchie, J. (1984). Induction of labor using high dose or low dose prostaglandin vaginal pessaries. *Obstet. Gynecol.*, **63**, 418–420

40. MacLennan, A.H. and Green, R.C. (1979). Cervical ripening and induction of labour with intravaginal prostaglandin $F_{2\alpha}$. *Lancet*, **1**, 117–119

41. MacKenzie, I.Z. and Embrey, M.P. (1979). A comparison of PGE_2 and $PGF_{2\alpha}$ vaginal gel for ripening the cervix before induction of labour. *Br. J. Obstet. Gynaecol.*, **85**, 657–661

42. Neilson, D.R., Prins, R.P., Bolton, R.N., Mark, C. and Watson, P. (1983). A comparison of prostaglandin E_2 gel and prostaglandin $F_{2\alpha}$ gel for pre-induction cervical ripening. *Am. J. Obstet. Gynecol.*, **146**, 526–530

43. MacKenzie, I.Z., Jenkin, G. and Bradley, S.G. (1979). The relation between plasma oestrogen, progesterone and prolactin concentrations and the efficacy of vaginal prostaglandin E_2 gel in initiating labour. *Br. J. Obstet. Gynaecol.*, **86**, 171–174

44. Gordon, A.J. and Calder, A.A. (1977). Oestradiol applied locally to ripen the unfavourable cervix. *Lancet*, **2**, 1319–1321

45. Craft, I. and Yovich, J. (1978). Oestradiol and induction of labour. *Lancet*, **2**, 208

46. Thiery, M., de Gezelle, H., van Kets, H., Voorhoof, L., Verheugen, C., Smis, B., Gerris, J. and Martens, G. (1978). Extra-amniotic oestrogens for the unfavourable cervix. *Lancet*, **2**, 835–836

47. Stewart, P., Kennedy, J.M., Barlow, D.H. and Calder, A.A. (1981). A comparison of oestradiol and prostaglandin E_2 for ripening the cervix. *Br. J. Obstet. Gynaecol.*, **88**, 236–239

48. Tromans, P.M., Beazley, J.M. and Shenouda, P.I. (1981). Comparative study of oestradiol and prostaglandin E_2 vaginal gel for ripening the unfavourable cervix before induction of labour. *Br. Med. J.*, **282**, 679–681

49. Quinn, M.A., Murphy, A.J., Kuhn, R.J.P., Robinson, H.P. and Brown, J.B. (1981). A double blind trial of extra-amniotic oestriol and prostaglandin $F_{2\alpha}$ gel in cervical ripening. *Br. J. Obstet. Gynaecol.*, **88**, 644–649

50. Luther, E.R., Roux, J., Popat, R., Gardner, A., Gray, J., Soubiran, E. and Korcaz, Y. (1980). The effect of oestrogen priming on induction of labour with prostaglandins. *Am. J. Obstet. Gynecol.*, **137**, 351–354

51. Craft, I. (1973). Oral prostaglandin E_2 and amniotomy for induction of labour. *Adv. Biosci.*, **9**, 593–598

52. Thiery, M., de Hemptinne, D., Vanderheyden, K., Sian, A.Y.L., Derom, R., van Kets, H. and Martens, G. (1973). Elective induction of term labour with amniotomy and oral prostaglandin E_2. *Eur. J. Obstet. Gynecol. Reprod. Biol.*, **3**, 159–166

53. Thiery, M., Sian, A.Y.L., de Hemptinne, D., Derom, R., Martens, G., van Kets, H. and Amy, J.J. (1974). Induction of labour with prostaglandin E_2 tablets. *J. Obstet. Gynaecol. Br. Commonw.*, **81**, 303–306

54. Yip, S.K., Ma, M.K. and Ng, K.H. (1973). Induction of labour with oral prostaglandin E_2. *J. Obstet. Gynaecol. Br. Commonw.*, **88**, 442–445

55. Ang, L.T. and Firth, K.M. (1977). An appraisal of oral prostaglandin E_2 and intravenous oxytocin in the induction of labour. *Eur. J. Obstet. Gynecol. Reprod. Biol.*, **7**, 243–246

56. Mathews, D.D., Hossain, H., Bharga, A.S. and D'Souza, F. (1976). A randomised controlled trial of an oral solution of prostaglandin E_2 and oral oxytocin used immediately after low amniotomy for induction of labour in the presence of a favourable cervix. *Con. Med. Res. Opin.*, **4**, 233–240

57. Mundow, L.S. (1977). The induction of labour with prostaglandin E_2 tablets. *J. Ir. Med. Assoc.*, **70**, 280–281

58. MacKenzie, I.Z. and Embrey, M.P. (1978). The influence of pre-induction vaginal prostaglandin E_2 gel upon subsequent labour outcome. *Br. J. Obstet. Gynaecol.*, **85**, 657–661

59. Clarke, G.A., Letchworth, A.T. and Noble, A.D. (1980). Comparative trial of extra-amniotic and vaginal prostaglandin E_2 in tylose gel for induction of labour. *J. Perinat. Med.*, **8**, 236–240

60. MacKenzie, I.Z., Bradley, S. and Embrey, M.P. (1981). A simpler approach to labour induction using a lipid-based prostaglandin E_2 vaginal suppository. *Am. J. Obstet. Gynecol.*, **141**, 158–162

61. Khoo, P.P.T., Kalshekar, M., Jogee, M. and Elder, M.G. (1981). Induction of labour with prostaglandin E_2 vaginal tablets. *Eur. J. Obstet. Gynecol. Reprod. Biol.*, **11**, 313–318

62. Shepherd, J.H., Bennett, M., Laurence, D., Moore, F. and Sims, C.D. (1981). Prostaglandin

vaginal suppositories; a simple and safe approach to the induction of labour. *Obstet. Gynecol.*, **58**, 596–600

63. Kennedy, J.H., Stewart, P., Barlow, D.H., Hillan, E. and Calder, A.A. (1982). Induction of labour: a comparison of a single prostaglandin E₂ vaginal tablet with amniotomy and intravenous oxytocin. *Br. J. Obstet. Gynaecol.*, **89**, 704–707

64. Smith, I.D. and Shearman, R.P. (1974). Circadian aspects of prostaglandin $F_{2\alpha}$-induced termination of pregnancy. *J. Obstet. Gynaecol. Brit. Commonw.*, **81**, 841–848

65. Steiner, H., Zahradnik, H.P., Beckwoldt, M., Robrecht, D. and Hillemanns, H.G. (1979). Cervical ripening prior to induction of labour (intracervical application of PGE₂ viscous gel). *Prostaglandins*, **17**, 125–133

66. MacKenzie, I.Z. (1984). Induction of labour with prostaglandins. *Prostagl. Perspect.*, **1**, 6–9

67. Embrey, M.P., Graham, N.B. and McNeill, M.E. (1980). Induction of labour with a sustained release prostaglandin E₂ vaginal pessary. *Br. Med. J.*, **281**, 901–902

68. Brundin, J., Christensen, N.J., Fuchs, T. and Larsson, M. (1983). The A-rod – a new possibility for cervical dilatation and/or induction of uterine contractions for abortion or delivery by combined pharmacological and mechanical action. *Acta Obstet. Gynecol. Scand.*, **113**, (Suppl.), 159–162

69. Embrey, M.P., Graham, N.B., McNeil, M.E. and Hillier, K. (1986). In vitro release characteristics and long-term stability of poly (ethylene oxide) hydrogel vaginal pessaries containing prostaglandin E₂. *J. Controlled Release*, **3**, 39–45

70. MacKenzie, I.Z., Bradley, S. and Embrey, M.P. (1984). Vaginal prostaglandins and labour induction for patients previously delivered by Caesarean section. *Br. J. Obstet. Gynaecol.*, **91**, 7–10

71. O'Herlihy, C. (1981). Vaginal prostaglandin E₂ gel and breech presentation. *Eur. J. Obstet. Gynecol. Reprod. Biol.*, **11**, 299–303

72. Thiery, M., Parewijck, W. and Martens, G. (1982). Intravenous infusion of prostaglandin E₂ for management of premature rupture of membranes. *Z. Geburtsch. Perinat.*, **186**, 87–88

73. Hauth, J.C., Cunningham, F.G. and Whalley, P.J. (1977). Early labour initiation with oral PGE₂ after premature rupture of the membranes at term. *Obstet. Gynecol.*, **49**, 523–526

74. Lange, A.P., Secher, N.J., Nielsen, F.H. and Pederson, G.T. (1981). Stimulation of labor in cases of premature rupture of the membranes at or near term: a consective randomised study of prostaglandin E₂ tablets and intravenous oxytocin. *Acta Obstet. Gynecol. Scand.*, **60**, 207–210

75. Ekman-Ordeberg, G., Uldbjerg, N. and Ulmsten, U. (1985). Comparison of intravenous oxytocin and vaginal prostaglandin E₂ gel in women with unripe cervices and premature rupture of the membranes. *Obstet. Gynecol.*, **66**, 307–310

76. Magos, A.L., Noble, M.C.B., Wong Ten Yuen, A. and Rodeck, C.H. (1983). Controlled study comparing vaginal prostaglandin E₂ pessaries with intravenous oxytocin for the stimulation of labour after spontaneous rupture of membranes. *Br. J. Obstet. Gynaecol.*, **90**, 726–731

77. Chapman, M., Lawrence, D., Sims, C. and Bennett, M. (1984). Induction of labour by prostaglandin pessaries or oxytocin infusion after spontaneous rupture of membranes. *J. Obstet. Gynecol.*, **4**, 185–187

78. Thiery, M., Parewyck, W., de Grezelle, H., van Kets, H., Smis, B., Verheugen, C., Gervis, J., Vorhoof, L., Derom, R. and Martens, G. (1978). Pre-induction ripening of the cervix with extra-amniotic prostaglandin E₂ gel. *Z. Geburtsh. Perinat.*, **182**, 251–357

79. MacKenzie, I.Z. and Embrey, M.P. (1981). Prostaglandins in obstetrics. *Br. Med. J.*, **283**, 142

80. MacKenzie, I.Z., Bradley, S. and Mitchell, M.D. (1980). Prostaglandin levels in cord venous plasma at delivery or related to labour. In Samuelsson, B., Ramwell, P.W. and Paoletti, R. (eds.) *Advances in Prostaglandin and Thromboxane Research*, Vol. 8, pp. 1401–1405. (New York: Raven Press)

81. Beazley, J.M. and Weekes, A.R.L. (1976). Neonatal hyper-bilirubinaemia following the use of prostaglandin E₂ in labour. *Br. J. Obstet. Gynaecol.*, **83**, 62–67

82. Conway, D.I., Read, M.D., Baver, C. and Martin, R.H. (1976). Neonatal jaundice - a comparison between intravenous oxytocin and oral prostaglandin E₂. *J. Int. Med. Res.*, **4**, 241–246

83. Chew, W.C. (1977). Neonatal hyperbilirubinaemia: a comparison between prostaglandin E_2 and oxytocin inductions. *Br. Med. J.*, **2**, 679–680
84. Saruta, T. and Kaplan, N.M. (1972). Adrenocortical steroidogenesis: the effects of prostaglandins. *J. Clin. Invest.*, **51**, 2246–2251
85. Flack, J.D., and Ramwell, P.W. (1972). A comparison of the effects of ACTH, cyclic AMP, Dibutyryl cyclic AMP, and PGE_2 on corticosteroidogenesis in vitro. *Endocrinology*, **90**, 371–377
86. Calder, A.A., MacKenzie, I.Z. and Embrey, M.P. (1976). Intrauterine (extra-amniotic) prostaglandins in the management of unsuccessful pregnancy. *J. Reprod. Med.*, **16**, 271–275
87. Lippert, T.H. and Luthi, A. (1978). Induction of labour with prostaglandin E_2 gel in cases of intrauterine fetal death. *Prostaglandins*, **15**, 533–542
88. Rutland, A. and Ballard, C. (1977). Vaginal prostaglandin E_2 for missed abortion and intrauterine fetal death. *Am. J. Obstet. Gynecol.*, **128**, 503–505
89. El-Demarawy, H., El-Sahwi, S. and Toppozada, M. (1977). Management of missed abortion and fetal death in utero. *Prostaglandins*, **14**, 583–590
90. MacKenzie, I.Z., Davies, A.J. and Embrey, M.P. (1979). Fetal death in utero managed with vaginal prostaglandin E_2 gel. *Br. Med. J.*, **2**, 1764–1765
91. Toppozada, M., Warda, A., Ramadan, M. (1979). Intramuscular 15 phenoxy PGE_2 ester for pregnancy termination. *Prostaglandins*, **17**, 461–467
92. Wallenburg, H.C.S., Keirse, M.J.N.C., Freie, H.M.P. and Blacquiere, J.F. (1980). Intramuscular administration of 15(S)-15-methyl prostaglandin $F_{2\alpha}$ for induction of labour in patients with fetal death. *Br. J. Obstet. Gynecol.*, **87**, 203–209
93. Sher, G. (1976). Intra-amniotic use of urea and prostaglandin $F_{2\alpha}$ to induce labour in pregnancies complicated by death of the fetus. *S. Afr. Med. J.*, **50**, 510–512
94. MacKenzie, I.Z. (1979). Induction of labour and post-partum haemorrhage. *Br. Med. J.*, **1**, 750
95. Takagi, S., Yoshida, T., Yogo, T., Abe, M., Tochigi, H., Sakata, H. and Takahasho, H. (1976). The effects of intramyometrial injection of $PGF_{2\alpha}$ on severe postpartum haemorrhage. *Prostaglandins*, **12**, 565–579
96. Corson, S.L. and Bolognese, R.J. (1977). Postpartum uterine atony treated with prostaglandins. *Am. J. Obstet. Gynecol.*, **129**, 918–919
97. Hertz, R.H., Sokol, R.J. and Dierker, L.J. (1980). Treatment of postpartum uterine atony with prostaglandin E_2 vaginal suppositories. *Obstet. Gynecol.*, **56**, 129–139
98. Henson, G., Gough, J.D. and Gillmer, M.D. (1983). Control of persistent primary postpartum haemorrhage due to uterine atony with intravenous prostaglandin E_2: Case Report. *Br. J. Obstet. Gynaecol.*, **90**, 280–282
99. Heyl, P.S., Stubblefield, P.G. and Phillippe, M. (1984). Recurrent inversion of the puerperal uterus managed with 15(S)-15-methyl prostaglandin $F_{2\alpha}$ and uterine packing. *Obstet. Gynecol.*, **63**, 263–264
100. Andrinopoulos, G.C. and Dendenhall, H.W. (1983). Prostaglandin $F_{2\alpha}$ in the management of delayed postpartum haemorrhage. *Am. J. Obstet. Gynecol.*, **146**, 217–218
101. Kerekes, L. and Domokos, N. (1979). The effects of prostaglandin $F_{2\alpha}$ on the third stage of labour. *Prostaglandins*, **18**, 161–166
102. Selinger, M., Gillmer, M.D., Phipps, S. and MacKenzie, I.Z. (1986). Midtrimester myometrial sensitisation following antiprogesterone therapy. Abstracts for *23rd British Congress of Obstetrics and Gynaecology*, Cardiff

11
Prostaglandins and leukotrienes and the fetal and perinatal circulations

M.A. Heymann

INTRODUCTION

Several metabolites of arachidonic acid are important in maintaining the integrity of the fetal and neonatal circulations. The cyclo-oxygenase mediated metabolites, the prostaglandins (PGs) and thromboxane (Tx) have received most attention. However, recent studies indicate that the leukotrienes (LTs), the 5′-lipoxygenase mediated products of arachidonic acid, play an equally important role, both groups perhaps affecting different fetal structures or vascular beds, as well as perhaps interacting in the regulation of flow in some.

Although PGs are generally locally synthesized and therefore locally active substances that do not normally circulate in adult blood, in the fetus this is not the case and readily detectable concentrations are present in plasma[1-4]. It is likely that these circulating PGs are derived mainly from the placenta. However, the fetal vasculature does produce PGs, and the umbilical vessels, ductus arteriosus, and pulmonary artery and aorta produce significant amounts of PGE and particularly prostacyclin (PGI_2)[4,5-8]. Exogenous PGs or LTs, administered to the fetus or newborn have diverse and extensive cardiovascular effects and likewise inhibitors of PG or LT synthesis or blockers of LT action affect the circulation suggesting at least some intrinsic role for endogenous PGs and LTs in cardiovascular homeostasis in the fetus and newborn.

GENERAL CIRCULATORY EFFECTS

Infusing PGE_1 into fetal sheep has no significant effect on fetal cardiac output, heart rate, or systemic arterial blood pressure. Blood flow to the myocardium, adrenals, gastrointestinal tract, lungs and peripheral tissues increases[9]. The possible role of endogenous PG production in overall regulation of the fetal circulation has been evaluated by administering inhibitors of PG synthesis to fetal lambs *in utero*. Aspirin administration was associated with a small decrease in blood flow to the brain, gastrointestinal tract, liver, peripheral circulation and kidneys and a small increase in blood flow to the myocardium, adrenal glands and placenta[10]. However, since aspirin constricts the ductus arteriosus (see below) and in these studies pulmonary blood flow increased probably secondarily to the ductus arteriosus constriction, it is not clear whether or not the relatively small changes in specific organ blood flows reflect a true physiological regulation or not.

Meclofenamate, also an inhibitor of PG synthesis, has no significant effect on the renal circulation in normal fetal calves but with hypoxaemia renal vasoconstriction is potentiated[11] suggesting perhaps a role in circulatory responses to stress. Although inhibition of PG synthesis may not have a significant biological effect on resting renal blood flow renal PG production may modulate salt and water homeostasis in the fetus[12] and administration of indomethacin to rhesus monkeys is associated with oligohydramnios[13] most certainly related to a reduction in fetal urinary output. Similar effects may occur in human pregnancy where oligohydramnios is thought to be associated with the administration of indomethacin to inhibit premature labour[14]. In both fetal and neonatal lambs mesenteric arterial vasoconstriction in response to catecholamines is enhanced by indomethacin suggesting an interplay between PGs and catecholamines in controlling vascular tone in the gastrointestinal tract[15].

UMBILICAL PLACENTAL CIRCULATION

In fetal lambs both PGE_2 and $PGF_{2\alpha}$ reduce umbilical blood flow[16–19]. The selective injection of PGE_2 or $PGF_{2\alpha}$ directly into the intact umbilical circulation of fetal lambs decreases umbilical placental blood flow associated with an increase in umbilical placental vascular resistance[20]. Both substances also constrict human umbilical arteries *in vitro*[21,22]. Only prostacyclin (PGI_2) relaxes the umbilical arteries[22] and this effect is best in a low O_2 environment. Perhaps PGI_2 production is an important mechanism for maintaining umbilical placental flow during fetal stress.

However, in intact fetal sheep the increase in umbilical placental flow with PGI_2 is relatively little[23]. Rankin and several co-workers have suggested that PGs may play a regulatory role in maintaining a fetal–maternal perfusion–perfusion balance[17,24] either directly or by modulating the effects of other vasoactive substances.

DUCTUS ARTERIOSUS

It is now clearly established that in the fetus the ductus arteriosus is maintained in an open, relaxed state by the action of PGs[25–27]. Circulating PGE_2 is likely the most important in this respect; however, locally produced PGI_2 may have some effect as well. In pregnant rats and rabbits, maternal administration of sodium salicylate or indomethacin constricts the ductus arteriosus of the fetuses as assessed by direct visualization and measurement after rapidly freezing the fetuses[28,29]. More direct physiological evaluation of this effect has been performed in chronically instrumented fetal lambs[10]. Pulmonary and systemic arterial blood pressures and blood flow across the ductus arteriosus (with radionuclide-labelled microspheres) were measured. After administration of aspirin to the fetus, pulmonary arterial but not systemic arterial blood pressure rose significantly and blood flow across the ductus arteriosus fell significantly indicating an increase in resistance to flow across the ductus arteriosus and therefore constriction of the ductus arteriosus. This was confirmed by direct visualization *in situ* and by section of tissue fixed *in situ*. Similar physiological fetal effects have been reported with indomethacin given to the pregnant ewe[30].

In fetal lamb ductus arteriosus rings studied *in vitro* the magnitude of the effect of indomethacin is clearly different at different gestational ages; greater ductus arteriosus constriction occurs in the immature fetus than in the mature fetus[26,27,31,32]. Arachidonic acid relaxes oxygen constricted ductus arteriosus rings and this effect too is related to gestation, the relaxation being greater in the ductus arteriosus from immature fetuses.

Arachidonic acid metabolism produces several vasoactive products whose generation can be blocked by indomethacin: thromboxane A_2 (TXA_2), PGI_2, the primary PGs (PGE_2, $PGF_{2\alpha}$ and PGD_2) and the intermediate compounds, the PG endoperoxides (PGG_2 and PGH_2). In the fetal lamb, the ductus arteriosus is not affected by physiologic concentrations of TXA_2 and $PGF_{2\alpha}$, both generally vasoconstrictive metabolites of arachidonic acid[25,27,33]. The other products of arachidonic acid metabolism (PGE_2, PGH_2, and PGI_2) cause relaxation of the ductus arteriosus[25,27,33,34].

Tissue homogenates or intact rings of fetal lamb or calf ductus arteriosus synthesize mainly PGE_2, PGI_2, and $PGF_{2\alpha}$[4-6,35-37]. Measurement of the intrinsic rate of endogenous PG production in the isolated fetal lamb ductus arteriosus is complicated since the rate of release is accelerated by damage to or manipulation of the vessel wall and even transient changes in wall tension may increase the amounts of PGs produced. To compare changes in production rates of PGI_2 and PGE_2 with changes in active tension in the ductus arteriosus, the amounts of PGE_2 and PGI_2 released from isolated rings incubated under similar conditions have been measured[26,37]; rings of ductus arteriosus from immature fetal lambs released twice as much PGI_2 as did rings from fetal animals near term. The opposite is true for PGE_2, however.

At both these gestational ages the endogenous production of PGE_2 by the ductus arteriosus is significantly lower than that of PGI_2. However, at any given gestational age, oxygen plus indomethacin constricted fetal lamb ductus arteriosus rings are two to three orders of magnitude more sensitive to the relaxing effects of equimolar amounts of PGE_2 than they are to PGI_2[26,27,38,39]. Further there also is a marked gestational-age related difference in response to either PGE_2 or PGI_2. The immature ductus arteriosus is significantly more sensitive to the same concentration of either PG than is the mature ductus arteriosus, a phenomenon that very likely explains the differences in response to indomethacin between the immature and mature ductus arteriosus. This 'maturation' of sensitivity, i.e. a developmental fall in sensitivity to PGE_2 or PGI_2, appears to be triggered by corticosteroids and also very likely plays a significant role in persistent patency of the ductus arteriosus in preterm infants.

As indicated before, circulating concentrations of PGE_2 are high in the fetus; this is probably related to placental production and also the normally very low fetal pulmonary blood flow and consequent reduced catabolism of any placentally produced material. It is likely, therefore, that although local production of PGE_2 in the fetal ductus arteriosus is markedly less than that of PGI_2, the circulating PGE_2 concentrations and the significantly greater sensitivity of the fetal ductus arteriosus to PGE_2 make PGE_2 the most important endogenous PG in regulation of ductus arteriosus patency in the fetus. The good correlation between the magnitude of constriction of the ductus arteriosus, as measured with sonomicrometer dimension crystals chronically implanted on the fetal lamb ductus arteriosus, and circulating PGE_2 concentrations would seem to confirm this thesis[40].

All these findings, together with those which have shown that pharmacological inhibition of prostaglandin synthesis in fetal animals produces ductus arteriosus constriction, suggest strongly that patency of the fetal ductus arteriosus is not a passive phenomenon but rather a balance between constriction and relaxation with relaxation and dilatation sustained by prostaglandins. Both PGI_2 and PGE_2 are probably involved, however, it also is most likely that PGE_2 is the dominant prostaglandin involved in this function.

Shortly after birth the concentration of PGE_2 in blood falls dramatically, probably associated with increased pulmonary blood flow and greater metabolism of PGE_2 as well as removal of the placenta which produces PGE_2,[41]. The effect of removal of a circulating substance that maintains dilatation will allow the ductus arteriosus to constrict in response to the other known stimuli such as an increase in oxygen and perhaps the release of other constricting vasoactive substances.

In lambs delivered by caesarean section and then mechanically ventilated during the first several hours of postnatal life, circulating plasma concentrations of PGE_2 were significantly higher in severely ill animals (with respiratory distress syndrome of prematurity) requiring aggressive ventilatory support and high inspired oxygen concentrations, than in those animals that required only minimal ventilatory support. Plasma PGE_2 concentrations in the animals requiring less than 25% O_2 were similar to maternal plasma concentrations within three hours after delivery, whereas the concentrations in the severely ill animals were greater than those found as fetuses. Both a decreased plasma clearance, due most likely to reduced pulmonary blood flow, and increased PGE_2 production appear to be responsible for the elevated concentrations in the lambs with severe respiratory distress[44]. The ductus arteriosus was more widely patent in the animals with the higher plasma PGE_2 concentrations. In clinical situations in which pulmonary blood flow is likely to be reduced, the increased circulating plasma concentrations of PGE_2 may contribute to the pathogenesis of persistent patent ductus arteriosus.

The potentially adverse effects of constriction of the ductus arteriosus in the normally developing fetus *in utero* requires some consideration. Many pharmacological agents of the non-steroidal anti-inflammatory group (e.g.

aspirin, indomethacin, ibuprofen) inhibit the cyclo-oxygenase step in arach-idonic acid metabolism. By so doing PG production is inhibited and potentially the ductus arteriosus constricts. As described above this could lead to reorientation of the fetal circulation with increased pulmonary blood flow and an elevation of pulmonary arterial blood pressure[10,30]. Several secondary phenomena may occur.

Pulmonary hypertension (*in utero*) and thereby increased right ventricular afterload, caused by ductus arteriosus constriction, may have generalized haemodynamic effects. Two clinical reports have linked congestive heart failure presenting before or at birth and *in utero* closure of the ductus arteriosus, in one possibly associated with aspirin ingestion[42,43]. Increased right ventricular afterload may lead to right ventricular myocardial subendocardial ischaemia because of the elevation of right ventricular end-diastolic pressure and perhaps also increased work and metabolic demands. In fetal sheep exposed to maternally-administered indomethacin, morphological changes similar to those described clinically in transient tricuspid insufficiency syndrome and compatible with ischaemia were observed in the right ventricular myocardium, particularly the tricuspid valve papillary muscle[44]. Similar, more extensive morphological changes in the myocardium were found in an infant, exposed *in utero* to salicylates, who died from persistent pulmonary hypertension syndrome[45]. That infant also had clinical evidence of tricuspid insufficiency. The similarity between the animal and human findings further suggests clinical implications of *in utero* exposure to non-steroidal anti-inflammatory analgesics.

In normally developing fetal lamb lungs, medial smooth muscle development in individual resistance arteries remains relatively unchanged during the latter half of gestation, and medial muscle thickness remains constant in relationship to external diameter of the artery[46]. Similar observations on the amount and distribution of the medial smooth muscle have been made in human lungs[47,48]. An abnormal increase in the amount of medial smooth muscle occurs in association with pulmonary hypertension *in utero* in fetal lambs[49]. Of significant clinical importance is the pulmonary hypertension and possible morphological changes which could occur *in utero* following constriction of the ductus arteriosus by inhibitors of prostaglandin synthesis. Indomethacin administered maternally for several days was associated with an increase in pulmonary arterial medial smooth muscle in the fetal lambs when compared to control animals[44]. Similar observations were subsequently made in rats[50]. In these circumstances the increased amount of pulmonary vascular medial smooth muscle could interfere with the normal postnatal fall in pulmonary vascular resistance as suggested by the studies of Cassin[51] who showed that following exposure to indomethacin for 9–23 days prior to delivery near term, the normal postnatal fall in pulmonary vascular resistance associated with ventilation of the lambs did not occur. The baseline pulmonary vascular resistance was also significantly higher than in control lambs. Whether this occurs in human infants exposed *in utero* to non-steroidal anti-inflammatory analgesics is not established. Infants dying from the syndrome of persistent pulmonary hypertension of the newborn (persistent fetal circulation syndrome) do have both an increased medial smooth muscle mass as well as an ontogenetically-accelerated peripheral distribution of smooth muscle in the small pulmonary arteries[52-54]. In those studies, the possible role of non-steroidal anti-inflammatory analgesics was not evaluated. Levin *et al.*[45], however, found an increase in small pulmonary artery medial smooth muscle mass in two infants who died with the syndrome of persistent pulmonary hypertension of the newborn and in whom *in utero* exposure to inhibitors of prostaglandin synthesis was established. Several other clinical studies have suggested but not proven the association[55-59]. Evaluation of cord blood salicylate concentrations and the severity of disease have shown the highest concentrations in the infants with the most severe disease[60]. This latter study also underscores the problem of uncovering drug ingestion as a cause of these types of conditions as many over the counter, non-prescription agents contain non-steroidal anti-inflammatory agents and are taken in considerable quantity without the realization that a major pharmacological agent is in fact being used.

The relatively high incidence of tricuspid valve insufficiency in infants with the syndrome of persistent pulmonary hypertension of the newborn may also point to previous, *in utero* pulmonary hypertension as described above. Although these studies have suggested the association of persistent pulmonary hypertension syndrome and the use of non-steroidal anti-inflammatory analgesics during pregnancy, several large studies, particularly those in which indomethacin was used to inhibit premature labour, have failed to support this as an absolute association[61-65].

PULMONARY CIRCULATION

In the fetus, since gas exchange occurs in the placenta, pulmonary vascular resistance is high and pulmonary blood flow is low. Near term in the fetal lamb (140–145 days gestation) this is about 100 ml/min per 100 g of lung tissue or 30–40 ml/min per kg fetal body weight and represents about 8% of the combined left and right ventricular output of the heart (about 450 ml/min per kg). Shortly after birth with initiation of pulmonary ventilation, pulmonary vascular resistance falls rapidly, associated with an eight- to ten-fold increase in pulmonary blood flow. In lambs born at term this is about 300–400 ml/min per kg of body weight shortly after birth.

Many factors likely regulate pulmonary blood flow in the fetus and in the postnatal period. The O_2 environment certainly plays a role during both periods and the release at birth of vasoactive substances such as bradykinin or angiotensin II also likely plays a direct role in the rapid pulmonary vasodilatation. Probably more important is their interactive role with the products of arachidonic acid metabolism since it is rapidly becoming apparent that these substances play a key role in regulation of the pulmonary circulation.

Prostaglandins are potent vasoactive substances and their role in perinatal pulmonary vascular changes has been studied quite extensively. In fetal goats or lambs, prostaglandin E_1 and prostaglandin E_2 are both modest pulmonary vasodilators[66,67]. PGI_2 is also a pulmonary vasodilator and is somewhat more potent than PGE_2[68,69]. None of these PGs is specific for the fetal pulmonary circulation, and they all generally affect the systemic vascular resistance to the same or even a greater degree[9,70].

It is possible that local production and release of these substances in the fetus may modulate the constrictor effects of, for example, the normally low pO_2, or perhaps thromboxane but this has not been established. $PGF_{2\alpha}$ produces only pulmonary vasoconstriction in fetal goats[71] and therefore together with thromboxane may play some role in active pulmonary vasoconstriction. The non-specific systemic effects also does not exclude the possibility that local production and metabolism occurs in the perinatal period and there is strong evidence that PGI_2 does play a physiological role in causing postnatal pulmonary vasodilatation. Lung distension or mechanical stimulation of the lungs lead to 'prostaglandin' or PGI_2 production[72–74] and ventilation of fetal lungs, even without changing O_2, is associated with the net production and release into left atrial or pulmonary venous blood of small amounts of the stable metabolite of PGI_2 (6-keto-$PGF_{1\alpha}$)[75–77]. The concentration of the metabolite falls to very low concentrations after several hours, further suggesting a definite role for PGI_2 in the immediate postnatal period.

PGD_2 also has been shown to be a pulmonary vasodilator in perfused fetal lungs[78]. In intact newly delivered term lambs with hypoxia-induced pulmonary hypertension, PGD_2 produced a specific fall in pulmonary arterial blood pressure and calculated pulmonary vascular resistance with an increase in both pulmonary and systemic blood flows; there was no change in systemic arterial blood pressure[79]. Beyond about ten days of age this effect is no longer present and PGD_2 produces pulmonary vasoconstriction[80]. These specific perinatal effects suggest a physiological role for PGD_2 in establishing a normal pulmonary circulation in the immediate newborn period. This is further supported by studies in rhesus monkeys which showed an increase in the number of mast cells in the lungs in the latter part of gestation with significantly fewer mast cells present after birth[81]. Since PGD_2 is released from mast cells, degranulation of these cells with the release of PGD_2 may be one important aspect of the perinatal pulmonary vascular changes.

The positive role of vasodilating prostaglandins in the immediate postnatal period has been further substantiated by studies using inhibition of cyclo-oxygenase activity[51,82,83]. The fall in calculated pulmonary vascular resistance that normally occurred when fetal lungs were ventilated was shown to have two separate phases. There was an initial rapid fall within 30–60 seconds after the onset of ventilation, followed by a slower fall that occurred over about 15 minutes. In fetal goats, this latter, second phase was inhibited or attenuated by pretreatment with indomethacin. These studies also suggest that if indomethacin is administered shortly before delivery in humans, the normal fall in pulmonary vascular resistance might not occur and respiratory distress may result.

It has recently been considered that the 5-lipoxygenase products of arachidonic acid metabolism, the leukotrienes, are responsible, at least in part, for mediating hypoxic pulmonary vasoconstriction in adults[83–85]. We have shown similar effects of LT antagonism in newborn lambs[86]. We therefore considered that leukotrienes could be actively involved in regulating the normal pulmonary vasoconstriction found in the fetus. End organ antagonism of leukotriene effect in fetal lambs using FPL 57231 (Fisons plc) increased pulmonary blood flow to the level expected with normal ventilation after birth[87]. These studies strongly suggest a physiological role for LTs in maintaining pulmonary vasoconstriction and thereby a low pulmonary blood flow in the fetus. Further studies have shown that these effects of LTs are direct and not through the secondary stimulation of thromboxane production[88].

It is probable therefore that control of the perinatal pulmonary circulation reflects a balance between factors producing active pulmonary vasoconstriction and those leading to pulmonary vasodilatation. The dramatic increase in pulmonary blood flow after birth most likely reflects a major shift from active pulmonary vasoconstriction to active pulmonary vasodilatation. It is possible that arachidonic acid or even phospholipid precursor metabolism shifts from lipoxygenase products (LTs) in the low oxygen environment of the fetal animal towards cyclo-oxygenase products (PGs) either with mechanical stimulation due to lung expansion or in the higher oxygen environment after birth.

REFERENCES

1. Challis, J.R.G., Osathanondh, R., Ryan, K.J., et al. (1974). Maternal and fetal plasma prostaglandin levels at vaginal delivery and caesarean section. Prostaglandins, 6, 281−288
2. Challis, J.R.G., Dilley, S.R., Robinson, J.S. et al. (1976). Prostaglandins in the circulation of the fetal lamb. Prostaglandins, 11, 1041
3. Mitchell, M.D., Flint, A.P., Bibby, J. et al. (1978). Plasma concentrations of prostaglandins during late human pregnancy: Influence of normal and preterm labor. J. Clin. Endocrinol. Metab., 46, 947−951
4. Challis, R.G. and Patrick, J.E. (1980). The production of prostaglandins and thromboxanes in the feto-placental unit and their effects on the developing fetus. Semin. Perinatol., 4, 23−33
5. Pace-Asciak, C.R. and Rangaraj, G. (1977). The 6-ketoprostaglandin $F_{1\alpha}$ pathway in the lamb ductus arteriosus. Biochim. Biophys. Acta, 486, 583−585
6. Powell, W.S. and Solomon, S. (1977). Formation of 6-oxoprostaglandin $F_{1\alpha}$ by arteries of the fetal calf. Biochem. Biophys. Res. Commun., 75, 815−822
7. Terragno, N.A. and Terragno, A. (1979). Prostaglandin metabolism in the fetal and maternal vasculature. Fed. Proc., 38, 75−77
8. Terragno, N.A., Terragno, A. and McGiff, J.C. (1980). Role of prostaglandins in blood vessels. Semin. Perinatol., 4, 85−90
9. Tripp, M.E., Heymann, M.A., Rudolph, A.M. (1978). Hemodynamic effects of prostaglandin E_1 on lambs in utero. In Coceani, F. and Olley, P.M. (eds.) Prostaglandin and Perinatal Medicine. Advances in Prostaglandin and Thromboxane Research, Vol. 4, pp. 221−229 (New York: Raven Press)
10. Heymann, M.A. and Rudolph, A.M. (1976). Effects of acetylsalicylic acid on the ductus arteriosus and circulation of fetal lambs in utero. Circ. Res., 38, 418−422
11. Millard, R.W., Baig, H. and Vatner, S.F. (1979). Prostaglandin control of the renal circulation in response to hypoxemia in the fetal lamb in utero. Circ. Res., 45, 172−179
12. Walker, D.W. and Mitchell, M.D. (1978). Prostaglandins in urine of fetal lambs. Nature, 271, 161−162
13. Novy, M.J. (1978). Effects of indomethacin on labor, fetal oxygenation, and fetal development in rhesus monkeys. In Coceani, F. and Olley, P.M. (eds.) Advances in Prostaglandin and Thromboxane Research, Vol. 4, pp. 285−300. (New York: Raven Press)
14. Itskovitz, J., Abramovici, H. and Brandes, J.M. (1980). Oligohydramnios, meconium and perinatal death concurrent with indomethacin treatment in human pregnancy. J. Reprod. Med., 24, 137−140
15. Yabek, S.M. and Avner, B.P. (1979). Effects of prostaglandin E_1 and indomethacin on fetal

and neonatal lamb mesenteric artery responses to norepinephrine. *Prostaglandins*, **17**, 227–233

16. Novy, M.J., Piasecki, G. and Jackson, B.T. (1974). Effect of prostaglandin E_2 and $F_{2\alpha}$ on umbilical blood flow and fetal hemodynamics. *Prostaglandins*, **5**, 543–555

17. Rankin, J.H.G. (1976). A role for prostaglandins in the regulation of the placental blood flows. *Prostaglandins*, **11**, 343–353

18. Rankin, J.H.G. and Phernetton, T.M. (1976). Circulatory responses of the near-term sheep fetus to prostaglandin E_2. *Am. J. Physiol.*, **231**, 760–765

19. McLaughlin, M.K., Brennan, S.C. and Chez, R.A. (1978). Vasoconstrictive effects of prostaglandins in sheep placental circulations. *Am. J. Obstet. Gynecol.*, **130**, 408–413

20. Berman, W. Jr, Goodlin, R.C., Heymann, M.A. *et al.* (1978). Effects of pharmacologic agents on umbilical blood flow in fetal lambs in utero. *Biol. Neonate*, **33**, 225–235

21. Tuvemo, T. (1978). Action of prostaglandins and blockers of prostaglandin synthesis on the isolated human umbilical artery. In Coceani, F. and Olley, P.M. (eds.) *Advances in Prostaglandin and Thromboxane Research*, Vol. 4, pp. 271–274. (New York: Raven Press)

22. Tuvemo, T. (1980). Role of prostaglandins, prostacyclin, and thromboxanes in the control of the umbilical-placental circulation. *Semin. Perinatol.*, **4**, 91–95

23. Rankin, J.H.G., Phernetton, T.M., Anderson, D.F. *et al.* (1979). Effect of prostaglandin I_2 on ovine placental vasculature. *J. Dev. Physiol.*, **1**, 151–160

24. Rankin, J.H.G. and McLaughlin, M.K. (1979). The regulation of placental blood flows. *J. Dev. Physiol.*, **1**, 3–30

25. Coceani, F. and Olley, P.M. (1980). Role of prostaglandins, prostacyclin and thromboxanes in the control of prenatal patency and postnatal closure of the ductus arteriosus. *Semin. Perinatol.*, **4**, 109–113

26. Clyman, R.I. (1980). Ontogeny of the ductus arteriosus response to prostaglandins and inhibitors of their synthesis. *Semin. Perinatol.*, **4**, 115–124

27. Clyman, R.I. and Heymann, M.A. (1981). Pharmacology of the ductus arteriosus. *Pediatr. Clin. N. Am.*, **28**, 77–93

28. Sharpe, G.L., Thalme, B. and Larsson, K.S. (1974). Studies on closure of the ductus arteriosus: XI. Ductal closure in utero by a prostaglandin synthetase inhibitor. *Prostaglandins*, **8**, 363–368

29. Sharpe, G.L., Larsson, K.S. and Thalme, B. (1975). Studies on closure of the ductus arteriosus: XII. In utero effect of indomethacin and sodium salicylate in rats and rabbits. *Prostaglandins*, **9**, 585–596

30. Levin, D.L., Mills, L.J., Parkey, *et al.* (1979). Constriction of the fetal ductus arteriosus after administration of indomethacin to the pregnant ewe. *J. Pediatr.*, **94**, 647–650

31. Clyman, R.I. (1978). Developmental responses to oxygen, arachidonic acid and indomethacin in the fetal lamb ductus arteriosus in vitro. *Prostagl. Med.*, **1**, 167–174

32. Clyman, R.I., Mauray, F., Rudolph, A.M. *et al.* (1980). Age dependent sensitivity of the lamb ductus arteriosus to indomethacin and prostaglandins. *J. Pediatr.*, **96**, 94

33. Coceani, F., Bishai, I., White, E. *et al.* (1978). Actions of prostaglandins, endoperoxides and thromboxanes on the lamb ductus arteriosus. *Am. J. Physiol.*, **234**, H117–H122

34. Olley, P.M., Bodach, E., Heaton, J. *et al.* (1975). Further evidence implicating E-type prostaglandins in the patency of the lamb ductus arteriosus. *Eur. J. Pharmacol.*, **34**, 247–250

35. Terragno, N.A., Terragno, A. McGiff, J.C. *et al.* (1977). Synthesis of prostaglandins by the ductus arteriosus of the bovine fetus. *Prostaglandins*, **14**, 721–727

36. Pace-Asciak, C.R. and Rangaraj, G. (1978). Prostaglandin biosynthesis and catabolism in the lamb ductus arteriosus, aorta, and pulmonary artery. *Biochim. Biophys. Acta*, **529**, 13–20

37. Clyman, R.I., Mauray, F., Koerper, M.A. *et al.* (1978). Formation of prostacyclin (PGI_2) by the ductus arteriosus of fetal lambs at different stages of gestation. *Prostaglandins*, **16**, 633–642

38. Clyman, R.I., Mauray, F., Roman, C. *et al.* (1978). PGE_2 is a more potent vasodilator of the lamb ductus arteriosus than either PGI_2 or 6-keto-$PGF_{1\alpha}$. *Prostaglandins*, **16**, 259–264

39. Coceani, F., Bodach, E., White, E. *et al.* (1978). Prostaglandin I_2 is less relaxant than prostaglandin E_2 on the lamb ductus arteriosus. *Prostaglandins*, **15**, 551–556

40. Friedman, W.F., Molony, D.A. and Kirkpatrick, S.E. (1978). Prostaglandins: Physiological

and clinical correlations. In Barness, L.A. (ed.) *Advances in Pediatrics*, Vol. 25, pp. 151–204 (Chicago: Year Book Medical Publishers)

41. Clyman, R.I., Mauray, F., Roman, C. *et al.* (1980). Circulatory prostaglandin E_2 concentrations and patent ductus arteriosus in fetal and neonatal lambs. *J. Pediatr.*, **97**, 455–461

42. Kohler, H.G. (1967). Intrauterine cardiac failure associated with premature closure of the ductus arteriosus. *Arch. Dis. Child.*, **42**, 335

43. Arcilla, R.A., Thilenius, O.G. and Ranniger, K. (1969). Congestive heart failure from suspected ductal closure in utero. *J. Pediatr.*, **75**, 74–78

44. Levin, D.L., Mills, L.J., Weinberg, A.G. *et al.* (1979). Hemodynamic, pulmonary vascular, and myocardial abnormalities secondary to pharmacologic constriction of the fetal ductus arteriosus: A possible mechanism for persistent pulmonary hypertension and transient tricuspid insufficiency in the newborn infant. *Circulation*, **60**, 360–364

45. Levin, D.L., Fixler, D.E., Morriss, F.C. *et al.* (1978). Morphologic analysis of the pulmonary vascular bed in infants exposed in utero to prostaglandin synthetase inhibitors. *J. Pediatr.*, **92**, 478–483

46. Levin, D.L., Rudolph, A.M. Heymann, M.A. *et al.* (1976). Morphological development of the pulmonary vascular bed in fetal lambs. *Circulation*, **53**, 144–151

47. Hislop, A. and Reid, L. (1972). Intra-pulmonary arterial development during fetal life – branching pattern and structure. *J. Anat.*, **113**, 35–48

48. Reid, L. (1979). The pulmonary circulation: Remodelling in growth and disease. *Am. Rev. Respir. Dis.*, **119**, 531–546

49. Levin, D.L., Hyman, A.I., Heymann, M.A. *et al.* (1978). Fetal hypertension and the development of increased pulmonary vascular smooth muscle: A possible mechanism for persistent pulmonary hypertension of the newborn infant. *J. Pediatr.*, **92**, 265–269

50. Harker, L.C., Kirkpatrick, S.E., Friedman, W.F. *et al.* (1981). Effects of indomethacin on fetal rat lungs: A possible cause of persistent fetal circulation. *Pediatr. Res.*, **15**, 147–151

51. Cassin, S. (1982). Humoral factors affecting pulmonary blood flow in the fetus and newborn infant. In Peckham, G. and Heymann, M.A. (eds.) *Cardiovascular Sequelae of Asphyxia in the Newborn*, pp. 10–18. (Columbus, Ohio: Ross Laboratories)

52. Haworth, S.G. and Reid, L. (1976). Persistent fetal circulation: Newly recognized structural features. *J. Pediatr.*, **88**, 614–620

53. Murphy, J.D., Rabinovitch, M., Goldstein, J.D. *et al.* (1981). The structural basis of persistent pulmonary hypertension of the newborn infant. *J. Pediatr.*, **98**, 962–967

54. Reid, L. (1982). The development of the pulmonary circulation. In Peckham, G. and Heymann, M.A. (eds.) *Cardiovascular Sequelae of Asphyxia in the Newborn*, pp. 2–10. (Columbus, Ohio: Ross Laboratories)

55. Manchester, D., Margolis, H.S. and Sheldon, R.E. (1976). Possible association between maternal indomethacin therapy and primary pulmonary hypertension of the newborn. *Am. J. Obstet. Gynecol.*, **126**, 467–469

56. Csaba, I.F., Sulyok, E. and Ertl, T. (1978). Relationship of maternal treatment with indomethacin to persistence of fetal circulation syndrome. *J. Pediatr.*, **92**, 484–488

57. Grella, P. and Zanor, P. (1978). Premature labour and indomethacin. *Prostaglandins*, **16**, 1007–1017

58. Rubaltelli, F.F., Chiozza, M.L., Zanardo, V. *et al.* (1979). Effect on neonate of maternal treatment with indomethacin. *J. Pediatr.*, **94**, 161–172

59. Wilkinson, A.R., Aynsley-Green, A. and Mitchell, M.D. (1979). Persistent pulmonary hypertension and abnormal PGE levels in preterm infants after maternal treatment with naproxen. *Arch. Dis. Child*, **54**, 942–945

60. Perkin, R.M., Levin, D.L. and Clark, R. (1980). Serum salicylate levels and right-to-left ductal shunts in newborn infants with persistent pulmonary hypertension. *J. Pediatr.*, **96**, 721–726

61. Zuckerman, H., Reiss, U. and Rubinstein, I. (1974). Inhibition of human premature labor by indomethacin. *Obstet. Gynecol.*, **44**, 787–792

62. Kumor, K.M., White, R.D., Blade, D.A. *et al.* (1979). Indomethacin as a treatment for premature labor. Neonatal outcome. *Pediatr. Res.*, **13**, 370–375

63. Van Kets, H., Thiery, M., Derom, R., *et al.* (1979). Perinatal hazards of chronic antenatal tocolysis with indomethacin. *Prostaglandins*, **18**, 893–907

64. Niebyl, J.R., Blake, D.A., White, R.D., Kumor, K.M. *et al.* (1980). The inhibition of premature labor with indomethacin. *Am. J. Obstet. Gynecol.*, **136**, 1014–1019

65. Wiqvist, N. (1981). Preterm labour: Other drug possibilities including drugs not to use. In Elder, M.G. and Hendricks, C.H. (eds.) *Butterworths International Medical Reviews Obstetrics and Gynecology 1: Preterm Labor*, pp. 148–175. (London: Butterworths)

66. Cassin, S., Tyler, T.L. and Wallis, R. (1975). The effects of prostaglandin E_1 on fetal pulmonary vascular resistance. *Proc. Soc. Exp. Biol. Med.*, **148**, 584–587

67. Tyler, T.L., Leffler, C.W. and Cassin, S. (1977). Effects of prostaglandin precursors, prostaglandins, and prostaglandin metabolites on pulmonary circulation in perinatal goats. *Chest*, **71**, 271S–273S

68. Leffler, C.W. and Hessler, J.R. (1979). Pulmonary and systemic vascular effects of exogenous prostaglandin I_2 in fetal lambs. *Eur. J. Pharmacol.*, **54**, 37–42

69. Cassin, S., Winikor, I., Tod, M. *et al.* (1981). Effects of prostacyclin on the fetal pulmonary circulation. *Pediatr. Pharmacol.*, **1**, 197–207

70. Tripp, M.E., Drummond, W.H., Heymann, M.A. *et al.* (1980). Hemodynamic effects of pulmonary arterial infusion of vasodilators in newborn lambs. *Pediatr. Res.*, **14**, 1311–1315

71. Tyler, T.L., Leffler, C.W. and Cassin, S. (1977). Effects of prostaglandin precursors, prostaglandins, and prostaglandin metabolites on pulmonary circulation in perinatal goats. *Chest*, **72**, 271S–273S

72. Edmonds, J.F., Berry, E. and Wyllie, J.H. (1969). Release of prostaglandins by distension of the lungs. *Br. J. Surg.*, **56**, 622–623

73. Gryglewski, R.J., Korbut, R. and Ocetkiewicz, A. (1978). Generation of prostacyclin by lungs in vivo and its release into the arterial circulation. *Nature*, **273**, 765–767

74. Gryglewski, R.J. (1980). The lung as a generator of prostacyclin. *Ciba Found. Symp.*, **78**, 147–164

75. Leffler, C.W., Hessler, J.R. and Terragno, N.A. (1980). Ventilation-induced release of prostaglandin-like material from fetal lungs. *Am. J. Physiol.*, **238**, H282–H286

76. Leffler, C.W., Hessler, J.R. and Green, R.S. (1984). Mechanism of stimulation of pulmonary prostaglandin synthesis at birth. *Prostaglandins*, **28**, 877–887

77. Leffler, C.W., Hessler, J.R. and Green, R.S. (1984). The onset of breathing at birth stimulates pulmonary vascular prostacyclin synthesis. *Pediatr. Res.*, **18**, 938–942

78. Cassin, S., Tod, M., Philips, J., Frisinger, J. *et al.* (1981). Effects of prostaglandin D_2 in perinatal circulation. *Am. J. Physiol.*, **240**, H755–H760

79. Soifer, S.J., Morin, F.C. III and Heymann, M.A. (1982). Prostaglandin D_2 reverses induced pulmonary hypertension in the newborn lamb. *J. Pediatr.*, **100**, 458–463

80. Soifer, S.J., Morin, F.C. III, Kaslow, D.C. and Heymann, M.A. (1983). The developmental effects of PGD_2 on the pulmonary and systemic circulations in the newborn lamb. *J. Dev. Physiol.*, **5**, 237–250

81. Schwartz, L.W., Osburn, B.I. and Frick, O.L. (1974). An ontogenic study of histamine and mast cells in the fetal rhesus monkey. *J. Allerg. Clin. Immunol.*, **56**, 381–386

82. Leffler, C.W, Tyler, T.L. and Cassin, S. (1978). Effect of indomethacin on pulmonary vascular response to ventilation of fetal goats. *Am. J. Physiol.*, **234**, H346–H351

83. Cassin, S. (1980). Role of prostaglandins and thromboxanes in the control of the pulmonary circulation in the fetus and newborn. *Semin. Perinatol.*, **4**, 101–107

84. Ahmed, T. and Oliver, W. Jr (1983). Does slow-reacting substance of anaphylaxis mediate hypoxic pulmonary vasoconstriction? *Am. Rev. Respir. Dis.*, **127**, 566–571

85. Morganroth, M.L., Reeves, J.T., Murphy, R.C. *et al.* (1984). Leukotriene synthesis and receptor blockers block hypoxic pulmonary vasoconstriction. *J. Appl. Physiol.*, **56**, 1340–1346

86. Schreiber, M.D., Heymann, M.A. and Soifer, S.J. (1985). Leukotriene inhibition prevents and reverses hypoxic pulmonary vasoconstriction in newborn lambs. *Pediatr. Res.*, **19**, 437–441

87. Soifer, S.J., Loitz, R.D., Roman, C. *et al.* (1985). Leukotriene end organ antagonists increase pulmonary blood flow in fetal lambs. *Am. J. Physiol.*, **249**, H570–H576

88. Clozel, M., Clyman, R.I., Soifer, S.J. *et al.* (1985). Thromboxane is not responsible for the high pulmonary vascular resistance in fetal lambs. *Pediatr. Res.*, **19**, 1254–1257

Index